T0226795

Biliary Tract and Primary Liver Tumors

Editor

T. CLARK GAMBLIN

SURGICAL ONCOLOGY CLINICS OF NORTH AMERICA

www.surgonc.theclinics.com

Consulting Editor
TIMOTHY M. PAWLIK

October 2019 • Volume 28 • Number 4

ELSEVIER

1600 John F. Kennedy Boulevard ● Suite 1800 ● Philadelphia, Pennsylvania, 19103-2899

http://www.theclinics.com

SURGICAL ONCOLOGY CLINICS OF NORTH AMERICA Volume 28, Number 4
October 2019 ISSN 1055-3207, ISBN-13: 978-0-323-70882-1

Editor: John Vassallo (j.vassallo@elsevier.com)
Developmental Editor: Laura Kavanaugh

Surgical Oncology Clinics of North America (ISSN 1055-3207) is published quarterly by Elsevier Inc., 360 Park Avenue South, New York, NY 10010-1710. Months of publication are January, April, July, and October. Business and Editorial Offices: 1600 John F. Kennedy Blvd., Ste. 1800, Philadelphia, PA 19103-2899. Customer Service Office: 3251 Riverport Lane, Maryland Heights, MO 63043. Periodicals postage paid at New York, NY and additional mailing offices. Subscription prices are $306.00 per year (US individuals), $533.00 (US institutions) $100.00 (US student/resident), $352.00 (Canadian individuals), $674.00 (Canadian institutions), $205.00 (Canadian student/resident), $422.00 (foreign individuals), $674.00 (foreign institutions), and $205.00 (foreign student/resident). Foreign air speed delivery is included in all *Clinics* subscription prices. All prices are subject to change without notice. **POSTMASTER**: Send address changes to *Surgical Oncology Clinics of North America*, Elsevier Health Science Division, Subscription Customer Service, 3251 Riverport Lane, Maryland Heights, MO 63043. **Customer Service: 1-800-654-2452 (US and Canada). 314-447-8871 (outside US and Canada). Fax: 314-447-8029. E-mail: journalscustomerservice-usa@elsevier.com (for print support); journalsonline support-usa@elsevier.com (for online support).**

Reprints. For copies of 100 or more, of articles in this publication, please contact the Commercial Reprints Department, Elsevier Inc., 360 Park Avenue South, New York, New York 10010-1710. Tel. 212-633-3874; Fax: 212-633-3820; E-mail: reprints@elsevier.com.

Surgical Oncology Clinics of North America is covered in *MEDLINE/PubMed (Index Medicus)* and *EMBASE/ Excerpta Medica, Current Contents/Clinical Medicine, and ISI/BIOMED.*

Contributors

CONSULTING EDITOR

TIMOTHY M. PAWLIK, MD, MPH, PhD, FACS, FRACS (Hon.)
Professor and Chair, Department of Surgery, The Urban Meyer III and Shelley Meyer Chair for Cancer Research, Professor of Surgery, Oncology, and Health Services Management and Policy, Surgeon in Chief, The Ohio State University, Wexner Medical Center, Columbus, Ohio

EDITOR

T. CLARK GAMBLIN, MD, MS, MBA, FACS
Professor of Surgery, Stuart D. Wilson Chair in Surgical Oncology, Vice-Chair, Off Campus Clinical Operations, Chief, Division of Surgical Oncology, Medical College of Wisconsin, Milwaukee, Wisconsin

AUTHORS

THOMAS A. ALOIA, MD, MHCM, FACS
Professor, Department of Surgical Oncology, The University of Texas MD Anderson Cancer Center, Houston, Texas

BLAIRE ANDERSON, MD
Abdominal Transplant Surgery Fellow, Division of Transplantation Surgery, Department of Surgery, University of Nebraska Medical Center, Omaha, Nebraska

ANTHONY BEJJANI, MD
Fellow, Department of Medicine, Division of Hematology/Oncology, David Geffen School of Medicine at UCLA, Jonsson Comprehensive Cancer Center at UCLA, Los Angeles, California

MORGAN BONDS, MD
Division of HPB Surgery, Digestive Diseases Institute, Virginia Mason Medical Center, Seattle, Washington

AKHIL CHAWLA, MD
Complex General Surgical Oncology Fellow, Department of Surgery, Massachusetts General Hospital, Harvard Medical School, Boston, Massachusetts

LEONID CHERKASSKY, MD
Clinical Fellow in Complex General Surgical Oncology, Department of Surgical Oncology, Memorial Sloan Kettering Cancer Center, New York, New York

DAVID COY, MD, PhD
Department of Radiology, Virginia Mason Medical Center, Seattle, Washington

MICHAEL D'ANGELICA, MD
Enid A. Haupt Chair in Surgery, Vice Chair of Education, Department of Surgery, Memorial Sloan Kettering Cancer Center, Professor of Surgery, Weill Cornell Medical Center, New York, New York

M.B. MAJELLA DOYLE, MD, MBA
Section of Abdominal Organ Transplant, Professor, Department of Surgery, Washington University, Washington University School of Medicine, St Louis, Missouri

ASLAM EJAZ, MD, MPH
Department of Surgery, The Ohio State University, Columbus, Ohio

RAMY EL-DIWANY, MPH
Department of Surgery, Johns Hopkins University, Baltimore, Maryland

CRISTINA R. FERRONE, MD
Associate Professor, Department of Surgery, Massachusetts General Hospital, Harvard Medical School, Boston, Massachusetts

RICHARD S. FINN, MD
Professor, Department of Medicine, Division of Hematology/Oncology, David Geffen School of Medicine at UCLA, Jonsson Comprehensive Cancer Center at UCLA, Los Angeles, California

T. CLARK GAMBLIN, MD, MS, MBA, FACS
Professor of Surgery, Stuart D. Wilson Chair in Surgical Oncology, Vice-Chair, Off Campus Clinical Operations, Chief, Division of Surgical Oncology, Medical College of Wisconsin, Milwaukee, Wisconsin

DAVID A. GELLER, MD
Department of Surgery, Liver Cancer Center, University of Pittsburgh Medical Center, Pittsburgh, Pennsylvania

BENJAMIN L. GREEN, MD
Department of Surgery, Indiana University School of Medicine, IU Health University Hospital, Indianapolis, Indiana

SCOTT HELTON, MD
Division of HPB Surgery, Digestive Diseases Institute, Virginia Mason Medical Center, Seattle, Washington

ALAN W. HEMMING, MD, MSc
Professor, Department of Surgery, Division of Transplantation and HPB Surgery, University of Iowa, Iowa City, Iowa USA

MICHAEL G. HOUSE, MD, FACS
Chief, Division of Surgical Oncology, Department of Surgery, Indiana University School of Medicine, IU Health University Hospital, Indianapolis, Indiana

NANCY E. KEMENY, MD
Gastrointestinal Oncology Service, Division of Solid Tumor Oncology, Department of Medicine, Memorial Sloan Kettering Cancer Center, New York, New York

GEOFFREY W. KRAMPITZ, MD, PhD
Assistant Professor, Division of Surgical Oncology, Department of Surgery, Thomas Jefferson University, Philadelphia, Pennsylvania

RACHEL M. LEE, MD, MSPH
Division of Surgical Oncology, Department of Surgery, Postdoctoral Research Fellow, Winship Cancer Institute, Emory University School of Medicine, Atlanta, Georgia

TIFFANY C. LEE, MD
General Surgery Resident, Cincinnati Research on Outcomes and Safety in Surgery (CROSS), Department of Surgery, University of Cincinnati College of Medicine, Cincinnati, Ohio

DILIP MADDIRELA, PhD
Department of Radiology, Medical College of Wisconsin, Milwaukee, Wisconsin

SHISHIR K. MAITHEL, MD
Division of Surgical Oncology, Professor, Department of Surgery, Scientific Director, Emory Liver and Pancreas Center, Winship Cancer Institute, Emory University School of Medicine, Atlanta, Georgia

SOPHIA K. McKINLEY, MD, EdM
General Surgery Resident, Department of Surgery, Massachusetts General Hospital, Harvard Medical School, Boston, Massachusetts

SEBASTIAN MONDACA, MD
Gastrointestinal Oncology Service, Division of Solid Tumor Oncology, Department of Medicine, Memorial Sloan Kettering Cancer Center, New York, New York

MACKENZIE C. MORRIS, MD
General Surgery Resident, Cincinnati Research on Outcomes and Safety in Surgery (CROSS), Department of Surgery, University of Cincinnati College of Medicine, Cincinnati, Ohio

SAMEER H. PATEL, MD
Assistant Professor, Cincinnati Research on Outcomes and Safety in Surgery (CROSS), Department of Surgery, University of Cincinnati College of Medicine, Cincinnati, Ohio

TIMOTHY M. PAWLIK, MD, MPH, PhD, FACS, FRACS (Hon.)
Professor and Chair, Department of Surgery, The Urban Meyer III and Shelley Meyer Chair for Cancer Research, Professor of Surgery, Oncology, and Health Services Management and Policy, Surgeon in Chief, The Ohio State University, Wexner Medical Center, Columbus, Ohio

JANELLE F. REKMAN, MD, MAEd, FRCSC
Division of HPB Surgery, Digestive Diseases Institute, Virginia Mason Medical Center, Seattle, Washington

SAEED SADEGHI, MD
Associate Professor, Department of Medicine, Division of Hematology/Oncology, David Geffen School of Medicine at UCLA, Jonsson Comprehensive Cancer Center at UCLA, Los Angeles, California

SHIMUL A. SHAH, MD, MHCM
Cincinnati Research on Outcomes and Safety in Surgery (CROSS), James and Catherine Orr Chair of Liver Transplantation, Professor, Department of Surgery, University of Cincinnati College of Medicine, Cincinnati, Ohio

PHILIP SMITH, MD
Department of Radiology, Virginia Mason Medical Center, Seattle, Washington

AMY C. TAYLOR, MD
Radiology Consultants of Little Rock, Little Rock, Arkansas

SUSAN TSAI, MD, MHS
Associate Professor, Division of Surgical Oncology, Department of Surgery, Medical College of Wisconsin, Milwaukee, Wisconsin

SARAH B. WHITE, MD, MS, FSIR
Department of Radiology, Division of Vascular and Interventional Radiology, Medical College of Wisconsin, Milwaukee, Wisconsin

GREGORY C. WILSON, MD
Department of Surgery, Liver Cancer Center, University of Pittsburgh Medical Center, Pittsburgh, Pennsylvania

HOOMAN YARMOHAMMADI, MD
Interventional Radiology Service, Department of Radiology, Memorial Sloan Kettering Cancer Center, New York, New York

Contents

> Biliary tract and primary liver tumors can be divided into intrahepatic and extrahepatic sites. Hepatocellular carcinoma (HCC) and intrahepatic cholangiocarcinoma are the most common primary liver malignancies, making up 75% and 15% of cases, respectively. In the United States, there has been an increase in incidence of HCC and cholangiocarcinoma over the last 2 decades, and it is probable that the incidence of both will continue to climb. Gallbladder cancer, however, is the most frequent biliary tract cancer, comprising 80% to 90% of biliary tract cancers worldwide. Underlying epidemiology and cause are discussed.

> The accurate diagnosis of a liver mass can usually be established with a thorough history, examination, laboratory inquiry, and imaging. The necessity of a liver biopsy to determine the nature of a liver mass is rarely necessary. Contrast-enhanced computed tomography and magnetic resonance are the standard of care for diagnosing liver lesions and high-quality imaging should be performed before performing a biopsy. This article discusses current consensus guidelines for imaging of liver masses, as well as masses found on surveillance imaging. The ability to accurately characterize lesions requires proper use and understanding of the technology and expert interpretation.

> Endoscopic and percutaneous therapies have been shown to prolong life and reduce morbidity for patients with unresectable advanced stages of primary hepatobiliary malignances. This article reviews pertinent studies published within the last 5 years that involve locoregional techniques to manage hepatocellular carcinoma, perihilar and distal cholangiocarcinoma. A major emphasis is placed on photodynamic therapy, radiofrequency ablation, irreversible electroporation, and microwave ablation. Technical advances, combinational therapies, and postintervention outcomes are discussed. Despite widespread application, high-quality

evidence does not show superiority of any particular locoregional technique for treating advanced hepatobiliary cancers.

Intrahepatic cholangiocarcinoma (ICC) arises from the epithelial cells of the intrahepatic and extrahepatic bile ducts and occurs proximal to the segmental biliary ducts. Risk factors include chronic hepatitis and cirrhosis, biliary inflammatory diseases, and hepatobiliary flukes, although in most cases, no known risk factor is identified. ICC is highly aggressive, with long-term survival only observed in patients with a complete R0 surgical resection. Technical and physiologic resectability should be considered when performing an operative plan. Nodal involvement is among the most important prognostic factors associated with survival and a porta hepatis lymphadenectomy should be performed at the time of resection. Adjuvant chemotherapy can provide a significant survival benefit for patients with more advanced or aggressive tumors. Systemic, locoregional, and targeted therapies exist for patients with unresectable or metastatic disease.

Cholangiocarcinoma is an aggressive malignancy of the extrahepatic bile ducts. Hilar lesions are most common. Patients present with obstructive jaundice and intrahepatic bile duct dilation. Cross-sectional imaging reveals local, regional, and distant extent of disease, with direct cholangiography providing tissue for diagnosis. The consensus of a multidisciplinary committee dictates treatment. Resection of the extrahepatic bile duct and ipsilateral hepatic lobe with or without vascular resection and transplantation after neoadjuvant protocol are options for curative treatment. The goal of surgery is to remove the tumor with negative margins. Patients with inoperable tumors or metastatic disease are best served with palliative chemoradiotherapy.

Managing patients with incidental gallbladder cancer requires stratifying patients risk for recurrence and an appreciation for the recurrence patterns characterizing this malignancy. Although standard management includes reresection to remove sites at risk of harboring residual disease and to achieve negative resection margin status, the decision to perform surgery is tempered by an early and frequent distant recurrence, the most common cause of surgical failure. High-risk patients may benefit from neoadjuvant chemotherapy before reresection. The goal of curative-intent reresection is achieving R0 margin status and optimal staging while limiting morbidity and mortality.

Distal cholangiocarcinoma is a rare malignancy with a dismal prognosis. Because of its location and aggressive nature, patients often present with locally advanced or metastatic disease, and effective treatment options are limited. For patients with resectable disease, surgery is the only chance for cure, but achieving an R0 resection is paramount. Optimal adjuvant therapy in resectable disease remains under investigation. Randomized controlled trials investigating neoadjuvant therapy and its impact on resectability and long-term outcomes are needed to continue to improve the outcomes of patients with distal cholangiocarcinoma.

Surgical resection and liver transplant remain the cornerstones of curative treatment options for hepatocellular carcinoma. Determining the best treatment option for each patient is a complex decision based on degree of liver cirrhosis, extent of tumor, and overall patient performance status. A multidisciplinary approach is best. With widespread adoption, the role of laparoscopic liver resection for hepatocellular carcinoma continues to expand. Long-term oncologic outcomes are similar for laparoscopic and open resection, with improved short-term results, mainly blood loss and hospital length of stay. Liver transplant remains the ideal treatment of cirrhotic patients with signs of portal hypertension and hepatocellular carcinoma.

Hepatobiliary malignancies are a diverse group of neoplasms involving the liver, gallbladder, and bile ducts. Although intrahepatic cholangiocarcinoma, perihilar cholangiocarcinoma, hepatocellular carcinoma, and gallbladder adenocarcinoma share many biological and anatomic features, they have distinct clinical presentations and natural histories that require individual consideration. Here, we discuss the incidence, outcomes, patient presentation, initial workup, pathologic diagnoses, staging classification, imaging and surgical staging, and determinants of resectability for each malignancy.

With the recent decline in cost of high-throughput next-generation sequencing, detailed characterization of biliary tract and primary liver tumors continues to evolve. Recent studies have elucidated molecular signatures that reflect distinct pathways of carcinogenesis reflective of viral, parasitic, and toxin-related etiologic factors. With greater elucidation of the molecular pathogenesis of disease, novel targets that may be potential clinically actionable continue to be identified.

In the past decade, there has been significant progress in the treatment of primary liver cancer. There has been increasing knowledge of the molecular alterations occurring in these tumors, which is now being translated into patient care. Ongoing clinical trials will further advance the therapeutic options available to patients, including the introduction of molecular targeted therapeutics and immunotherapy approaches. Critical to the success of these new drugs, is the appropriate use of them in the clinic to maximize efficacy and limit toxicity.

Locally advanced hepatocellular carcinoma and intrahepatic cholangio-carcinoma are associated with a grim prognosis. The development of high-ly effective systemic therapies for these tumors has been challenging; however, numerous locoregional treatment alternatives have emerged, including transarterial hepatic embolization (TAE), transarterial chemoem-bolization (TACE), drug-eluting bead TACE (DEB-TACE), hepatic arterial infusion chemotherapy (HAI), radioembolization, and stereotactic body ra-diation therapy. Although there is potential for long-term disease control for these therapies, the evidence to guide adequate patient selection and choose among different treatment alternatives is still limited. This re-view focuses on the rationale and data supporting TAE, TACE, DEB-TACE, and HAI in hepatobiliary cancers.

Hepatocellular carcinoma and intrahepatic cholangiocarcinoma are often amenable to locoregional therapy, including percutaneous ablation, trans-arterial chemoembolization (TACE), or transarterial radioembolization (TARE). TARE is a technique that delivers a high dose of radiation to the tumor, while limiting the dose to the normal liver parenchyma and the adja-cent organs. It has been shown to effectively provide disease control with relatively few toxicities, and in certain cases results in a complete response. It is the preferred therapy as a bridge to liver transplant and can provide necessary compensatory future liver remnant hypertrophy before planned surgical resection.

Primary liver tumors are most commonly hepatocellular carcinoma and intrahepatic cholangiocarcinoma. Although surgical resection offers a chance for cure, these tumors generally present at a late, inoperable stage, necessitating an understanding of noncurative and palliative treatment options. These options include ablative therapies, including ra-diofrequency ablation; intra-arterial therapies, including transcatheter chemoembolization; biliary decompression; radiotherapy; systemic ther-apies, including traditional chemotherapeutic agents; and molecular therapies, such as sorafenib. Selection of nonoperative treatment de-pends on patient and tumor factors as well as institutional resources and expertise.

Surgical management of primary liver and biliary tract tumors has evolved over the past several decades, resulting in improved outcomes in these malignancies with historically poor prognoses. Expansion of patient selection criteria, progress in neoadjuvant and adjuvant therapies, development of techniques to increase future liver remnant, and the select utilization of liver transplantation have all contributed to increasing the patient pool for surgical intervention. Ongoing and future studies need to focus on improving multimodality treatment regimens and further refining the selection criteria for transplantation in order to optimize utilization of limited organ resources.

SURGICAL ONCOLOGY CLINICS OF NORTH AMERICA

SERIES OF RELATED INTEREST

Surgical Clinics of North America
http://www.surgical.theclinics.com
Thoracic Surgery Clinics
http://www.thoracic.theclinics.com
Advances in Surgery
http://www.advancessurgery.com

THE CLINICS ARE AVAILABLE ONLINE!
Access your subscription at:
www.theclinics.com

Foreword

Biliary Tract and Primary Liver Tumors

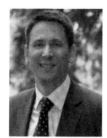

Timothy M. Pawlik, MD, MPH, PhD, FACS, FRACS (Hon.)
Consulting Editor

This issue of the *Surgical Oncology Clinics of North America* is devoted to the topic of biliary tract and primary liver tumors under the guest editorship of T. Clark Gamblin, Professor of Surgery and Division Chief of Surgical Oncology at the Medical College of Wisconsin. As the Stuart D. Wilson Chair in Surgical Oncology, Dr Gamblin has extensive expertise in the treatment of patients with biliary tract and primary liver cancers. In fact, Dr Gamblin is a nationally and internationally recognized hepatobiliary surgeon who has published over 100 papers on this topic. Dr Gamblin's research has played a pivotal role in providing important data to help better understand how to treat this challenging group of patients. As such, Dr Gamblin is a perfect individual to be the guest editor of this important issue of the *Surgical Oncology Clinics of North America*.

The issue covers a number of important topics on biliary tract and primary liver tumors. Cholangiocarcinoma and hepatocellular carcinoma are two of the most common malignancies worldwide. Despite being diagnosed with greatest frequency in Eastern Asian countries, the diagnosis of biliary tract and liver tumors is generally on the rise worldwide, including in Western countries. Risk factors are varied and include infectious causes, such as hepatitis, hepatobiliary flukes, primary sclerosing cholangitis, as well as cirrhosis. In addition, the epidemic of obesity has resulted in an increase in nonalcoholic fatty liver disease and nonalcoholic steatohepatitis with an associated greater risk of liver tumors. In general, surgery remains the cornerstone of therapy for biliary tract and primary liver cancers in the form of resection and, in select patients, transplantation. Selection of patients for surgery necessitates high-quality, state-of-the art imaging and often cholangioscopy/cholangiography. Unfortunately, despite surgical intervention, recurrence is not uncommon, and long-term prognosis remains guarded for many patients with biliary tract and primary liver cancer. In turn, there is a need for more effective systemic and targeted therapies that can be delivered to patients in the neoadjuvant or adjuvant setting.

Surg Oncol Clin N Am 28 (2019) xiii–xiv
https://doi.org/10.1016/j.soc.2019.07.002
1055-3207/19/© 2019 Published by Elsevier Inc.

surgonc.theclinics.com

The current issue touches on such important topics as imaging, biliary drainage, as well as surgical options for various biliary tract and primary liver cancers, ranging from intrahepatic cholangiocarcinoma to gallbladder cancer to hepatocellular carcinoma. In addition, the issue highlights the role of both systemic and targeted agents as well as the important role that locoregional therapy can play in treating patients with primary liver tumors. To accomplish such a comprehensive and thorough state-of-the-art review on this wide range of topics, Dr Gamblin employed an incredible group of authors who are the respective leaders in their field. As you will note in reading this issue, Dr Gamblin and his colleagues have done an outstanding job of thoroughly covering such a complex disease process. I would like to thank Dr Gamblin and all the authors who contributed to this excellent issue of the *Surgical Oncology Clinics of North America*.

Timothy M. Pawlik, MD, MPH, PhD, FACS, FRACS (Hon.)
Department of Surgery
The Ohio State University
Wexner Medical Center
395 West 12th Avenue, Suite 670
Columbus, OH 43210, USA

E-mail address:
tim.pawlik@osumc.edu

Preface

Hepatobiliary Malignancies: The Changing Landscape

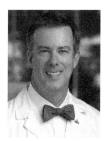

T. Clark Gamblin, MD, MS, MBA, FACS
Editor

This issue of *Surgical Oncology Clinics of North America* is focused on the management of primary liver cancer and biliary malignancies. Management of these challenging diseases requires a multidisciplinary approach in a field that has made substantial advances in recent years. A panel of experts has contributed to this topic with articles ranging from epidemiology, liver-directed therapy, and systemic therapy to genetic profiling and management options for inoperable patients. Authors have provided an in-depth review of topics and pointed to the patient of tomorrow as the field rapidly expands.

Topics describing molecular profiling of hepatobiliary tumors and the evolution of targeted therapy are coupled with an update on first- and second-line systemic therapy as well as current clinical trials. State-of-the-art imaging and subsequent staging are focused on specific anatomic tumor locations, and the role of endoscopic and percutaneous approaches is considered. With safer surgery and evolving technology, the group eligible for surgical intervention has continued to expand. This text is organized into specific diseases and challenges to guide the reader regarding unique biology and treatment options.

It is with true gratitude to the contributors and publishers that I invite you to explore the current state of hepatobiliary management.

T. Clark Gamblin, MD, MS, MBA, FACS
Division of Surgical Oncology
8701 Watertown Plank Road
Milwaukee, WI 53226, USA

E-mail address:
tcgamblin@mcw.edu

Biliary Tract and Primary Liver Tumors
Who, What, and Why?

Alan W. Hemming, MD, MSc

KEYWORDS

- Hepatocellular carcinoma • Cholangiocarcinoma • Gallbladder carcinoma
- Epidemiology • Cause

KEY POINTS

- Primary liver cancer (hepatocellular carcinoma [HCC] and intrahepatic cholangiocarcinoma) continues to increase in incidence in the last decade and is projected to continue to increase in the next decade.
- The incidence of biliary tract and primary liver malignancy varies worldwide because of both environmental and genetic factors.
- Hepatitis B and hepatitis C are well known to contribute to the development of both HCC and cholangiocarcinoma.
- Gallbladder cancer is the most common biliary malignancy, and the most common etiologic agent is the chronic inflammation from various causes.

INTRODUCTION

Biliary tract and primary liver tumors can be divided into intrahepatic and extrahepatic sites. Hepatocellular carcinoma (HCC) and intrahepatic cholangiocarcinoma (ICC) are the most common primary liver malignancies, making up 75% and 15% of cases, respectively.[1] In the United States, there has been an increase in the incidence of HCC and likely ICC over the last 2 decades, and it is probable that the incidence of both will continue to climb.[2–6] Extrahepatic biliary tumors can be divided into cholangiocarcinoma and gallbladder cancer. Extrahepatic cholangiocarcinoma (eCC) is classified into proximal or perihilar cholangiocarcinoma (pCC) and distal cholangiocarcinoma (dCC) with approximately two-thirds of cases occurring in the perihilar region and one-third occurring in the distal duct. Gallbladder cancer, however, is the most frequent biliary tract cancer, comprising 80% to 90% of biliary tract cancers worldwide.[7] The purpose of this article is to review the epidemiology, risk factors, and

Disclosure Statement: The authors have nothing to disclose.
Department of Surgery, University of Iowa, University of Iowa Hospitals & Clinics, 200 Hawkins Drive, SE427 GH, Iowa City, IA 52242, USA
E-mail address: alan-hemming@uiowa.edu

potential mechanisms underlying the development of primary liver and biliary tract malignancy.

Hepatocellular Carcinoma

HCC is the most common primary liver malignancy in the world with wide geographic variation largely based on the incidence of viral hepatitis in the observed population[8–10] (**Fig. 1**). HCC is the sixth most common cancer worldwide and the second deadliest cancer for men and sixth deadliest cancer for women. The incidence of HCC is highest in men, with a male-to-female ratio of approximately 2.5 or 3 to 1. The overall HCC incidence increases with advancing age with a peak at the age of 70.[11] There are more than 700,000 deaths per year from HCC worldwide. High areas of incidence are found in Southeast Asia and Africa, the populations of which have high rates of hepatitis B, whereas North America and westernized Europe have a considerably lower incidence.[12] Even in the United States, however, the incidence of HCC has been increasing in the last 4 decades, and it is currently among the most commonly diagnosed new cancers and one of the fastest increasing causes of cancer-related deaths.[13] Current estimates from the Surveillance, Epidemiology, and End Results (SEER) population-based cancer registry suggest there has been a nearly 4-fold increase in HCC incidence in the United States over the last 4 decades (1.6 per 100,000 in 1975–1977 to 4.8 per 100,000 in 2005–2007) and that this increasing incidence may continue further into the future.[3,6] In addition, the mortality from HCC is very nearly the same as its incidence, making HCC a major cause of cancer-related mortality.[13]

Hepatocellular carcinoma risk factors

Risk factors for the development of HCC are shown in **Box 1**. The dominant risk factors are discussed later.

Cirrhosis The association between cirrhosis and the development of HCC is well described, and cirrhosis is associated with more than a 30-fold increase in the

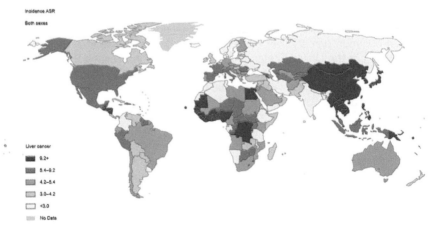

Fig. 1. Global incidence of HCC per 100,000. *Abbreviations*: ASR, Age standardized incidence rates. (*Adapted with permission from* Ferlay J., Soerjomataram I., Ervik M., Dikshit R., Eser S., Mathers C., Rebelo M., Parkin D.M., Forman D., Bray, F. GLOBOCAN 2012 v1.0, Cancer Incidence and Mortality Worldwide: IARC CancerBase No. 11 [Internet]. Lyon, France: International Agency for Research on Cancer; 2013. Available from: http://gco.iarc.fr/today/home, accessed on May 8, 2018.)

Box 1
Hepatocellular carcinoma risk factors

Cirrhosis
  Viral hepatitis
    HBV
    HCV
  Toxins
    Alcohol
    Tobacco
    Aflatoxins
  Hereditary liver disease
    Hemochromatosis
    Alpha-1 antitrypsin

Autoimmune hepatitis
  States of insulin resistance
    Obesity
    Diabetes
    Nonalcoholic fatty liver disease
    Nonalcoholic steatohepatitis

---

development of HCC.[14,15] Cirrhosis however is the common end result of liver disease caused by a variety of agents that result in inflammation, hepatocellular damage, and subsequent fibrosis. Because cirrhosis is associated with differing degrees of liver dysfunction, the assessment of liver function plays a key role in subsequent selection of treatment with HCC in well-compensated cirrhosis being amenable to a wide variety of therapies, including liver resection, whereas advanced decompensated cirrhosis may preclude any therapy. In fact, in many patients with advanced decompensated cirrhosis, the end cause of mortality is due to the dysfunction from the underlying liver disease and cirrhosis rather than from the progression of HCC.

Viral hepatitis Hepatitis B virus (HBV) and hepatitis C virus (HCV) are the most common HCC risk factors worldwide and 40% to 50% of incident cases are attributable to HBV or HCV. Although worldwide HBV is the most common etiologic agent accounting for approximately 50% of cases, in the United States, HBV is much less common, accounting for only 10% to 15% of cases, and HCV accounting for 45% to 55% of cases, whereas 5% are coinfected patients and 30% to 35% are not infected with either.[13,16,17]

Hepatitis B Hepatitis B and its role in the development have been well studied. Hepatitis B is a double stranded, hepatotrophic DNA virus. Hepatitis B infection confers a 15-20 times risk over the average uninfected individual and is believed to account for half of all cases of HCC diagnosed worldwide.[17–19] Specific HBV genotypes and various mutations in genomic regions have been associated with the development of clinical manifestations, such as cirrhosis and/or HCC.[20,21] HBV has 9 genotypes (A to I) and 1 additional proposed genotype J.[22–24] The distribution of the genotypes is geographic and correlates with the distribution of the different ethnic populations worldwide.[22,24–26]

Most reports on the effect of genotype come from the Asia Pacific regions, where HBV genotype B and/or C predominate. HBV genotype B is thought to be less aggressive than genotype C.[21,27,28] HBV genotype C reportedly has a higher tendency to induce DNA double-strand breaks and accumulate reactive oxygen species that increase the risk of chromosomal rearrangements and DNA damage, leading to the formation and development of HCC.[29]

Several reports suggest that a double mutation in the basal core promoter region of HBV genome (A1762T/G1764A) is associated with up to a 10-fold increased risk of HCC and that this is more frequent in those infected with HBV genotype C compared with genotype B.[28,30,31] In combination with other point mutations, these core promoter mutations are associated with an even higher risk of HCC in HBeAg-positive patients.[28,32]

Mutations in other regions of HBV genome have also been linked with disease progression; in particular, the PreS region is associated with the progression of chronic hepatitis and is associated with a significant increase in HCC risk.[28,33] A mutation in codon 38 of X gene was found at an increased frequency in patients with HCC and has been used as an independent risk factor for the development of HCC.[34]

Integration of HBV DNA into the human genome may explain the incidence of noncirrhotic HCC.[35] This insertion can involve deletions, cis/trans-activations, translocations, production of fusion transcripts, and generalized genomic instability.[36] However, noncirrhotic HCC with low-grade fibrosis can also be found in non-HBV-related HCC.[37,38] HBV DNA integration is present in most HBV-related HCC but can also be identified in nontumor tissue and chronic hepatitis B without HCC.[39]

Integration of HBV X sequence into host genome is a common event in HCC. It has been reported that HBV X integration occurs more often in HCC than in cirrhosis.[40] Whole-genome sequencing of HCC samples has demonstrated HBV X DNA integration within or upstream of the sequence of telomerase reverse transcriptase (TERT), epigenetic regulator MLL4, and cell-cycle gene CCNE1.[41–43] DNA integration was observed in approximately 80% of tumors but was present in only 30% of adjacent liver tissues.[43]

Both PreS1 and PreS2 regions are variable and prone to genetic mutations. In animal models, the insertion of PreS/S gene regions expressed high levels of HBsAg, showed inflammation and appearance of preneoplastic lesions, and finally, led to HCC in most animals, suggesting a direct oncogenic effect.[44] A recent study reported that HCC patients with occult hepatitis B had HBV DNA integration in approximately 75% of cases. The inserted viral genes were mainly X and PreS/S, followed by C and polymerase sequences.[45]

Hepatitis C HCV is a hepatotrophic RNA virus. Patients infected with HCV carry a 15- to 20-fold increase in HCC with the annual incidence of HCC in cirrhotics estimated at 1% to 4%.[46] A total of 170,000 new cancer cases, or approximately 7.8% of all new cancers, were attributable to HCV in 2012.[47] Over the past decade, deaths from HCV-attributable HCC increased by 21%, during which time deaths from HCC secondary to causes other than HCV and alcohol remained stable.[48,49] Although HBV is the most common etiologic agent for HCC in the world, HCV is the most common cause of HCC in the United States, Europe, Japan, and South America.[49] It is estimated that 2.5% of the world's population is infected with HCV (177 million). HCV prevalence is approximately 3% in Japan, and 85% of HCC patients are infected with HCV, whereas in the United States, the prevalence of HCV is 1.8% and approximately 50% to 60% of cases of HCC are infected with HCV.[50,51]

HCV genotype appears to be a risk factor for the development of HCC with genotype 3 carrying an 80% increased risk of developing HCC as compared with genotype 1.[52]

HCV is thought to induce carcinogenesis through a complex interplay between host, viral, and environmental factors (**Fig. 2**).[53] The process of hepatocarcinogenesis may take more than 20 to 30 years and is mediated by viral factors and host immune response. Studies have shown that HCV core protein may drive lipogenesis and impair oxidative stress metabolism.[54] In addition, viral proteins can act directly on cell-

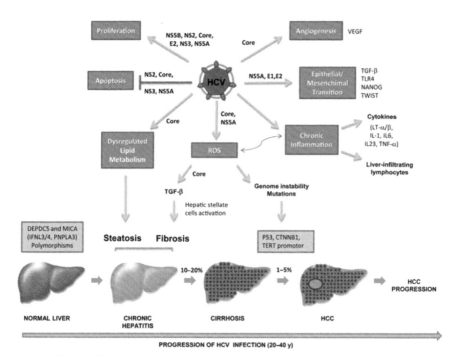

Fig. 2. HCV-related mechanisms of carcinogenesis from HCV infection to HCC. Hepatocarcinogenesis is a multistep process that involves progressive accumulation of different genetic alternations, which lead to malignant transformation. Malignant transformation of hepatocytes occurs through increased liver cell turnover, induced by chronic liver injury and regeneration, in the context of inflammation and oxidative stress. LT α/β, Lymphotoxin alpha/beta; IL-1, interleukin-1; ROS, reactive oxygen species; TGF, transforming growth factor B; TNF-α, tumor necrosis factor-α; VEGF, vascular endothelial growth factor. (*From* Vescovo T, Refolo G, Vitagliano G, Fimia GM, Piacentini M. Molecular mechanisms of hepatitis C virus-induced hepatocellular carcinoma. *Clin Microbiol Infect.* 2016;22(10):853-861; with permission.)

signaling pathways to promote HCC by inhibiting tumor suppressor genes and cell-cycle check points or by causing activation of signaling pathways that upregulate growth and division.[55] Host-induced immunologic response is mediated by tumor necrosis factor, interferons, and chronic inflammation secondary to HCV. Repeated cell cycles are associated with accumulation of mutations that may transform hepatocytes to malignant cells.[49]

Alcohol The association of alcohol with HCC development is well known and yet there remains uncertainty as to whether alcohol itself is a direct carcinogen or whether it exerts its effect on hepatocarcinogenesis through the effect of cirrhosis development.[13] The effect of alcohol is also potentiated by other concurrent risk factors for chronic liver disease, especially viral hepatitis, and probably obesity.[13] Although the estimate of increased risk for development of HCC attributable to alcohol is relatively low (1.5–3) as compared with viral hepatitis (15–25), alcohol abuse remains a pervasive problem in the United States and therefore a significant contributor to HCC development.[56,57]

Metabolic factors The prevalence of obesity in the United States has increased dramatically.[58] Associated with increased obesity is a constellation of conditions that include disorders of lipid and glucose metabolism with underlying insulin resistance that has increasingly been implicated in the development of a variety of malignancies.[56] Nonalcoholic fatty liver disease is now the most common cause of cirrhosis in the United States and accounts for 30% to 40% of new cases of HCC.[15,59] Although the intrahepatic molecular changes and the exact mechanism by which metabolic syndrome leads to chronic liver disease and/or HCC are yet to be defined, development of steatosis and nonalcoholic steatohepatitis undoubtedly plays a role.

Cholangiocarcinoma

Cholangiocarcinoma is a malignancy that can arise from any portion of the biliary tree from the canals of Hering to the main bile duct and can be classified into iCC or eCC. Tumors that arise above the second-order branching of the biliary tree are classified as iCC, whereas eCC tumors arise below the second-order branching and can extend down the main bile duct to the ampulla. Extrahepatic bile duct tumors are subsequently divided into proximal or pCC that occurs above the cystic duct and dCC that occurs below the cystic duct.[60] Approximately 50% to 60% of cholangiocarcinomas are pCC, 30% are dCC, whereas 10% are iCC.[61] ICC can also be classified by its growth pattern into mass-forming (MF-iCC), periductal infiltrating, and intraductal growing, in which the MF-iCC largely represents the most frequent form[62,63] (**Fig. 3**)

Epidemiologic assessment of trends in different countries has largely reported an increase in cholangiocarcinoma (**Fig. 4**).[60] There are consistent reports of an increasing incidence of iCC and a decreasing or stable incidence of eCC from the World Health Organization database, from US cancer registries, and also from Japanese and European cohorts.[5,64–66] An analysis from the SEER database confirmed that the incidence of iCC has risen by 128% in the United States between 1973 and 2012, whereas the incidence of eCC remained stable.[67]

Cholangiocarcinoma occurs largely after the fourth decade of life and more frequently in men than women.[68] This sex difference is reported to become more pronounced with increasing age in an analysis of the SEER database. The same analysis also demonstrates that the highest incidence among all ethnic groups and cholangiocarcinoma types was in Asians.[2] The incidence rates of cholangiocarcinoma most likely vary in different geographic regions because of environmental and genetic

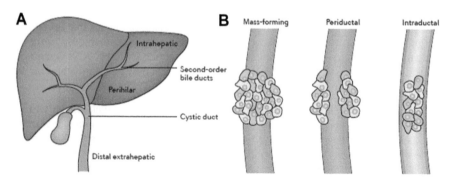

Fig. 3. (*A*) Cholangiocarcinomas are classified according to the anatomic location into iCC, pCC, and dCC. (*B*) Concerning the gross appearance, the iCCA can present 3 different patterns of growth: mass-forming, periductal infiltrating, and intraductal growth. (*From* Rahnemai-Azar AA, Weisbrod A, Dillhoff M, Schmidt C, Pawlik TM. Intrahepatic cholangiocarcinoma: Molecular markers for diagnosis and prognosis. *Surg Oncol.* 2017;26(2):125-137; with permission.)

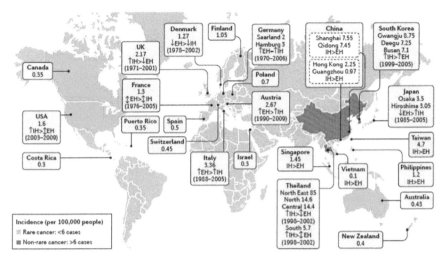

Fig. 4. Worldwide incidence of cholangiocarcinoma per 100,000. EH, extrahepatic cholangiocarcinoma; IH, intrahepatic cholangiocarcinoma. ↑, increasing trend; ↔, stable trend; ↓, decreasing trend. (*From* Banales JM, Cardinale V, Carpino G, et al. Expert consensus document: Cholangiocarcinoma: current knowledge and future perspectives consensus statement from the European Network for the Study of Cholangiocarcinoma (ENS-CCA). Nat Rev Gastroenterol Hepatol. 2016;13(5):261-280; with permission.)

differences. The highest incidence rates of intrahepatic choloangiocarcinoma have been reported in the north of Thailand (113 per 100,000 person-years in men and 50 per 100,000 person-years in women), where the liver fluke *Opisthorchis viverrini* is endemic. In this area, cholangiocarcinoma make up 89% of primary liver cancers.[69]

Risk factors

Worldwide, approximately 70% of cholangiocarcinoma occurs without apparent cause; however, there are clearly identifiable risk factors. Parasitic infections, bile duct disorders, toxins, and viral hepatitis have all been demonstrated to be strong risk factors for cholangiocarcinoma development. Risk factors thought to play a role in cholangiocarcinoma development with somewhat less evidence are inflammatory bowel disease, diabetes, obesity, gallstone disease, alcohol, smoking, and genetic polymorphisms.[70] A summary of risk factors for cholangiocarcinoma is shown in **Box 2**).

Southeast Asia and the Far East are areas that are endemic for the liver flukes *O viverrini* and *Clonorchis sinensis*, flatworms that infect humans via ingestion of raw or pickled fish.[71] The parasite lives in the bile duct for years feeding on biliary epithelial cells, causing chronic ductal inflammation and increasing the risk of cholangiocarcinoma. *O viverrini* is endemic in northeast Thailand, Laos, and Cambodia, whereas the endemic areas for *C sinensis* are China, Taiwan, Korea, and Vietnam.[72] A metaanalysis of case-control studies demonstrates a strong association (odds ratio [OR] 4.7, 95% confidence interval 2.2–9.8) between the infection of *O viverrini* or *C sinensis* and cholangiocarcinoma.[73]

Biliary disorders, such as primary sclerosing cholangitis (PSC), biliary cysts, or ductal stone disease, are also risk factors for cholangiocarcinoma development.

PSC has a well-known association with cholangiocarcinoma marked by chronic inflammation of the biliary tree and liver injury. The lifetime incidence of

---

Box 2
Cholangiocarcinoma risk factors

General
- Age greater than 65 years
- Obesity
- Diabetes mellitus

Inflammatory diseases
- Primary sclerosing cholangitis
- Hepatolithiasis (Oriental cholangiohepatitis)
- Biliary tract stone disease
- Biliary-enteric anastomosis
- Liver cirrhosis

Infectious diseases
- O viverrini (liver flukes)
- C sinensis (liver flukes)
- Hepatitis C
- Hepatitis B

Drugs, toxins, or chemicals
- Alcohol
- Smoking
- Thorotrast
- Dioxin
- Vinyl chloride
- Nitrosamines
- Asbestos
- Oral contraceptive pills
- Isoniazid

Congenital
- Choledochal cysts (type 1, solitary, extrahepatic, type IV, extrahepatic and intrahepatic)
- Caroli disease
- Congenital hepatic fibrosis

Data from Bergquist A, von Seth E. Epidemiology of cholangiocarcinoma. Best Pract Res Clin Gastroenterol. 2015;29(2):221-232.

---

cholangiocarcinoma in this patient population is between 5% and 10%.[74,75] About 50% of patients with PSC who develop cholangiocarcinoma are diagnosed with cholangiocarcinoma within 2 years of diagnosis of PSC.[75,76] The mean age of cholangiocarcinoma diagnosis in patients with PSC is in the fourth decade of life compared with the seventh decade in the general population.[68,75,77,78] The development of cholangiocarcinoma in PSC patients has a dismal prognosis because of both the malignancy and the underlying liver disease with median survival of about 5 months after diagnosis.[76] In a Swedish cohort study of PSC patients, 44% of deaths were caused by cancer during a median follow-up of 5.7 years.[79]

Choledochal cysts are relatively rare congenital abnormalities of the biliary tree characterized by dilations of portions of the biliary tree. Most cases are identified in children, but up to 20% of cases are identified in adults. The presence of particular subtypes of choledochal cysts implies a field change in the biliary epithelium, and cholangiocarcinoma can occur in either the cyst or nondilated portions of the biliary tree with cases of cholangiocarcinoma occurring even after resection of the biliary cyst. The lifetime risk for the development of cholangiocarcinoma in adult patients is 10% to 30%.[80,81]

Hepatolithiasis is thought to predispose to malignancy by causing bile stasis, recurrent cholangitis, and chronic inflammation. A 2% to 13% incidence of cholangiocarcinoma in hospital-based cohorts of patients with hepatolithiasis in Asian countries has been reported.[82,83] Intrahepatic stones are unusual in Western countries with an incidence of 0.6% to 1.3% but more common in parts of Asia with an incidence of 17% to 39%.[84,85] Other aspects of biliary tract stone disease have also been linked to the development of cholangiocarcinoma. A Swedish population-based study in patients with gallstones demonstrated a 2-fold increased risk of cholangiocarcinoma in noncholecystectomized individuals.[86] Choledocholithiasis has also shown a strong positive association with CCA in studies from the United States and Denmark with risk estimates ranging from 4 to 34.[87,88]

Cirrhosis and viral hepatitis C and B are recognized as risk factors for cholangiocarcinoma, particularly intrahepatic cholangiocarcinoma. In western countries, hepatitis C contributes more to tumor development, whereas in Asian countries hepatitis B has a stronger contribution.[89] Reports from the United States and Europe demonstrate that hepatitis C was a risk factor for cholangiocarcinoma with the strongest association for ICC.[78,88,90,91] Studies from South Korea and China have more frequently shown hepatitis B as a risk factor for ICC, whereas Japanese studies are more similar to western studies reporting that hepatitis C exposure had a stronger association than with hepatitis B.[92–94] Cirrhosis of different causes was also identified in most of these studies. Pathogenically, release of inflammatory cytokines, cell death along with increases in cell proliferation, as well as changes in the liver in fibrosis predispose to carcinogenesis.[89] However, the presence of cirrhosis is not uniformly shown in all patients with viral hepatitis who develop cholangiocarcinoma.[95] A metaanalysis of risk factors for ICC showed that cirrhosis had a combined OR of 23, hepatitis C of 4.8, and hepatitis B of 5.1.[74]

Obesity, type II diabetes mellitus, and metabolic syndrome have been linked to development of CCA. In a large study from US SEER and Medicare databases, metabolic syndrome was significantly associated with iCC (OR 1.6).[96] In another metaanalysis, both obesity and diabetes were identified as risk factors for iCC.[74] Studies evaluating alcohol and smoking are inconsistent.[68] However, in a metaanalysis including studies in which alcohol exposure was defined as alcoholic liver disease, alcohol use was associated with iCC with an OR of 2.8.[74] Several genetic polymorphisms, alone or in interaction with other risk factors, have also been studied in cholangiocarcinoma. Genes involved in DNA repair, cellular protection against toxins, and immunologic response have been associated with cholangiocarcinoma development.[89,96,97]

Many of the underlying causes of cholangiocarcinoma are related to chronic inflammation. Sia and colleagues[98] examined the pathogenesis of cholangiocarcinoma, and 2 classes of cholangiocarcinoma, inflammatory and proliferative, were identified. The inflammatory classes were characterized by activation of inflammatory pathways, and the proliferation class was characterized by activation of oncogenic signaling pathways, such as mitogen-activated protein kinase and K-ras.[98] Molecular analysis demonstrated the relationship between inflammation and the development of cholangiocarcinoma. The genes involved in the inflammatory subtype were often related to cytokines, including interleukin-6.[99] These cancers had chromosomal instability and were reasonably well differentiated. Inflammatory cells are associated with oxidative stress, which can lead to genetic mutations, produce soluble factors, such as vascular endothelial growth factor, which can promote angiogenesis, and generate cytokines, which can aid in evasion of apoptosis and promotion of cell proliferation.[99]

Gallbladder Carcinoma

Gallbladder carcinoma is the most common biliary tract malignancy, making up 85% to 90% of all biliary tract cancer, and is the sixth most common gastrointestinal malignancy.[7] The global rates for gallbladder cancer show marked geographic variation, reaching epidemic levels for some regions and ethnicities (**Fig. 5**).[10] Gallbladder cancer has a particularly high incidence in Chile, Japan, and northern India.[7] The basis for this variance likely resides in differences in environmental exposure and genetic predisposition to carcinogenesis. Several conditions associated with chronic inflammation are considered risk factors, which include gallstone disease, gallbladder polyps, chronic Salmonella infection, congenital biliary cysts, and abnormal pancreaticobiliary duct junction.[7]

In most instances, gallbladder cancer develops over 5 to 15 years, when metaplasia progresses to dysplasia, carcinoma in situ, and then, invasive cancer.[100] Progression is frequently rapid with disease presentation generally occurring at advanced stage. Cure depends on an early diagnosis and surgical resection. Despite this potential for cure, less than 10% of patients have tumors that are resectable at the time of surgery, whereas nearly 50% have lymph node metastasis.[101] Gallbladder cancer found incidentally at the time of cholecystectomy occurs at a rate of 0.5% to 1.5%[101–103] Gallbladder cancer is a highly lethal disease with an overall 5-year survival of less than 5%.[104] The overall mean survival rate for patients with gallbladder cancer is 6 months.[102]

As is the case with most malignancies, the incidence of gallbladder cancer increases with age with the mean age at diagnosis being 65 years.[104] In contrast to other primary malignancies of the liver and biliary tract, there is a strong predilection for gallbladder cancer in women, with female-to-male ratios varying from 1.3 to 3.5:1.[7,105]

Risk Factors

Most gallbladder cancers are adenocarcinomas arising from the gallbladder mucosa.

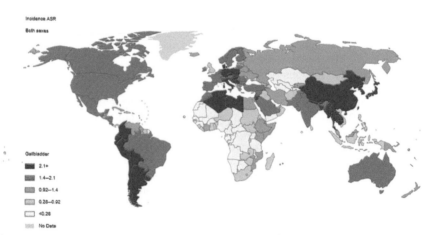

Fig. 5. Global incidence of gallbladder carcinoma per 100,000. (*Adapted with permission from Ferlay J., Soerjomataram I., Ervik M., Dikshit R., Eser S., Mathers C., Rebelo M., Parkin D.M., Forman D., Bray, F. GLOBOCAN 2012 v1.0, Cancer Incidence and Mortality Worldwide: IARC CancerBase No. 11 [Internet]. Lyon, France: International Agency for Research on Cancer; 2013. Available from: http://gco.iarc.fr/today/home, accessed on May 8, 2018.)*

The pathogenesis of gallbladder carcinoma is thought to be that chronic inflammation of the gallbladder mucosa leads to progression from dysplasia to carcinoma in susceptible patients. Most of the known risk factors for gallbladder cancer are related to inflammation.[7,106] Chronic inflammation is linked to malignant transformation, being a major factor in carcinogenesis at many sites. Recurrent inflammatory insults can promote DNA damage, inducing proliferation for tissue repair, releasing cytokines and growth factors, and predisposing cells to oncogenic transformation. Mediators, such as nuclear factor kappa B, reactive oxygen and nitrogen species, inflammatory cytokines, prostaglandins, and specific microRNAs might be oncogenic, acting through changes in cell proliferation, cell death (apoptosis), DNA mutation rates, DNA methylation, and angiogenesis.[7,107] Cholelithiasis can lead to repeated epithelial trauma, chronic inflammation, and oncogenesis.

Gallstones
The development of cholelithiasis is multifactorial in nature. Age, sex, race, parity, and rapid weight loss are all risk factors for the development of gallstones. Cholesterol stones are the predominant stone type in the United States and are formed as a result of cholesterol supersaturation of bile, accelerated cholesterol crystal nucleation, and impaired gallbladder motility.[108]

There is a definite association between benign gallstones and gallbladder cancer.[109,110] In 1 classic review of more than 2000 patients with gallbladder cancer, 73.9% of patients had stones present.[111] Other reports demonstrate similar results with 70% to 80% of patients who present with gallbladder cancer having a history or presence of stones. The incidence of gallbladder cancer among patients with stones, however, is only 1% to 3%.[112,113] Stone size greater than 3 cm and increased burden/volume of stones are risk factors for malignancy with stone size greater than 3 cm having a 10 times risk of malignancy and stone volume greater than 10 mL having a relative risk of malignancy of 11.[113,114] Increased rates for both gallbladder cancer incidence and gallstone prevalence occur in Chilean Pima Indian women (21/100,000 cancer incidence and 75.8% gallstone prevalence), North American Indian women (7.1/100,000 and 64.1%), Chilean Mapuche Indian women (27.3/100,000 and 49.4%), and East Indian women (22/10%,000 and 21.6%).[7,115–118]

Gallbladder polyps
Most gallbladder polyps are not adenomatous, and most gallbladder cancers do not arise from polyps; however, removal of gallbladders containing polyps greater than 1 cm is recommended for cancer risk reduction.[119,120] There are no particular risk factors like age, sex, or the metabolic syndrome, for gallbladder polyps. In asymptomatic individuals, there is no association between polyps and stones.[121] Benign adenomas constitute approximately 4% of all gallbladder polyps. Features that predict malignancy are polyp size greater than 1.0 cm, a solitary or sessile mass, associated gallstones, patient's age greater than 50, or rapid polyp growth.[103,118] In 1 particular report of 100 cases of gallbladder polyps, in patients with polyps greater than 10 mm, 85% were found to harbor malignancy and 15% were thought to be benign.[122]

Porcelain gallbladder
In the past, porcelain gallbladder was thought to increase the risk of gallbladder cancer tremendously. Over the last 2 decades, the magnitude of the risk that is associated with a porcelain gallbladder has been demonstrated to be less with reports showing a lower incidence of cancer associated with a calcified gallbladder of approximately 5% to 6%.[123,124] In 1 report of greater than 10,000 cholecystectomy patients, 15 were

found to have porcelain gallbladder, but none of the 15 had any evidence of malignancy.[125] A stippled, noncontinuous pattern of calcification is thought to be a greater indicator of underlying malignant potential than a completely calcified gallbladder. Although it is true that there is an increased risk associated with calcified gallbladders, the risk is more likely secondary to epithelial inflammation, resulting in the porcelain gallbladder as opposed to the porcelain gallbladder itself.[126]

Infections

Chronic bacterial cholangitis is a definite risk for biliary tract malignancy. Salmonella (eg, *Salmonella typhi and Salmonella paratyphi*) and Helicobacter (eg, *Helicobacter bilis*) are the organisms that have been associated with gallbladder cancer.[127,128] Approximately 6% of typhoid carriers develop gallbladder cancer, a 12-fold increase in risk. Bacterial colonization may affect malignant transformation, through degradation of bile constituents via bacterial hydrolysis of primary bile acids forming carcinogens and/or the action of β-glucuronides. Malignant transformation is further promoted by chronic inflammation itself, along with alterations of tumor suppressor genes, such as p53, or protooncogenes, such as mutations of *K-ras*.[107,129]

Anomalous junction

Anomalous junction of the pancreaticobiliary duct has also been implicated as a potential risk factor for gallbladder cancer.[130] This anomaly consists of a long common channel of the pancreatic duct and bile duct before entering the ampulla. The common channel may allow reflux of pancreatic secretions into the common bile duct. This reflux can lead to inflammation and metaplasia within the gallbladder and represents a possible mechanism for carcinogenesis.[131,132] Roughly 10% of patients with gallbladder cancer have this junction anomaly, and the development of cancer occurs at a younger age.[101,133] The gallbladder cancer associated with an anomalous junction is often histologically a papillary carcinoma, which tends to be less aggressive in nature than standard adenocarcinoma of the gallbladder.[103]

Genetics Gallbladder cancer arises from the interaction between genetic predisposition and exposure to environmental risk factors. Genetic factors have some role to play in the wide variability of the frequency of gallbladder cancer worldwide. One linked genetic risk is gallstone disease and gallbladder cancer. A family history of gallbladder disease increases the risk of developing gallbladder cancer.[134] The genetic background for gallstone disease accounts for approximately 25% of the total gallstone disease risk.[118] Subsequently, stones become a major risk factor for the development of gallbladder cancer. The molecular pathogenesis of gallbladder cancer, like many others, involves an accumulation of mutations, eventually leading to malignancy. The common genetic alterations are in the oncogenes, tumor suppressor genes, microsatellite instability, and methylation of gene promoter areas.[135] Pathways that have been suggested to be involved in the development of gallbladder carcinoma include (1) gallstone-mediated inflammation, p53 mutation, and eventual carcinoma; (2) *K-ras* point mutations contributing to atypical epithelium and eventually carcinoma in patients with anomalous pancreaticobiliary junctions; and (3) the potential for neoplastic foci in gallbladder polyps, arising secondarily to *K-ras* mutations. Tumor growth, as a result of neovascularization, is further promoted through interactions between p53 mutations and upregulated vascular endothelial growth factor.[7,129,135]

More than 1281 gene mutations associated with gallbladder cancer have been discovered, and yet genetic determinants in gallbladder carcinogenesis remain unclear.[136] These mutations range from monogenic mutations, in which environmental triggers play only a small role, to polymorphisms that only slightly increase the risk that is driven by environmental exposure. Carcinoma of the gallbladder is likely a multistep sequence involving cumulative genetic and epigenetic alterations.[7]

Others Body mass index (BMI) greater than 30 kg/m^2 is a risk factor for developing gallbladder cancer.[118,137] For each 5-point increase in BMI, the relative risk of developing gallbladder cancer increases by approximately 1.6 for women and 1.1 for men.[138] Obesity and the metabolic syndrome also pose other health concerns, some of which might predispose to gallbladder cancer. Diabetes, for example, is a risk factor for stone formation. Even in the absence of gallstones, however, the risk of developing gallbladder cancer in those with diabetes mellitus exists.[139]

Environmental exposure to specific toxins has also been shown to increase the risk of gallbladder cancer. Several studies have demonstrated that there is an increased incidence of gallbladder cancer in patients who work in the petroleum refining, textile, paper mill, and shoemaking industries.[140,141] There was 3.8 increased relative risk of gallbladder cancer in petroleum refining workers, and a 1.8 increased relative risk in paper mill workers compared with control cohorts.[140] Female workers in the textile industry had an increased relative risk of gallbladder cancer development of 3.2.[141] Additional associated risk factors include cigarette smoking, drugs, chemical exposure, postmenopausal state, autoimmune disorders, and inflammatory bowel disease.[100,126] Most of the nonepidemiologic risk factors seem to be related to the potential for mucosal inflammation and dysplasia.

REFERENCES

1. Altekruse SF, Devesa SS, Dickie LA, et al. Histological classification of liver and intrahepatic bile duct cancers in SEER registries. J Registry Manag 2011;38(4): 201–5.
2. Mosadeghi S, Liu B, Bhuket T, et al. Sex-specific and race/ethnicity-specific disparities in cholangiocarcinoma incidence and prevalence in the USA: an updated analysis of the 2000-2011 Surveillance, Epidemiology and End Results registry. Hepatol Res 2016;46(7):669–77.
3. Petrick JL, Kelly SP, Altekruse SF, et al. Future of hepatocellular carcinoma incidence in the United States forecast through 2030. J Clin Oncol 2016;34(15): 1787–94.
4. Rahib L, Smith BD, Aizenberg R, et al. Projecting cancer incidence and deaths to 2030: the unexpected burden of thyroid, liver, and pancreas cancers in the United States. Cancer Res 2014;74(11):2913–21.
5. Shaib YH, Davila JA, McGlynn K, et al. Rising incidence of intrahepatic cholangiocarcinoma in the United States: a true increase? J Hepatol 2004;40(3):472–7.
6. Valery PC, Laversanne M, Clark PJ, et al. Projections of primary liver cancer to 2030 in 30 countries worldwide. Hepatology 2018;67(2):600–11. [Epub ahead of print].
7. Hundal R, Shaffer EA. Gallbladder cancer: epidemiology and outcome. Clin Epidemiol 2014;6:99–109.
8. Forner A, Llovet JM, Bruix J. Hepatocellular carcinoma. Lancet 2012;379(9822): 1245–55.
9. Siegel R, Ma J, Zou Z, et al. Cancer statistics, 2014. CA Cancer J Clin 2014; 64(1):9–29.
10. Ferlay JSI, Ervik M, Dikshit R, et al. GLOBOCAN 2012 v1.0 cancer incidence and mortality worldwide: IARC CancerBase No.11 2013. Available at: http://globocan.iarc.fr. Accessed June 1, 2018.

11. El-Serag HB, Mason AC. Rising incidence of hepatocellular carcinoma in the United States. N Engl J Med 1999;340(10):745–50.
12. El-Serag HB. Epidemiology of hepatocellular carcinoma in USA. Hepatol Res 2007;37(Suppl 2):S88–94.
13. Massarweh NN, El-Serag HB. Epidemiology of hepatocellular carcinoma and intrahepatic cholangiocarcinoma. Cancer Control 2017;24(3). 1073274817729245.
14. Thiele M, Gluud LL, Fialla AD, et al. Large variations in risk of hepatocellular carcinoma and mortality in treatment naive hepatitis B patients: systematic review with meta-analyses. PLoS One 2014;9(9):e107177.
15. Makarova-Rusher OV, Altekruse SF, McNeel TS, et al. Population attributable fractions of risk factors for hepatocellular carcinoma in the United States. Cancer 2016;122(11):1757–65.
16. Mittal S, El-Serag HB. Epidemiology of hepatocellular carcinoma: consider the population. J Clin Gastroenterol 2013;47(Suppl):S2–6.
17. Parkin DM. The global health burden of infection-associated cancers in the year 2002. Int J Cancer 2006;118(12):3030–44.
18. Donato F, Boffetta P, Puoti M. A meta-analysis of epidemiological studies on the combined effect of hepatitis B and C virus infections in causing hepatocellular carcinoma. Int J Cancer 1998;75(3):347–54.
19. Shi J, Zhu L, Liu S, et al. A meta-analysis of case-control studies on the combined effect of hepatitis B and C virus infections in causing hepatocellular carcinoma in China. Br J Cancer 2005;92(3):607–12.
20. Pollack HJ, Kwon SC, Wang SH, et al. Chronic hepatitis B and liver cancer risks among Asian immigrants in New York City: results from a large, community-based screening, evaluation, and treatment program. Cancer Epidemiol Biomarkers Prev 2014;23(11):2229–39.
21. Chan HL, Wong ML, Hui AY, et al. Hepatitis B virus genotype C takes a more aggressive disease course than hepatitis B virus genotype B in hepatitis B e antigen-positive patients. J Clin Microbiol 2003;41(3):1277–9.
22. Kramvis A. Genotypes and genetic variability of hepatitis B virus. Intervirology 2014;57(3–4):141–50.
23. Pourkarim MR, Amini-Bavil-Olyaee S, Kurbanov F, et al. Molecular identification of hepatitis B virus genotypes/subgenotypes: revised classification hurdles and updated resolutions. World J Gastroenterol 2014;20(23):7152–68.
24. Kurbanov F, Tanaka Y, Mizokami M. Geographical and genetic diversity of the human hepatitis B virus. Hepatol Res 2010;40(1):14–30.
25. Thedja MD, Muljono DH, Nurainy N, et al. Ethnogeographical structure of hepatitis B virus genotype distribution in Indonesia and discovery of a new subgenotype, B9. Arch Virol 2011;156(5):855–68.
26. Hemming AW, Berumen J, Mekeel K. Hepatitis B and hepatocellular carcinoma. Clin Liver Dis 2016;20(4):703–20.
27. Orito E, Mizokami M. Hepatitis B virus genotypes and hepatocellular carcinoma in Japan. Intervirology 2003;46(6):408–12.
28. Liu S, Zhang H, Gu C, et al. Associations between hepatitis B virus mutations and the risk of hepatocellular carcinoma: a meta-analysis. J Natl Cancer Inst 2009;101(15):1066–82.
29. Datta S, Roychoudhury S, Ghosh A, et al. Distinct distribution pattern of hepatitis B virus genotype C and D in liver tissue and serum of dual genotype infected liver cirrhosis and hepatocellular carcinoma patients. PLoS One 2014;9(7): e102573.

30. Constantinescu I, Dinu AA, Boscaiu V, et al. Hepatitis B virus core promoter mutations in patients with chronic hepatitis B and hepatocellular carcinoma in bucharest, romania. Hepat Mon 2014;14(10):e22072.
31. Kao JH, Chen PJ, Lai MY, et al. Basal core promoter mutations of hepatitis B virus increase the risk of hepatocellular carcinoma in hepatitis B carriers. Gastroenterology 2003;124(2):327–34.
32. Chen CJ, Yang HI, Su J, et al. Risk of hepatocellular carcinoma across a biological gradient of serum hepatitis B virus DNA level. JAMA 2006;295(1):65–73.
33. Oba U, Koga Y, Hoshina T, et al. An adolescent female having hepatocellular carcinoma associated with hepatitis B virus genotype H with a deletion mutation in the pre-S2 region. J Infect Chemother 2015;21(4):302–4.
34. Muroyama R, Kato N, Yoshida H, et al. Nucleotide change of codon 38 in the X gene of hepatitis B virus genotype C is associated with an increased risk of hepatocellular carcinoma. J Hepatol 2006;45(6):805–12.
35. Nault JC. Pathogenesis of hepatocellular carcinoma according to aetiology. Best Pract Res Clin Gastroenterol 2014;28(5):937–47.
36. Ringelhan M, O'Connor T, Protzer U, et al. The direct and indirect roles of HBV in liver cancer: prospective markers for HCC screening and potential therapeutic targets. J Pathol 2015;235(2):355–67.
37. Albeldawi M, Soliman M, Lopez R, et al. Hepatitis C virus-associated primary hepatocellular carcinoma in non-cirrhotic patients. Dig Dis Sci 2012;57(12): 3265–70.
38. Kawada N, Imanaka K, Kawaguchi T, et al. Hepatocellular carcinoma arising from non-cirrhotic nonalcoholic steatohepatitis. J Gastroenterol 2009;44(12): 1190–4.
39. Tsai WL, Chung RT. Viral hepatocarcinogenesis. Oncogene 2010;29(16): 2309–24.
40. Peng Z, Zhang Y, Gu W, et al. Integration of the hepatitis B virus X fragment in hepatocellular carcinoma and its effects on the expression of multiple molecules: a key to the cell cycle and apoptosis. Int J Oncol 2005;26(2):467–73.
41. Fujimoto A, Totoki Y, Abe T, et al. Whole-genome sequencing of liver cancers identifies etiological influences on mutation patterns and recurrent mutations in chromatin regulators. Nat Genet 2012;44(7):760–4.
42. Jiang Z, Jhunjhunwala S, Liu J, et al. The effects of hepatitis B virus integration into the genomes of hepatocellular carcinoma patients. Genome Res 2012; 22(4):593–601.
43. Sung WK, Zheng H, Li S, et al. Genome-wide survey of recurrent HBV integration in hepatocellular carcinoma. Nat Genet 2012;44(7):765–9.
44. Chisari FV, Klopchin K, Moriyama T, et al. Molecular pathogenesis of hepatocellular carcinoma in hepatitis B virus transgenic mice. Cell 1989;59(6):1145–56.
45. Saitta C, Tripodi G, Barbera A, et al. Hepatitis B virus (HBV) DNA integration in patients with occult HBV infection and hepatocellular carcinoma. Liver Int 2015; 35(10):2311–7.
46. El-Serag HB. Epidemiology of viral hepatitis and hepatocellular carcinoma. Gastroenterology 2012;142(6):1264–73.e1.
47. Plummer M, de Martel C, Vignat J, et al. Global burden of cancers attributable to infections in 2012: a synthetic analysis. Lancet Glob Health 2016;4(9):e609–16.
48. Mortality GBD, Causes of Death C. Global, regional, and national life expectancy, all-cause mortality, and cause-specific mortality for 249 causes of death, 1980-2015: a systematic analysis for the Global Burden of Disease Study 2015. Lancet 2016;388(10053):1459–544.

49. Axley P, Ahmed Z, Ravi S, et al. Hepatitis C virus and hepatocellular carcinoma: a narrative review. J Clin Transl Hepatol 2018;6(1):79–84.
50. Sievert W, Altraif I, Razavi HA, et al. A systematic review of hepatitis C virus epidemiology in Asia, Australia and Egypt. Liver Int 2011;31(Suppl 2):61–80.
51. Altekruse SF, Henley SJ, Cucinelli JE, et al. Changing hepatocellular carcinoma incidence and liver cancer mortality rates in the United States. Am J Gastroenterol 2014;109(4):542–53.
52. Kanwal F, Kramer JR, Ilyas J, et al. HCV genotype 3 is associated with an increased risk of cirrhosis and hepatocellular cancer in a national sample of U.S. Veterans with HCV. Hepatology 2014;60(1):98–105.
53. Vescovo T, Refolo G, Vitagliano G, et al. Molecular mechanisms of hepatitis C virus-induced hepatocellular carcinoma. Clin Microbiol Infect 2016;22(10): 853–61.
54. Li Y, Boehning DF, Qian T, et al. Hepatitis C virus core protein increases mitochondrial ROS production by stimulation of Ca2+ uniporter activity. FASEB J 2007;21(10):2474–85.
55. Okuda M, Li K, Beard MR, et al. Mitochondrial injury, oxidative stress, and antioxidant gene expression are induced by hepatitis C virus core protein. Gastroenterology 2002;122(2):366–75.
56. Welzel TM, Graubard BI, Quraishi S, et al. Population-attributable fractions of risk factors for hepatocellular carcinoma in the United States. Am J Gastroenterol 2013;108(8):1314–21.
57. Grant BF, Stinson FS, Dawson DA, et al. Prevalence and co-occurrence of substance use disorders and independent mood and anxiety disorders: results from the National Epidemiologic Survey on Alcohol and Related Conditions. Arch Gen Psychiatry 2004;61(8):807–16.
58. Flegal KM, Kruszon-Moran D, Carroll MD, et al. Trends in obesity among adults in the United States, 2005 to 2014. JAMA 2016;315(21):2284–91.
59. Younossi ZM, Otgonsuren M, Henry L, et al. Association of nonalcoholic fatty liver disease (NAFLD) with hepatocellular carcinoma (HCC) in the United States from 2004 to 2009. Hepatology 2015;62(6):1723–30.
60. Banales JM, Cardinale V, Carpino G, et al. Expert consensus document: cholangiocarcinoma: current knowledge and future perspectives consensus statement from the European Network for the Study of Cholangiocarcinoma (ENS-CCA). Nat Rev Gastroenterol Hepatol 2016;13(5):261–80.
61. DeOliveira ML, Cunningham SC, Cameron JL, et al. Cholangiocarcinoma: thirty-one-year experience with 564 patients at a single institution. Ann Surg 2007; 245(5):755–62.
62. Blechacz B, Komuta M, Roskams T, et al. Clinical diagnosis and staging of cholangiocarcinoma. Nat Rev Gastroenterol Hepatol 2011;8(9):512–22.
63. Rahnemai-Azar AA, Weisbrod A, Dillhoff M, et al. Intrahepatic cholangiocarcinoma: molecular markers for diagnosis and prognosis. Surg Oncol 2017; 26(2):125–37.
64. Taylor-Robinson SD, Toledano MB, Arora S, et al. Increase in mortality rates from intrahepatic cholangiocarcinoma in England and Wales 1968-1998. Gut 2001; 48(6):816–20.
65. Alvaro D, Crocetti E, Ferretti S, et al. Descriptive epidemiology of cholangiocarcinoma in Italy. Dig Liver Dis 2010;42(7):490–5.
66. Utada M, Ohno Y, Tamaki T, et al. Long-term trends in incidence and mortality of intrahepatic and extrahepatic bile duct cancer in Japan. J Epidemiol 2014; 24(3):193–9.

67. Saha SK, Zhu AX, Fuchs CS, et al. Forty-year trends in cholangiocarcinoma incidence in the U.S.: intrahepatic disease on the rise. Oncologist 2016;21(5): 594–9.
68. Tyson GL, El-Serag HB. Risk factors for cholangiocarcinoma. Hepatology 2011; 54(1):173–84.
69. Sriamporn S, Pisani P, Pipitgool V, et al. Prevalence of Opisthorchis viverrini infection and incidence of cholangiocarcinoma in Khon Kaen, Northeast Thailand. Trop Med Int Health 2004;9(5):588–94.
70. Bergquist A, von Seth E. Epidemiology of cholangiocarcinoma. Best Pract Res Clin Gastroenterol 2015;29(2):221–32.
71. Kaewpitoon N, Kaewpitoon SJ, Pengsaa P, et al. Opisthorchis viverrini: the carcinogenic human liver fluke. World J Gastroenterol 2008;14(5):666–74.
72. Sithithaworn P, Yongvanit P, Duenngai K, et al. Roles of liver fluke infection as risk factor for cholangiocarcinoma. J Hepatobiliary Pancreat Sci 2014;21(5): 301–8.
73. Shin HR, Oh JK, Masuyer E, et al. Epidemiology of cholangiocarcinoma: an update focusing on risk factors. Cancer Sci 2010;101(3):579–85.
74. Palmer WC, Patel T. Are common factors involved in the pathogenesis of primary liver cancers? A meta-analysis of risk factors for intrahepatic cholangiocarcinoma. J Hepatol 2012;57(1):69–76.
75. Chapman MH, Webster GJ, Bannoo S, et al. Cholangiocarcinoma and dominant strictures in patients with primary sclerosing cholangitis: a 25-year single-centre experience. Eur J Gastroenterol Hepatol 2012;24(9):1051–8.
76. Boberg KM, Bergquist A, Mitchell S, et al. Cholangiocarcinoma in primary sclerosing cholangitis: risk factors and clinical presentation. Scand J Gastroenterol 2002;37(10):1205–11.
77. Chalasani N, Baluyut A, Ismail A, et al. Cholangiocarcinoma in patients with primary sclerosing cholangitis: a multicenter case-control study. Hepatology 2000; 31(1):7–11.
78. Shaib YH, El-Serag HB, Davila JA, et al. Risk factors of intrahepatic cholangiocarcinoma in the United States: a case-control study. Gastroenterology 2005; 128(3):620–6.
79. Bergquist A, Ekbom A, Olsson R, et al. Hepatic and extrahepatic malignancies in primary sclerosing cholangitis. J Hepatol 2002;36(3):321–7.
80. Soreide K, Korner H, Havnen J, et al. Bile duct cysts in adults. Br J Surg 2004; 91(12):1538–48.
81. Mabrut JY, Bozio G, Hubert C, et al. Management of congenital bile duct cysts. Dig Surg 2010;27(1):12–8.
82. Chijiiwa K, Yamashita H, Yoshida J, et al. Current management and long-term prognosis of hepatolithiasis. Arch Surg 1995;130(2):194–7.
83. Lee JY, Kim JS, Moon JM, et al. Incidence of cholangiocarcinoma with or without previous resection of liver for hepatolithiasis. Gut Liver 2013;7(4):475–9.
84. Su CH, Lui WY, P'Eng FK. Relative prevalence of gallstone diseases in Taiwan. A nationwide cooperative study. Dig Dis Sci 1992;37(5):764–8.
85. Tazuma S. Gallstone disease: epidemiology, pathogenesis, and classification of biliary stones (common bile duct and intrahepatic). Best Pract Res Clin Gastroenterol 2006;20(6):1075–83.
86. Nordenstedt H, Mattsson F, El-Serag H, et al. Gallstones and cholecystectomy in relation to risk of intra- and extrahepatic cholangiocarcinoma. Br J Cancer 2012; 106(5):1011–5.

87. Welzel TM, Graubard BI, El-Serag HB, et al. Risk factors for intrahepatic and extrahepatic cholangiocarcinoma in the United States: a population-based case-control study. Clin Gastroenterol Hepatol 2007;5(10):1221–8.

88. Welzel TM, Mellemkjaer L, Gloria G, et al. Risk factors for intrahepatic cholangiocarcinoma in a low-risk population: a nationwide case-control study. Int J Cancer 2007;120(3):638–41.

89. Razumilava N, Gores GJ. Cholangiocarcinoma. Lancet 2014;383(9935):2168–79.

90. Donato F, Gelatti U, Tagger A, et al. Intrahepatic cholangiocarcinoma and hepatitis C and B virus infection, alcohol intake, and hepatolithiasis: a case-control study in Italy. Cancer Causes Control 2001;12(10):959–64.

91. El-Serag HB, Engels EA, Landgren O, et al. Risk of hepatobiliary and pancreatic cancers after hepatitis C virus infection: a population-based study of U.S. veterans. Hepatology 2009;49(1):116–23.

92. Lee TY, Lee SS, Jung SW, et al. Hepatitis B virus infection and intrahepatic cholangiocarcinoma in Korea: a case-control study. Am J Gastroenterol 2008;103(7):1716–20.

93. Zhou YM, Yin ZF, Yang JM, et al. Risk factors for intrahepatic cholangiocarcinoma: a case-control study in China. World J Gastroenterol 2008;14(4):632–5.

94. Yamamoto S, Kubo S, Hai S, et al. Hepatitis C virus infection as a likely etiology of intrahepatic cholangiocarcinoma. Cancer Sci 2004;95(7):592–5.

95. Sekiya S, Suzuki A. Intrahepatic cholangiocarcinoma can arise from Notch-mediated conversion of hepatocytes. J Clin Invest 2012;122(11):3914–8.

96. Welzel TM, Graubard BI, Zeuzem S, et al. Metabolic syndrome increases the risk of primary liver cancer in the United States: a study in the SEER-Medicare database. Hepatology 2011;54(2):463–71.

97. Melum E, Karlsen TH, Schrumpf E, et al. Cholangiocarcinoma in primary sclerosing cholangitis is associated with NKG2D polymorphisms. Hepatology 2008;47(1):90–6.

98. Sia D, Tovar V, Moeini A, et al. Intrahepatic cholangiocarcinoma: pathogenesis and rationale for molecular therapies. Oncogene 2013;32(41):4861–70.

99. Rizvi S, Gores GJ. Molecular pathogenesis of cholangiocarcinoma. Dig Dis 2014;32(5):564–9.

100. Lazcano-Ponce EC, Miquel JF, Munoz N, et al. Epidemiology and molecular pathology of gallbladder cancer. CA Cancer J Clin 2001;51(6):349–64.

101. Sheth S, Bedford A, Chopra S. Primary gallbladder cancer: recognition of risk factors and the role of prophylactic cholecystectomy. Am J Gastroenterol 2000;95(6):1402–10.

102. Lai CH, Lau WY. Gallbladder cancer–a comprehensive review. Surgeon 2008;6(2):101–10.

103. Randi G, Franceschi S, La Vecchia C. Gallbladder cancer worldwide: geographical distribution and risk factors. Int J Cancer 2006;118(7):1591–602.

104. Duffy A, Capanu M, Abou-Alfa GK, et al. Gallbladder cancer (GBC): 10-year experience at Memorial Sloan-Kettering Cancer Centre (MSKCC). J Surg Oncol 2008;98(7):485–9.

105. Castro FA, Koshiol J, Hsing AW, et al. Biliary tract cancer incidence in the United States-demographic and temporal variations by anatomic site. Int J Cancer 2013;133(7):1664–71.

106. Albores-Saavedra J, Alcantra-Vazquez A, Cruz-Ortiz H, et al. The precursor lesions of invasive gallbladder carcinoma. Hyperplasia, atypical hyperplasia and carcinoma in situ. Cancer 1980;45(5):919–27.

107. Rashid A, Ueki T, Gao YT, et al. K-ras mutation, p53 overexpression, and micro-satellite instability in biliary tract cancers: a population-based study in China. Clin Cancer Res 2002;8(10):3156–63.

108. Venneman NG, van Erpecum KJ. Pathogenesis of gallstones. Gastroenterol Clin North Am 2010;39(2):171–83, vii.

109. Pilgrim CH, Groeschl RT, Christians KK, et al. Modern perspectives on factors predisposing to the development of gallbladder cancer. HPB (Oxford) 2013; 15(11):839–44.

110. Zatonski WA, Lowenfels AB, Boyle P, et al. Epidemiologic aspects of gallbladder cancer: a case-control study of the SEARCH Program of the International Agency for Research on Cancer. J Natl Cancer Inst 1997;89(15):1132–8.

111. Piehler JM, Crichlow RW. Primary carcinoma of the gallbladder. Surg Gynecol Obstet 1978;147(6):929–42.

112. Hsing AW, Gao YT, Han TQ, et al. Gallstones and the risk of biliary tract cancer: a population-based study in China. Br J Cancer 2007;97(11):1577–82.

113. Diehl AK. Gallstone size and the risk of gallbladder cancer. JAMA 1983;250(17): 2323–6.

114. Roa I, Ibacache G, Roa J, et al. Gallstones and gallbladder cancer-volume and weight of gallstones are associated with gallbladder cancer: a case-control study. J Surg Oncol 2006;93(8):624–8.

115. Everhart JE, Yeh F, Lee ET, et al. Prevalence of gallbladder disease in American Indian populations: findings from the Strong Heart Study. Hepatology 2002; 35(6):1507–12.

116. Miquel JF, Covarrubias C, Villaroel L, et al. Genetic epidemiology of cholesterol cholelithiasis among Chilean Hispanics, Amerindians, and Maoris. Gastroenterology 1998;115(4):937–46.

117. Singh V, Trikha B, Nain C, et al. Epidemiology of gallstone disease in Chandigarh: a community-based study. J Gastroenterol Hepatol 2001;16(5):560–3.

118. Stinton LM, Shaffer EA. Epidemiology of gallbladder disease: cholelithiasis and cancer. Gut Liver 2012;6(2):172–87.

119. Pilgrim CH, Groeschl RT, Pappas SG, et al. An often overlooked diagnosis: imaging features of gallbladder cancer. J Am Coll Surg 2013;216(2):333–9.

120. Gallahan WC, Conway JD. Diagnosis and management of gallbladder polyps. Gastroenterol Clin North Am 2010;39(2):359–67, x.

121. Jorgensen T, Jensen KH. Polyps in the gallbladder. A prevalence study. Scand J Gastroenterol 1990;25(3):281–6.

122. Terzi C, Sokmen S, Seckin S, et al. Polypoid lesions of the gallbladder: report of 100 cases with special reference to operative indications. Surgery 2000;127(6): 622–7.

123. Stephen AE, Berger DL. Carcinoma in the porcelain gallbladder: a relationship revisited. Surgery 2001;129(6):699–703.

124. Schnelldorfer T. Porcelain gallbladder: a benign process or concern for malignancy? J Gastrointest Surg 2013;17(6):1161–8.

125. Towfigh S, McFadden DW, Cortina GR, et al. Porcelain gallbladder is not associated with gallbladder carcinoma. Am Surg 2001;67(1):7–10.

126. Wernberg JA, Lucarelli DD. Gallbladder cancer. Surg Clin North Am 2014;94(2): 343–60.

127. Kumar S, Kumar S, Kumar S. Infection as a risk factor for gallbladder cancer. J Surg Oncol 2006;93(8):633–9.

128. Gonzalez-Escobedo G, Marshall JM, Gunn JS. Chronic and acute infection of the gall bladder by Salmonella typhi: understanding the carrier state. Nat Rev Microbiol 2011;9(1):9–14.

129. Saetta AA. K-ras, p53 mutations, and microsatellite instability (MSI) in gall-bladder cancer. J Surg Oncol 2006;93(8):644–9.

130. Pandey M. Risk factors for gallbladder cancer: a reappraisal. Eur J Cancer Prev 2003;12(1):15–24.

131. Nagata E, Sakai K, Kinoshita H, et al. The relation between carcinoma of the gallbladder and an anomalous connection between the choledochus and the pancreatic duct. Ann Surg 1985;202(2):182–90.

132. Nomura T, Shirai Y, Sandoh N, et al. Cholangiographic criteria for anomalous union of the pancreatic and biliary ducts. Gastrointest Endosc 2002;55(2): 204–8.

133. Kang CM, Kim KS, Choi JS, et al. Gallbladder carcinoma associated with anomalous pancreaticobiliary duct junction. Can J Gastroenterol 2007;21(6):383–7.

134. Dutta U, Nagi B, Garg PK, et al. Patients with gallstones develop gallbladder cancer at an earlier age. Eur J Cancer Prev 2005;14(4):381–5.

135. Dutta U. Gallbladder cancer: can newer insights improve the outcome? J Gastroenterol Hepatol 2012;27(4):642–53.

136. Itoi T, Watanabe H, Ajioka Y, et al. APC, K-ras codon 12 mutations and p53 gene expression in carcinoma and adenoma of the gall-bladder suggest two genetic pathways in gall-bladder carcinogenesis. Pathol Int 1996;46(5):333–40.

137. Calle EE, Rodriguez C, Walker-Thurmond K, et al. Overweight, obesity, and mortality from cancer in a prospectively studied cohort of U.S. adults. N Engl J Med 2003;348(17):1625–38.

138. Wolin KY, Carson K, Colditz GA. Obesity and cancer. Oncologist 2010;15(6): 556–65.

139. Lai HC, Chang SN, Lin CC, et al. Does diabetes mellitus with or without gall-stones increase the risk of gallbladder cancer? Results from a population-based cohort study. J Gastroenterol 2013;48(7):856–65.

140. Malker HS, McLaughlin JK, Malker BK, et al. Biliary tract cancer and occupation in Sweden. Br J Ind Med 1986;43(4):257–62.

141. Kuzmickiene I, Didziapetris R, Stukonis M. Cancer incidence in the workers cohort of textile manufacturing factory in Alytus, Lithuania. J Occup Environ Med 2004;46(2):147–53.

Current Imaging Standards for Nonmetastatic Benign and Malignant Liver Tumors

Janelle F. Rekman, MD, MAEd, FRCSC[a], Philip Smith, MD[b],
Morgan Bonds, MD[a], David Coy, MD, PhD[b], Scott Helton, MD[a],*

KEYWORDS

- Imaging • Nonmetastatic • Benign • Liver tumors • Malignant • Biopsy

KEY POINTS

- The accurate diagnosis of a liver mass can almost always be established in patients with a thorough history, physical examination, appropriate laboratory inquiry, and adequate imaging, usually without the need for a biopsy.
- Consensus guidelines, developed by the American College of Radiology (ACR), called the Appropriateness Criteria are publicly available and designed to help clinicians make bedside decisions for the best imaging tests in cases of incidentally discovered liver lesions.
- In most situations, contrast-enhanced MRI is considered the test of choice for characterization of a focal liver lesion. With MRI, additional phases are possible with contrast agents that are preferentially taken up by hepatocytes, (ie, hepatobiliary-specific contrast): the transitional and hepatobiliary phases. In situations in which MRI cannot be performed, 4-phase computed tomography of the abdomen is recommended as an alternative option.
- The decision as to which class of magnetic resonance contrast agent to use depends on the clinical scenario and should be made in consultation with a radiologist.
- In cirrhotic livers, the Liver Imaging Reporting and Data System (LiRADS) can provide a near-100% positive predictive value for hepatocellular carcinoma (HCC) if a label of LR-5 is assigned and has largely replaced biopsy as a diagnostic tool for HCC. The specifics of the LiRADS criteria are updated annually and LiRADS for contrast-enhanced ultrasonography is currently in development.

Disclosure: The authors have nothing to disclose.
Conflicts of Interest: J.F. Rekman, P. Smith, M. Bonds, and S. Helton have no commercial or financial conflicts of interest, and no funding sources.
Potential Conflicts: D. Coy: Textbook royalties from McGraw-Hill.
[a] Division of HPB Surgery, Digestive Diseases Institute, Virginia Mason Medical Center, 1100 Ninth Avenue, C6-GS, Seattle, WA 98101, USA; [b] Department of Radiology, Virginia Mason Medical Center, 1100 Ninth Avenue, C5-XR, Seattle, WA 98101, USA
* Corresponding author.
E-mail address: Scott.helton@virginiamason.org

Surg Oncol Clin N Am 28 (2019) 539–572
https://doi.org/10.1016/j.soc.2019.06.001
1055-3207/19/© 2019 Elsevier Inc. All rights reserved.

INTRODUCTION

The accurate diagnosis of a liver mass can almost always be established in patients with a thorough history, physical examination, appropriate laboratory inquiry, and adequate imaging. The necessity of a liver biopsy to determine the nature of a liver mass in 2019 is rarely necessary. This article discusses a clinical approach to patients who present with liver masses discovered incidentally and via screening based on American College of Radiology (ACR) and American Association for the Study of Liver Diseases (AASLD) guidelines, including discussion of current standards and upcoming methodologies.

CLINICAL PRESENTATION AND INITIAL IMAGING

The widespread use of cross-sectional imaging in the evaluation of patients with abdominal complaints has exponentially increased the number of incidentally discovered liver lesions.[1] In addition, screening programs to detect hepatocellular carcinoma (HCC) in patients with cirrhosis have been developed that require expert imaging interpretation. Patients with cirrhosis have an alternative differential diagnosis for a liver mass compared with patients without. The approaches to imaging for these disparate groups of patients differ (**Fig. 1**). The initial step in evaluating a patient with a liver mass always starts with an accurate history because there are many factors that influence the type of imaging modality chosen. Elements that may affect imaging choice include past exposure to chemotherapy, presence or history of other malignancies, presence of abdominal pain or symptoms, marginal renal function, and body habitus.

Most incidental liver lesions in noncirrhotic livers are benign,[2] independent of whether the patient has a known extrahepatic malignancy. Cysts, hemangiomas, focal nodular hyperplasia (FNH), and hepatocellular adenomas (HCAs) are the most common benign lesions in descending order of occurrence and are associated with different clinical patient histories.[3] The most common malignant lesions in the noncirrhotic liver are metastases, which are 40 times more likely than a primary liver tumor. In the case of a hypodense lesion on contrast-enhanced cross-sectional imaging, this possibility cannot be ignored. However, with the rapid development of imaging techniques and new contrast agents, cross-sectional imaging has become increasingly accurate at establishing a diagnosis, usually without a biopsy.

Consensus guidelines based on expert recommendations have been developed by the ACR, called the Appropriateness Criteria, and are publicly available online (https://www.acr.org/Clinical-Resources/ACR-Appropriateness-Criteria). These guidelines are designed to help clinicians make bedside decisions for best imaging tests in incidentally discovered liver lesions. In most situations, contrast-enhanced MRI is considered the test of choice for characterization of a focal liver lesion, as seen in the clinical algorithm in **Fig. 1**. In situations in which MRI cannot be performed, 4-phase computed tomography (CT) of the abdomen is recommended as an alternative option. It is key for clinicians to begin with a focused history and physical, as well as appropriate bloodwork (alpha fetoprotein [AFP], white blood cell count, cancer antigen 19-9 (Ca19-9), platelets, and so forth), to complement a properly performed cross-sectional imaging study.

MODERN IMAGING PROTOCOLS AND CONTRAST AGENTS

There are multiple cross-sectional imaging modalities available for the characterization of liver tumors, and, within each modality, multiple techniques can be used to obtain information about a tumor. The uses, advantages, and disadvantages of the

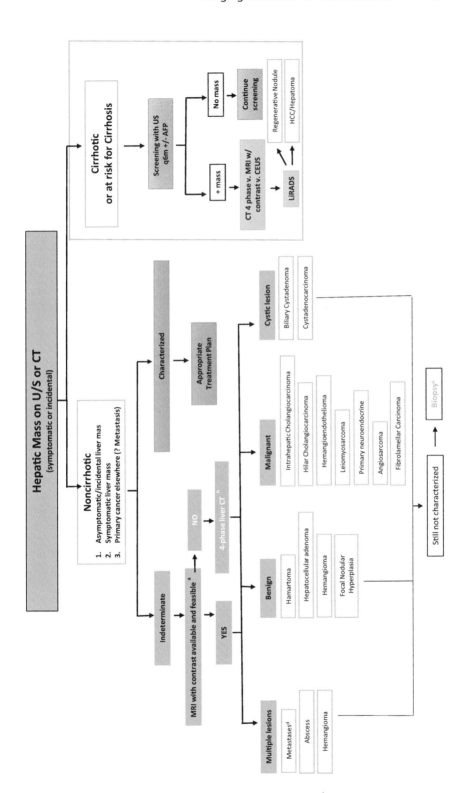

major modalities and techniques are described in **Table 1**. Particular attention is paid here to multiphase contrast-enhanced evaluation, which is the foundation of liver tumor characterization, as well as to the recent development of hepatobiliary-specific MRI contrast agents.

Multiphase Contrast-Enhanced Imaging

Multiphase contrast-enhanced imaging can be easily performed by CT or MRI. Contrast-enhanced ultrasonography (CEUS) also allows the characterization of enhancement characteristics but uses different technical parameters and is described separately. With CT and MRI, multiphase imaging refers to the serial acquisition of images of the liver at specific time intervals following intravenous contrast administration to evaluate the pattern of enhancement.

Precontrast (or noncontrast) images are helpful to evaluate the intrinsic imaging characteristics and provide a baseline with which contrast-enhanced images are compared. With CT, macroscopic fat or calcification may be evident. Noncontrast MRI is essential to determine the intrinsic signal characteristics of a lesion. Substances such as proteinaceous fluid, blood products, melanin, and macroscopic fat have intrinsic T1 hyperintensity and can be erroneously interpreted as enhancement without comparison with precontrast images.

Late arterial phase occurs approximately 30 to 35 seconds after contrast injection. There should be substantial enhancement of the hepatic artery and early enhancement of the portal vein[4] if this phase is performed correctly. Because the predominant blood supply to the liver is from the portal vein, during this phase there should be no or minimal enhancement of the hepatic parenchyma. Tumors that enhance conspicuously greater than the liver parenchyma in the late arterial phase are supplied by the hepatic artery and are said to be hypervascular.[5] Hypervascular tumors include HCC, regenerative nodules, HCC, FNH, and neuroendocrine tumor metastases.[6]

The portal venous phase occurs approximately 60 to 70 seconds after contrast injection and should show enhancement of the entire hepatic vasculature and diffuse liver parenchymal enhancement.[7] In this phase, there is maximum sinusoidal enhancement, allowing optimal visualization of hypovascular tumors. Portal venous phase imaging also allows determination of washout, which is defined as hypoenhancement of a lesion relative to the liver parenchyma. The physiology of washout appearance is not fully understood, but washout is a common feature in HCC and is seen in less than 1% of benign tumors.[8]

When using extracellular CT or magnetic resonance (MR) contrast agents (**Table 2** provides a description of the various MR contrast agents), the delayed phase is acquired between 3 and 8 minutes following contrast injection.[7] This phase allows visualization of slowly enhancing lesions or masses with fibrous characteristics, such as

---

Fig. 1. Approach to managing liver masses based on presentation and clinical history. [a] For some patients, MRI is not an optimal examination: inability to breath hold, difficulty holding still, volume ascites, and claustrophobic pacemakers (which are metallic objects in the body), wait times at center, obesity prohibiting fitting in machine, chronic kidney disease on displays caused by risk of nephrogenic systemic fibrosis. [b] See technical description of 4 phases in the text. [c] Despite best MRI technique and expert evaluation, sometimes lesions are not characterized. In this case, biopsy may be necessary if it will change the clinical management strategy. [d] Metastases from another primary tumor is much more likely than a primary liver tumor. AFP, alpha fetoprotein; CEUS, contrast-enhanced ultrasonography; CT, computed tomography; q6m, every 6 months; US, ultrasonography.

Table 1
Imaging for liver masses: indications, advantages, and disadvantages

Imaging Modality	Primary Use	Advantages	Disadvantages
MRI with conventional extracellular contrast agent (ie, Gadovist, Dotarem, Magnevist, Omniscan, Optimark, ProHance)	• Fist line, highest yield imaging modality in work-up of most liver tumors	• Excellent contrast resolution • No radiation • Highest yield diagnostic imaging technique for most scenarios	• Potential for contrast allergy • Pacemakers or other medical implants may be a contraindication • Claustrophobia or inability to remain motionless can be inhibitory • Renal failure (GFR<30) is a contraindication • Expensive
MRI with hepatobiliary-specific contrast agent (ie, Eovist/Primovist, MultiHance)	• Suspected pseudolesions such as perfusion anomalies • Differentiating FNH and adenoma • Most sensitive evaluation for very small liver metastases • Higher lesion detection rate in fatty livers and chemotherapy treated livers	• Excellent to rule out pseudolesions such as unusual fat deposition or perfusion anomalies • Highly sensitive for small nonhepatocyte lesions • Can be diagnostic for suspected FNH	• Diminished uptake in the early phases can limit evaluation for some types of tumors • Contraindications to MR as listed earlier • Hepatobiliary uptake is poor in severe hepatocellular dysfunction
Four-phase CT scan	• Next choice for primary evaluation when MRI is not available or not possible because of patient contraindications	• Quick and universally available • Few patient contraindications	• Contrast is contraindicated in renal failure • Less sensitive and lower diagnostic yield than MRI • Potential for contrast allergy
Ultrasonography	• First-line screening modality in most patients with chronic liver disease	• No radiation • Inexpensive	• Operator dependent • Large body habitus can limit visualization • Sensitivity of ultrasonography can be diminished in chronic liver disease • Ultrasonography findings are often nonspecific and rarely diagnostic

(continued on next page)

Table 1
(continued)

Imaging Modality	Primary Use	Advantages	Disadvantages
Contrast-enhanced ultrasonography	• Characterization of tumor enhancement pattern in patients unable to receive CT or MR contrast	• Can be used in renal failure and may be only opportunity for evaluation of enhancement characteristics in patients with severe renal insufficiency • Real-time enhancement evaluation	• Potential for contrast allergy • Same limitations as conventional ultrasonography • Evaluation of enhancement must be targeted to specific lesions
PET-CT	• Evaluation of distant metastatic disease	• Liver is included as part of whole-body scanning for metastatic disease	• Limited application in the work-up of an isolated liver mass • FDG-18 uptake is nonspecific; frequent false-positives and false-negatives in the liver • Rarely precludes biopsy
Tagged RBC scan	• Evaluation of suspected atypical or giant hemangioma, which is indeterminate by other modalities	• Can be helpful to confirm suspected atypical hemangioma	• Limited application • Angiosarcoma can also give a positive result
Angiography	• Not commonly used for diagnostic purposes	• Offers ability for endovascular treatment of some tumors	• Invasive with risk of complications • Rarely of primary diagnostic value

Abbreviations: CT, computed tomography; GFR, glomerular filtration rate; MR, magnetic resonance; RBC, red blood cell.

Table 2 Magnetic resonance contrast agents		
Conventional Extracellular Gadolinium-Based MR Contrast Agents		
Agent	**Trade Name**	
Gadoterate meglumine	Dotarem	
Gadobutrol	Gadavist/Gadovist	
Gadopentetate dimeglumine	Magnevist	
Gadodiamide	Omniscan	
Gadoversetamide	Optimark	
Gadoteridol	ProHance	
Hepatocyte-Specific MR Contrast Agents		
Agent	**Trade Name**	**Degree of Hepatocyte Uptake (%)**
Gadoxetate disodium	Eovist/Primovist	50
Gadobenate dimeglumine	MultiHance	3–5

intrahepatic cholangiocarcinoma. Washout appearance may also be evaluated in the delayed phase with extracellular contrast agents. With MRI, additional phases are possible with contrast agents that are preferentially taken up by hepatocytes (ie, hepatobiliary-specific contrast: the transitional and hepatobiliary phases). These additional phases and the specifics of hepatobiliary-specific contrast agents (HSCAs) are described in more detail later.

Magnetic Resonance Contrast Agents

MR contrast material comprises chelates of gadolinium, and there are currently multiple MR contrast agents available. The biodistribution of the contrast agent following injection allows broad categorization of the agents: exclusively extracellular (conventional gadolinium-based contrast agents) versus those with both extracellular and hepatobiliary-specific features.[9]

Conventional extracellular MR contrast agents behave similarly to iodine-containing CT contrast agents. That is, they are freely circulated and distributed into the extracellular space. As such, multiphase contrast-enhanced imaging with extracellular MR contrast agents provides similar enhancement information to multiphase CT. As on CT, typical extracellular contrast-enhanced phases include arterial, portal venous, and delayed/equilibrium phases.

In contrast with conventional extracellular contrast agents, a newer group of MR contrast agents that are taken up by hepatocytes have become available, allowing greater tissue differentiation. There are currently 2 available contrast agents (see **Table 2**) that show hepatobiliary activity: gadoxetic acid (Eovist in the United States and Primovist outside the United States) and gadobenate dimeglumine (MultiHance). HSCAs initially act similarly to the extracellular contrast agents, allowing arterial and portal venous phase imaging for assessment of hypervascularity and washout in the portal venous phase. However, because there is progressive accumulation of contrast material in hepatocytes, additional transitional (at 3–8 minutes) and hepatobiliary phases can be obtained. Notably, evaluation for washout appearance is possible in the portal venous phase with hepatocyte-specific contrast agents but not possible in the transitional or hepatobiliary phases, because the progressive normal, physiologic uptake of contrast by hepatocytes results in relative hypoenhancement of any nonhepatocellular tissue, mimicking washout appearance. Timing of the hepatobiliary phase depends on the degree of uptake by the agent. Gadoxetic acid shows 50% hepatobiliary uptake, whereas gadobenate dimeglumine only has 3% to 5% hepatocyte uptake.[10] Therefore, with gadoxetic acid, the hepatobiliary phase is traditionally acquired at 20 minutes, whereas the lower hepatocyte uptake of gadobenate dimeglumine requires a longer delay to acquire the hepatobiliary phase, and is typically acquired at 1 to 2 hours.

Because the degree of uptake of HSCA is directly related to the expression of hepatocyte-specific molecular transporters, the enhancement profile allows greater tissue characterization.[11] Specifically, enhancement of a focal liver lesion in the hepatobiliary phase indicates that the lesion is of primary liver origin, containing normally functioning hepatocytes connected to functioning bile ducts; the absence of enhancement implies the converse. For example, a common use case for HSCA is when FNH is suspected. FNH contains both normal hepatocytes and bile ducts and shows avid enhancement in the hepatobiliary phase. Alternatively, the absence of hepatobiliary phase enhancement in a focal liver lesion also provides important information, indicating that the lesion does not contain normal hepatocytes, bile ducts, or both. Non-hepatocyte lesions include metastases, cholangiocarcinoma, and dedifferentiated HCC, as well as benign entities such as simple cysts and hemangiomas. In addition, HSCAs can be particularly useful when problem solving in cases of suspected pseudolesions such as perfusion anomalies or unusual fat deposition.[10] Although these pseudolesions may have a masslike appearance on CT or MR with extracellular contrast, given that the underlying tissue contains normally functioning hepatocytes, enhancement is homogeneous in the hepatobiliary phase and a tumor can be confidently excluded.

The decision as to which class of MR contrast agent to use depends on the clinical scenario and should be made in consultation with a radiologist. Extracellular contrast agents and HSCAs can be complementary, and obtaining both types of examination may be of value in challenging cases. There are several specific indications when the use of gadoxetic acid is beneficial. These indications include the differentiation of HCA from FNH, evaluation of focal lesions in fatty livers, evaluation of the liver following treatment with irinotecan-based and oxaliplatin-based chemotherapy regimens, and preoperative planning for colorectal metastectomy.[12]

IMAGING FINDINGS OF COMMON PRIMARY LIVER MASSES BASED ON CLINICAL SCENARIO
Cirrhotic Livers

Regenerative nodules
Regenerative nodules are a form of benign mass that form in a cirrhotic liver, histologically characterized by micronodular or macronodular transformation of the hepatic parenchyma without fibrous septa between nodules. On arterial phase they hyperenhance and do not wash out on portal and delayed phases. MR imaging shows them to be hyperintense in T1-weighted and isointense to hyperintense on T2-weighted phases. Uptake and prolonged enhancement with hepatobiliary contrast MR proves their benign nature.

Hepatocellular carcinoma screening
The benefits of cancer screening in high-risk patients have been shown for multiple cancers,[13–15] including HCC. HCC arises from chronically inflamed liver parenchyma seen in diseases such as cirrhosis and viral hepatitis.[16] Patients with the predisposing

conditions listed in **Box 1** have an increased annual incidence of developing HCC and benefit from screening,[17] therefore patients known to have cirrhosis or these risk factors should enter into a screening program.

The AASLD recommends screening adult patients with cirrhosis, who are fit for therapeutic intervention, every 6 months with ultrasonography. Such screening has been shown to improve overall survival.[17] In certain situations, ultrasonography of the liver may not produce adequate images, either because of abdominal wall thickness or liver steatosis. Cross-sectional imaging can replace ultrasonography for screening in these scenarios.

Patients with negative imaging tests are returned to the routine screening schedule. Subthreshold lesions (<10 mm) are too small to characterize on diagnostic imaging and need to be closely followed with repeat imaging in 3 to 6 months. Increased levels of serum AFP increase the concern for malignancy in patients with subcentimeter lesions during screening.[18] Surveillance is considered positive when a mass greater than or equal to 10 mm is seen on ultrasonography or the serum AFP level is greater than or equal to 20 ng/mL. These patients should proceed to cross-sectional diagnostic imaging.

Update of Liver Imaging Reporting and Data System diagnostic criteria

The Liver Imaging Reporting and Data System (LiRADS) is designed to provide a uniform lexicon and guide image acquisition by creating an algorithm to definitively diagnose HCC and/or risk stratify liver lesions in high-risk patients.[19] This system has largely replaced biopsy as the diagnostic tool for HCC. LiRADS is routinely updated to clarify definitions and improve diagnostic accuracy, and updates to the specific criteria change yearly.

LiRADS can be applied in adult patients with high-risk features for HCC, including cirrhosis, chronic hepatitis B infection, and a current or previous history of HCC; this includes transplant candidates and recipients. LiRADS criteria should only be

---

Box 1
Conditions at risk for developing hepatocellular carcinoma

Clear surveillance benefit

Hepatitis B with cirrhosis

Hepatitis C with cirrhosis

Hemochromatosis with cirrhosis

Alpha-1 antitrypsin deficiency with cirrhosis

Other cirrhosis

Asian male hepatitis B carriers aged more than 40 years

Asian female hepatitis B carriers aged more than 50 years

Hepatitis B carrier with family history of HCC

Stage 4 primary biliary cirrhosis

Unclear surveillance benefit

Hepatitis B carriers younger than above

Hepatitis C and stage 3 fibrosis

Nonalcoholic fatty liver disease without cirrhosis

LR-1	Definitely benign
LR-2	Probably benign
LR-3	Intermediate probability of malignancy
LR-4	Probably HCC
LR-5	Definitely HCC
LR-M	Malignancy not consistent with typical HCC
LR-TIV	Tumor definitely in vein

APHE		No APHE		Non-Rim APHE		
Size (mm)		<20	>/= 20	<10	10–19	>/= 20
Additional	None	LR-3	LR-3	LR-3	LR-3	LR-4
Major	One	LR-3	LR-4	LR-4	LR-4/LR-5[a]	LR-5
Features	Two	LR-4	LR-4	LR-4	LR-5	LR-5

APHE- Arterial phase hyperenhancement; mm-millimeters; Additional major features include: Enhancing capsule, non-peripheral washout or threshold growth

Fig. 2. LiRADS categories and diagnostic criteria for CT/MR. Additional major features include enhancing capsule, nonperipheral washout, and threshold growth. [a] LR-4 if additional feature enhancing capsule. LR-5 if the additional feature is nonperipheral washout or threshold growth. TIV, tumor in vein. (*From* CT/MRI LI-RADS v2018 CORE. In: American College of Radiology. 2018; with permission.)

used when the presence of cirrhosis is confirmed.[20] Patients with variable degrees of liver disease (eg, patients with nonalcoholic steatohepatitis or nonalcoholic fatty liver disease) and chronic liver disease, but not cirrhosis, are not included in this category.

Diagnostic criteria for HCC on CT or MRI include the following major features: non-rim arterial phase hyperenhancement (APHE), size, enhancing capsule, nonperipheral washout, and threshold growth. The 2018 version (v2018) of LiRADS defines threshold growth as greater than or equal to 5 mm of growth in 6 months or less, but this is subject to change in future versions. Using these criteria, experienced radiologists risk stratify the lesion from category LR-1, definitely benign, to LR-5, definitely HCC (**Fig. 2**). Ancillary characteristics can be used at the radiologist's discretion to upgrade

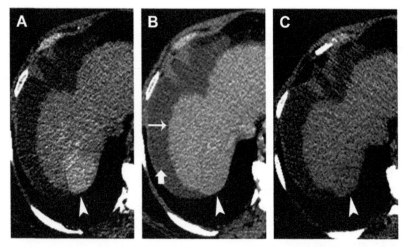

Fig. 3. Hepatocellular carcinoma. A 62-year-old woman with cirrhosis. Axial contrast-enhanced CT images in the arterial (*A*), portal venous (*B*), and 5-minute delay (*C*) phases show an arterially hyperenhancing mass (*arrowhead, A*) that is isodense to liver in the portal venous phase (*arrowhead, B*) and shows washout appearance in the delayed phase (*arrowhead, C*). These findings are characteristic of hepatocellular carcinoma in patients with cirrhosis, as indicated by liver surface nodularity (*thin arrow, B*) and ascites (*thick arrow, B*).

or downgrade the LiRADS category of a lesion. Note that these characteristics cannot be used to upgrade a lesion to an LR-5 lesion. When there is difficulty differentiating between two categories, the category of lower certainty is chosen.[20] Imaging can provide a near-100% positive predictive value for HCC in patients with cirrhosis if a label of LR-5 is assigned. The diagnosis of malignancies other than HCC can also be addressed by LiRADS. **Figs. 3–5** show examples of the typical CT and MR imaging findings of HCC.

Targetlike, rim APHE lesions are consistent with cholangiocarcinoma. However, these imaging findings can occur with atypical HCC. It is thus recommended that LR-M (malignant but not consistent with HCC) lesions undergo biopsy and pathologic diagnosis when found on screening for cirrhosis.

CEUS was added as an accepted diagnostic imaging modality to LiRADS in 2017, and readers are advised to review future LiRADS updates because the criteria are in evolution. This technique requires a high level of expertise but, because it is performed in real time and the contrast agent is purely intravascular, it allows better characterization of APHE and washout of a lesion, particularly if there is concern for contrast mistiming on cross-sectional imaging. The LiRADS diagnostic criteria for HCC on CEUS

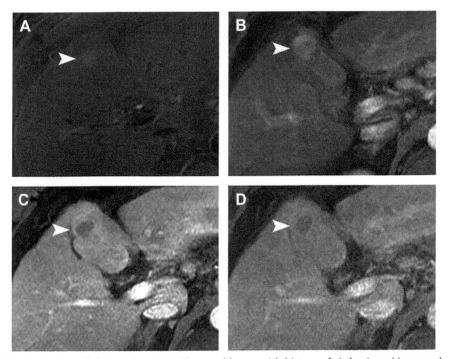

Fig. 4. Hepatocellular carcinoma. A 58-year-old man with history of cirrhosis and increased AFP level. Axial T2 (*A*) and T1 images with a conventional extracellular gadolinium-based contrast agent in the arterial (*B*), portal venous (*C*), and 5-minute delay (*D*) phases show a T2 mildly hyperintense mass (*arrowhead, A*) that has fairly homogeneous arterial phase hyperenhancement (*arrowhead, B*). There is washout (*arrowhead, C, D*) with an enhancing pseudocapsule appearance in the portal venous (*C*) and delayed (*D*) phases. This appearance is typical of HCC on MRI. Larger HCCs commonly show heterogeneous appearance, and washout appearance of any portion of the tumor is sufficient to qualify as washout.

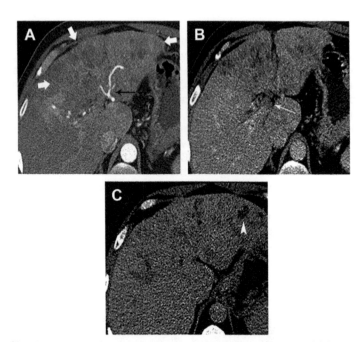

Fig. 5. Infiltrative HCC. Axial contrast-enhanced CT images in the arterial (*A*), portal venous (*B*), and 5-minute delay (*C*) phases show a large infiltrative mass (*thick arrows*) in the left lobe of the liver. There is enhancing tumor thrombus within the left portal vein (*thin white arrow, B*), and diffuse caliber enlargement of the left hepatic artery (*black arrow, A*). The mass contains macroscopic fat (*arrowhead, C*), which is a nonspecific finding associated with HCC.

are similar to those of CT or MR with a few exceptions. The presence of a capsule is not major criterion for HCC because CEUS does not depict a capsule. Rim-enhancing lesions or lesions with washout less than 60 seconds that is marked on CEUS are defined as LR-M. In addition, lesions that show globular discontinuous enhancement represent hemangiomas and are thus LR-1.[21] CEUS LiRADS categories are due to be changed in 2019 and therefore interested readers should refer to the ACR Web site for updates.

Noncirrhotic Livers

Advanced cross-sectional imaging is increasingly being used for patients without cirrhosis, resulting in an increased rate of incidentally found liver masses. Studies from the 1990s showed that 12% to 17% of CT examinations found incidental small liver lesions,[22,23] and, given continually improving technology, this number can be assumed to be even higher. Most of these lesions are benign, even in the case of extrahepatic malignancy. Distinguishing benign from malignant in a healthy liver is the focus of the remainder of this article. **Table 3** highlights specific imaging characteristics and strategies for diagnosis of specific primary tumors; some of the more common benign and malignant primary liver tumors have expanded explanations (discussed later). Examples of the imaging appearance of these tumors are shown in **Figs. 6–15**, and common liver imaging findings mimicking tumors are shown in **Figs. 16–19**.

Table 3
Specific liver masses broken down by most likely presenting clinical scenario, clinical features, and classic imaging features

Cirrhosis/Chronic Liver Disease at Risk for Cirrhosis

Clinical Scenario	Type of Mass	Common Clinical Features	MRI	CT	Enhancement Pattern (Gadolinium or Iodinated Contrast)	Ultrasonography/ CEUS
IVDU Incarceration Hepatitis B and C ETOH Obesity	Regenerative nodules	• Asymptomatic	T1 • Hyperintense T2 • Isointense to hyperintense	• Nodules 0.5–5 cm in size • Usually isoenhancing to normal liver	• Persistent enhancement on hepatobiliary-enhanced MR confirms benign nature • Hypervascular on arterial, portal venous, and delayed phase imaging (no washout)	• Often difficult to see on ultrasonography in a nodular/ fibrotic liver
	HCC/hepatoma	• Increased AFP level • Ascites • Low Platelets • Encephalopathy • Esophageal varices	T1 • Hypointense, isointense, or hyperintense to liver • Tumors with fat or hemorrhage are hyperintense T2 • Hyperintense to liver	• Look for invasion of portal or hepatic veins • Satellite nodules • Hyperenhancing capsule	LiRADS system • Hypervascular on arterial phase • Washout in venous and delayed phases • Hypointense lesion on hepatobiliary phase	• Lower sensitivity and specificity than CT or MR in diagnosing HCC • Especially in nodular, fibrotic, cirrhotic liver • CEUS: LiRADS system

(continued on next page)

Table 3
(continued)

Clinical Scenario	Type of Mass	Common Clinical Features	MRI	CT	Enhancement Pattern (Gadolinium or Iodinated Contrast)	Ultrasonography/ CEUS
Noncirrhotic						
Multiple lesions	Abscess	• Fever • Chills • RUQ pain • Weight loss	T1 • Hypointense • Diffusion-weighted imaging to determine metastasis vs abscess • Abscess shows greater restricted diffusion T2 • Hyperintense	• Internal septations are occasionally seen • Sharply marginated	• Conspicuous after contrast because of central nonenhancement • Intense early wall enhancement is characteristic • 2–5 mm uniform wall thickness • Wall enhancement persists on delayed images, with little to no perceptible change in thickness	• Early: hyperenhancing • Mature hypoenhancing or nonenhancing CEUS • Marginal enhancement in the arterial phase • Lack of enhancement in the liquefied portions
Single or Multiple Lesions						
Benign	Hamartomas	• Usually asymptomatic	• MR imaging can readily differentiate from metastases • Hypointense • Lack of restricted diffusion helps distinguish them from microabscesses T2 • Well-defined T2 hyperintense cystic lesions lack communication with the biliary tree	• Lobulated margins • Thin septations	• Characteristic thin rim of enhancement related to adjacent compressed liver parenchyma and inflammation	—

Hemangiomas	• Female predominance • Asymptomatic	T1 • Hypointense T2 • Very hyperintense	• Well circumscribed • Most remain stable in size on follow-up imaging	• Characteristic discontinuous peripheral nodular enhancement during arterial phase • Postcontrast images show progressive centripetal filling of the hemangioma • On Eovist, MRI can show potential pseudowashout that can be deceiving	• 2–10 cm, >10 = giant/cavernous • Homogeneous hyperechoic mass with acoustic enhancement CEUS • Improves diagnosis to nearly 95%
FNH	• Young and middle-aged women • Diagnosis cannot be made in cirrhotic liver	T1 • Homogeneous • Isointense to slightly hypointense T2 • Stellate central scar with T2 hyperintense signal	• Well circumscribed • Nonencapsulated • Called a stealth lesion for being invisible on noncontrast CT	• Intense uniform enhancement in arterial phase • Isointense or slightly hyperintense to the liver on portal venous and equilibrium phases; if present, the central scar shows delayed enhancement (especially in lesions larger than 3 cm)	• Difficult to detect on noncontrast ultrasonography CEUS: • Hyperenhancing in arterial and portovenous phases in wheel-spoke pattern of outward filling

(continued on next page)

Table 3
(continued)

Clinical Scenario	Type of Mass	Common Clinical Features	MRI	CT	Enhancement Pattern (Gadolinium or Iodinated Contrast)	Ultrasonography/CEUS
—	HCA	• Women • Oral contraceptives • Anabolic steroids • Diabetes • Glycogen storage diseases • Obesity • Rupture possible	MRI better than CT for diagnosis T1 • Well defined • Heterogeneous • Loss of signal on opposed-phase T1 (35%–77%) indicating fat T2 • Hyperintense	• Capsule (17%–30%) • Well defined • Range in size from <1 cm to >15 cm • Calcification: focal, present in ~5%	• Strong arterial hyperenhancement	• Highly variable • Complex, hyperechoic/hypoechoic, heterogeneous mass with anechoic areas • Capsule possible CEUS: • Useful for distinguishing from FNA (adenoma has centripetal filling on late phases, FNA centrifugal filling)
—	HNF1-α mutation	• Diffuse and homogenous signal dropout on opposed-phase T1 caused by intralesional fat • Homogeneous on other phases • Show washout on portal and/or delayed phase MRI with extracellular contrast agent • 87%–91% sensitivity and 89%–100% specificity of MRI for diagnosis				
—	Inflammatory	• Because of telangiectatic features, show strong hyperintensity on T2 • Markedly hypervascular and heterogeneous • Persistent enhancement on delayed phase • Combined findings have sensitivity of 85%–88% and 88%–100% specificity				

		B-catenin activated	No specific features			
Malignant	Fibrolamellar HCC	• Young women • Rarer than FNH	T1 • Mass: heterogeneous and slightly hypointense • Scar and septa: hypointense T2 • Mass is hyperintense • Hypointense central scar (compared with FNH)	• Large size (>10 cm) • Tumor heterogeneity • Large scar (width >2 cm) • Calcification • Invasion of adjacent vessels • Lymphadenopathy • Extrahepatic metastases	• Mass enhances on arterial phase and becomes more homogeneous enhancing on delayed phases • Central scar hypointense on all sequences and does not enhance, owing to collagen and/or coarse calcification	—
	Intrahepatic cholangiocarcinoma 1. Mass forming 2. Periductal infiltrating 3. Intraductal growth	• Weight loss • Increased Ca19-9 level	T1 • Heterogeneous • Low intensity, nonenhancing (fibrotic/necrotic areas) T2 • Mild hyperintensity • Hyperintense periphery + large central hypointensity • If hyperintense foci in center may represent necrosis or mucin	• Lobular margins • Parenchymal atrophy of affected segments • Dilated intrahepatic bile ducts • Capsular retraction over segments affected • Satellite lesions (65%) • Look for portal adenopathy with the same enhancement pattern	• Delayed images (5–20 min) show heterogeneous, persistent enhancement (caused by fibrous stroma) • Heterogeneous mild hyperintensity • Continuous peripheral ring enhancement	CEUS • Peripheral, rimlike enhancement

(continued on next page)

Table 3
(continued)

Clinical Scenario	Type of Mass	Common Clinical Features	MRI	CT	Enhancement Pattern (Gadolinium or Iodinated Contrast)	Ultrasonography/CEUS
—	Hilar cholangio-carcinoma	• Jaundice • Weight loss • Increased Ca19-9 level	• Similar to ICC but at the hilum • Often small masses, challenging to visualize	• Similar to ICC but at the hilum • Often small masses, challenging to visualize • Atrophy of hepatic segments shows long-standing obstruction	• Peripheral irregular rimlike enhancement • Heterogeneous central hypoenhancement	• Mixed echogenicity masses with biliary ductal dilatation CEUS: • Peripheral irregular rimlike enhancement with heterogeneous central hypoenhancement and washout on later phases
—	Epithelioid hemangioend-othelioma	—	• Target appearance	• Coalescent peripheral nodules • Target appearance • Capsular retraction	• Enhancing inner peripheral rim • Nonenhancing outer rim (halo appearance) • Delayed or unenhancing central portion (hyalinized stroma)	—

—	Hepatic angiosarcoma	• Highly aggressive • Weight loss • Early metastatic spread • Death within 1 y	• Hyperintense (less than hemangiomas)	• Heterogeneous • Hypervascular • Multifocal • Variable degrees of necrosis • May have masses in spleen as well	• May have peripheral and delayed enhancement that simulates hemangiomas	—
Cystic component	Biliary cystadenomas	• Rare • Middle-aged women • Ovarian stroma (histology)	T1 • Variable because of proteinaceous content or blood products T2 • Hyperintense	• Mural nodules • Septae	• Look for enhancement of capsule • Largely avascular therefore minimal enhancement seen • MR imaging can better evaluate the relationship of the mass to the bile ducts and also can help detect the unusual case of intraductal tumoral extension	• Large, well-defined, multiloculated anechoic mass • Highly echogenic septa • Nodular components may be present
—	Cystadenocarcinoma	• Similar to cystadenoma • Can have weight loss, jaundice, fatigue	• Difficult to distinguish from biliary cystadenomas on preoperative imaging	• Similar to biliary cystadenomas	• Abnormal enhancing vessels may be seen peripherally or within the septae	• Similar to biliary cystadenomas

(continued on next page)

Table 3
(continued)

Clinical Scenario	Type of Mass	Common Clinical Features	MRI	CT	Enhancement Pattern (Gadolinium or Iodinated Contrast)	Ultrasonography/ CEUS
Other primary cancer elsewhere	Metastatic lesions	• Usually multifocal disease in liver • Many times more common than primary liver tumors	• Variable appearance depending on location of primary tumor	• Variable appearance	Hyperenhancing metastases: • Neuroendocrine • Renal • Melanoma • Thyroid Hypoenhancing metastases: • Adenocarcinoma (colon, gastric, gallbladder, pancreas, lung) • Ovarian metastases almost always show washout on portal venous phase	• Hypoenhancing during the portal venous and late phases • Classic targetoid appearance (hypoechoic halo) CEUS: • Very helpful for detection

Abbreviations: ETOH, ethyl alcohol; FNA, fine-needle aspiration; HNF1-α, hepatocyte nuclear factor 1 alpha; ICC, intrahepatic cholangiocarcinoma; IVDU, intravenous drug user; RUQ, right upper quadrant.

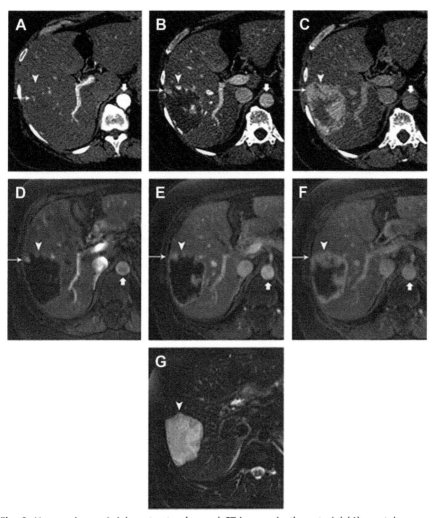

Fig. 6. Hemangioma. Axial contrast-enhanced CT images in the arterial (*A*), portal venous (*B*), and 5-minute delay phases (*C*), axial MR T1 images with a conventional extracellular gadolinium-based contrast agent in the arterial (*D*), portal venous (*E*), and 5-minute delay (*F*) phases; and axial MR T2 image (*G*). There is a mass (*arrowhead, G*) in the right lobe of the liver that is markedly T2 hyperintense and shows peripheral, nodular, discontinuous, and progressive enhancement (*thin arrow, A–F*) that follows blood pool (*thick arrow, A–F*). These findings are characteristic of a benign hemangioma, which is a slow-flow vascular malformation with the nodular enhancement representing slow filling in of the vascular channels that comprise the lesion.

Hemangioma

Hemangiomas are the most common primary benign liver mass. They are most commonly seen in women, asymptomatic, and incidentally found. Ultrasonography imaging typically shows a 2-cm to 10-cm homogeneously hyperechoic mass with acoustic enhancement. CEUS can achieve a correct diagnosis 95% of the time, compared with 75% for classic B-mode ultrasonography. On CT they are well circum-scribed and remain stable in size across follow-up studies. MRI shows a hypointense

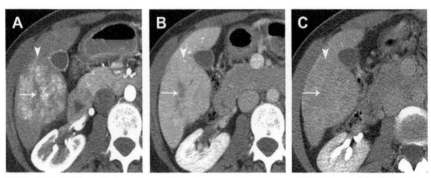

Fig. 7. FNH. Axial contrast-enhanced CT images in the arterial (*A*), portal venous (*B*), and 5-minute delay (*C*) phases show a lobulated mass (*arrowhead, A–C*) in the inferior aspect of the right lobe of the liver. There is a central hypoenhancing linear scar (*arrow, A, B*) in the arterial and portal venous phases, which shows enhancement in the delayed phase (*arrow, C*). These findings are highly suggestive of FNH, and MRI with hepatobiliary-specific contrast could be confirmatory.

lesion in T1 and very hyperintense one in T2. Their characteristic feature is discontinuous peripheral nodular enhancement during arterial phase CT or MRI with portal and delayed phases showing progressive centripetal filling over time (see **Fig. 6**). Hepatobiliary contrast MRI can show a potential pseudowashout that may be deceiving and of which radiologists need to be aware.[2]

Focal nodular hyperplasia

FNH is the second most common primary benign liver lesion and occurs mainly in young and middle-aged women, with a female predominance of 8:1. They are generally asymptomatic and once diagnosed do not require surgical management or surveillance. They are well-circumscribed, nonencapsulated, homogeneous lesions that are seldom larger than 5 cm. FNHs are challenging to detect on unenhanced ultrasonography and are called stealth lesions because of their nonvisualization on noncontrast CT. On contrast imaging, FNHs show strong, uniform, rapid enhancement in the arterial phase (see **Figs. 7** and **8**). The classic imaging feature of FNH is a central scar, most commonly seen in large lesions and present 50% to 70% of the time, which enhances in a delayed fashion because it is fibrous (in contrast with the central scar in fibrolamellar HCC, which is hypoenhancing).[24]

Hepatocellular adenoma

There are currently 4 commonly accepted molecular subtypes of HCAs, which portend a change in clinical management. When performed by an expert radiologist, MRI can often distinguish between these subtypes and may change whether a biopsy is indicated.[25] MR shows a lesion that is hyperintense on T1 with a marked decrease in signal intensity on opposed-phase sequencing suggesting presence of fat. T2 sequences often show a hypointense center. Adenomas show strong contrast enhancement on arterial phase, predominantly in the periphery (see **Fig. 9**).[26] Hepatocyte nuclear factor 1 alpha (HNF1-α) and the inflammatory subtypes are distinguishable on imaging (see **Box 1** for more information on specific imaging features).

Fibrolamellar hepatocellular carcinoma

Fibrolamellar HCC is an aggressive malignant primary liver tumor that primarily affects young woman and, in contrast with classic HCC, occurs in noncirrhotic livers. Differentiating fibrolamellar HCC from FNH can be challenging; however, radiologic features

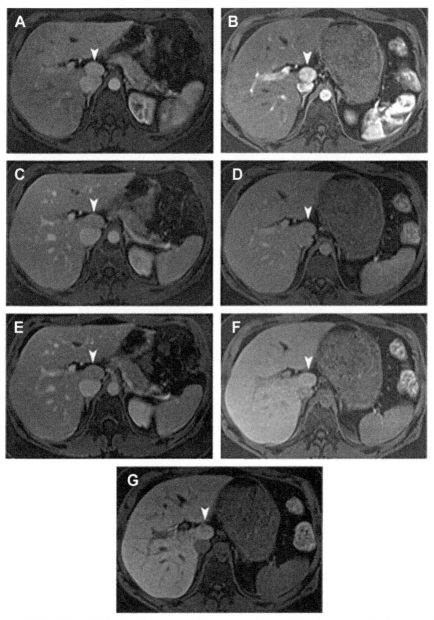

Fig. 8. FNH MRI. Axial MR T1 images with conventional extracellular gadolinium-based contrast agent in arterial (*A*), portal venous (*C*), and 5-minute delay (*E*) phases. Axial MR T1 with HSCAs in arterial (*B*), portal venous (*D*), 5-minute delayed images (*F*), and hepatobiliary (*G*) phases also obtained during a separate examination. There is an arterial phase hyperenhancing mass (*arrowheads*) in the caudate lobe. Note the similar degrees of enhancement in the arterial (*A, B*) and portal venous (*C, D*) phases with both contrast agents, because both conventional extracellular and hepatobiliary contrast agents result in similar arterial and portal venous phase enhancement. In the hepatobiliary phase (*G*), there is a similar degree of uptake in the mass compared with the normal liver parenchyma. Compare this degree of uptake with the hypointensity in hepatobiliary phase uptake of an adenoma (see **Fig. 5**E). FNH shows a central scar in approximately 50% to 70% of all cases, and is less common in lesions smaller than 3 cm, such as this one.

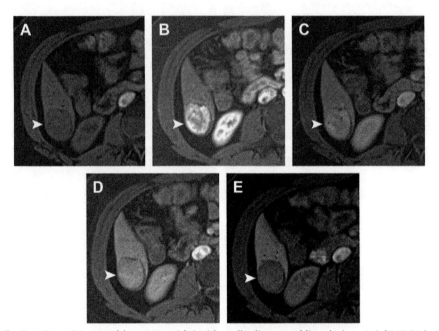

Fig. 9. HCA. A 34-year-old woman with incidentally discovered liver lesion. Axial MR T1 images with HSCA including precontrast (*A*) and postcontrast in arterial (*B*), portal venous (*C*), 5-minute delay (*D*), and hepatobiliary phase (*E*) images with a HSCA. There is a solid hypervascular mass (*arrowheads*) in the right lobe of the liver with avid arterial phase enhancement (*B*), no washout on portal venous phase (*C*), and signal loss on the hepatobiliary phase (*E*). The primary differential diagnosis is adenoma versus FNH; the signal loss on hepatobiliary phase is consistent with adenoma. FNH would be expected to have signal on the hepatobiliary phase.

consistent with aggressive malignant masses (large size, tumor heterogeneity, large central scar >2 cm, internal calcifications, invasion of adjacent vessels, lymphadenopathy, and extrahepatic metastases) are only present in the former.[27] Fibrolamellar HCC enhances on arterial phase imaging and becomes more homogeneously enhanced on delayed phases (see **Fig. 10**). Often a central scar occurs, but, in contrast with FNH, it is hypointense on all sequences and does not enhance because of collagenous deposits and/or coarse calcifications.[28]

Intrahepatic cholangiocarcinoma

There are 3 subtypes of intrahepatic cholangiocarcinoma (ICC) based on their histology and imaging behavior (mass forming, periductal infiltrating, and intraductal growth). What they all share in common in terms of imaging features is heterogeneous, persistent enhancement in delayed images (5–20 minutes) caused by their fibrous stroma (see **Fig. 11**). Portal lymphadenopathy resulting from an ICC should have a similar enhancement pattern. Mass-forming lesions show a more easily identifiable continuous peripheral ring enhancement[29] and a hyperintense periphery (cellular) with a large central area of hypointensity (fibrosis). Other imaging features include lobular margins, dilated intrahepatic ducts proximal to the lesion indicating bile duct involvement, capsular retraction over affected liver segments, and satellite lesions in 65% of ICCs.

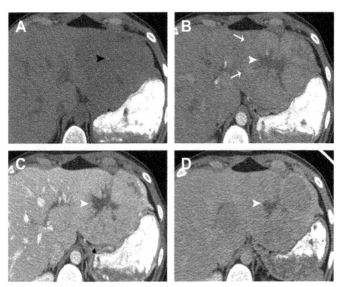

Fig. 10. Fibrolamellar HCC. A 19-year-old woman with increased AFP level. Axial CT noncontrast (A) and contrast-enhanced images in the arterial (B), portal venous (C), and 5-minute delay (D) phases show a large heterogeneous mass (*arrows*) occupying the left lateral segment. Punctate calcification (*black arrowhead*) and a large central scar (*white arrowhead*) are present. The scar shows progressive enhancement on subsequent postcontrast images, typical of fibrous tissue. Although FNH can also show a central scar (see **Fig. 1**), the presence of calcification and marked heterogeneity of this mass, as well as increased AFP level, indicate the diagnosis of fibrolamellar HCC.

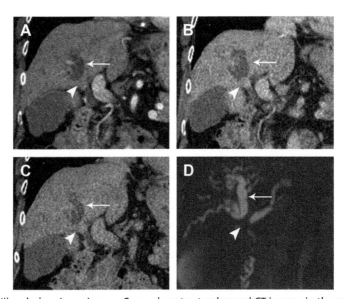

Fig. 11. Hilar cholangiocarcinoma. Coronal contrast-enhanced CT images in the arterial (A), portal venous (B), and 5-minute delay (C) phases, as well as a coronal MR cholangiopancreatography (MRCP) image (D), show an enhancing stricture in the biliary hilum (*arrowheads*) with obstruction of the intrahepatic biliary tree (*arrows*).

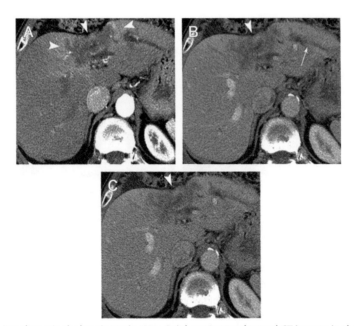

Fig. 12. Intrahepatic cholangiocarcinoma. Axial contrast-enhanced CT images in the arterial (*A*), portal venous (*B*), and 5-minute delay (*C*) phases show an ill-defined mass in the left hepatic lobe (*arrowheads*) with slow, progressive enhancement, typical of the fibrous tissue of an intrahepatic cholangiocarcinoma. There is biliary obstruction in the left lateral segment (*arrow, B*). Note the capsular retraction (*arrowhead, B*) which is a feature associated with cholangiocarcinoma.

Hilar cholangiocarcinoma

Hilar cholangiocarcinomas (Klatskin tumors) occur at the bifurcation of the right and left hepatic ducts and therefore most patients present with clinical jaundice and dilated intrahepatic ducts. MR, CT with intravenous contrast, and CEUS can show masses with similar enhancement patterns to that of ICC, and the masses can be small. MR cholangiopancreatography (MRCP) and endoscopic retrograde cholangiopancreatography (ERCP) cholangiograms can be helpful to differentiate levels of ductal involvement (see **Fig. 12**). Cross-sectional imaging showing hepatic segmental atrophy usually indicates long-standing biliary obstruction of that segment.

LESS COMMON INVESTIGATIONS FOR PRIMARY LIVER MASSES
PET Computed Tomography

PET-CT is useful for staging malignancies but is infrequently used for diagnosing primary liver cancers. The physiologic information of PET provides a functional map of abnormal versus normal tissue metabolism, and overlaying this on a CT image provides complementary anatomic detail, which can localize PET findings. These modalities are synergistic, with the diagnostic findings of PET-CT routinely outperforming PET alone.[30] Although PET-CT is not routinely used for imaging primary tumors of the liver, there are distinct indications for which it can add useful information.[31]

The most common isotope used for PET-CT is fludeoxyglucose F 18 (FDG-18). A well-differentiated HCC has mild FDG-18 uptake but, because the normal liver has physiologic mild FDG-18 uptake as well because of its extensive role in glucose

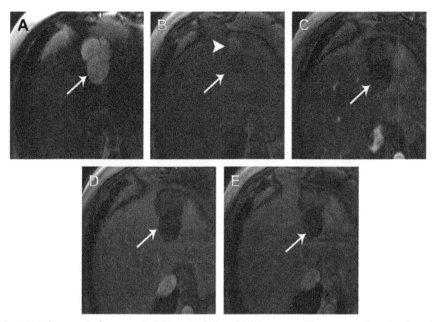

Fig. 13. Biliary cystadenoma. Axial MR T2 (*A*) and T1 images with a conventional extracellular gadolinium-based contrast agent, including precontrast (*B*) and postcontrast in the arterial (*C*), portal venous (*D*), and 5-minute delay (*E*) phases. There is a mildly complex cyst (*arrow, A–E*) in the left hepatic lobe with multiple thin septations. There is intermediate-intensity T1 material in the anterior aspect of the cyst (*arrowhead, B*) compatible with debris or hemorrhage but no enhancing component to increase suspicion for cystadenocarcinoma.

metabolism, uptake by HCC is obscured. Given that a well-differentiated HCC has similar physiology to normal liver, their degrees of glucose uptake are similar. Overall, the sensitivity of FDG-18–PET for a well-differentiated HCC is only 50%.[32] In contrast, poorly differentiated HCC shows increased uptake relative to surrounding liver on FDG-18–PET, but these tumors are also easily detected on other imaging modalities, which are quicker, less expensive, and have lower radiation exposure. Therefore, the yield of FDG-18–PET for HCC is low. Because FDG-18–PET has such limited sensitivity, another radioisotope, ^{11}C-acetate, has been shown to preferentially accumulate in well-differentiated HCC, and ^{11}C-acetate PET is an option for this lesion if offered by a center's nuclear medicine department.[33]

One example of the utility of PET-CT in hepatic lesions is in the diagnosis and staging of ICC. As with many other intrahepatic tumors, PET-CT has not been found to improve diagnostic accuracy of CT, MRI, or MRCP, despite ICC being FDG-18 avid.[34] An exception may be differentiating benign and malignant bile duct strictures because a significant difference in standardized uptake value units has been found.[35]

Contrast-Enhanced Ultrasonography

CEUS is increasingly being used to evaluate liver masses, with all the positive attributes of ultrasonography and avoidance of radiation and the contraindications of MRI. In addition, microbubble contrast agents are nonnephrotoxic. In order to use

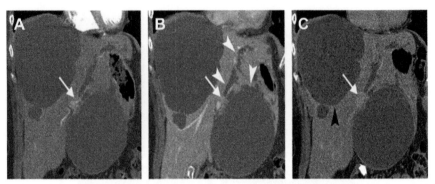

Fig. 14. Biliary cystadenocarcinoma. Coronal contrast-enhanced CT images in the arterial (*A*), portal venous (*B*), and 5-minute delayed (*C*) phases. Large complex cyst in the left hepatic lobe with a solid enhancing mural nodule (*thin arrow*) that extends into the central biliary tree and results in upstream biliary obstruction (*white arrowheads, B*). There is also wall thickening of the inferior aspect of the cyst (*thick arrow, C*). There are other simple cysts in the right lobe (*black arrowhead, C*) without any solid components representing benign hepatic cysts.

CEUS, the lesion must be able to be visualized on noncontrast ultrasonography. The study is initiated by injecting an approved microbubble contrast. The arterial phase occurs approximately 10 to 45 seconds after contrast injection. Portal venous phase then begins and lasts until 2 minutes postinjection. The late phase lasts until the

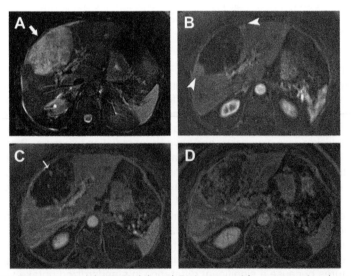

Fig. 15. Angiosarcoma. Axial MR T2 (*A*) and T1 images with a conventional extracellular gadolinium-based contrast agent in the arterial (*B*), portal venous (*C*), and 5-minute delay (*D*) phases. There is a hypervascular mass (*thick arrow, A*) in the right lobe of the liver that is T2 hyperintense, but more heterogeneous and lower signal intensity than a typical hemangioma. There is surrounding transient perfusion anomaly of the adjacent liver parenchyma in the arterial phase (*arrowheads, B*), commonly seen with hypervascular lesions. There is internal progressive heterogeneous enhancement (*thin arrow, C*) in the portal venous and delayed phases.

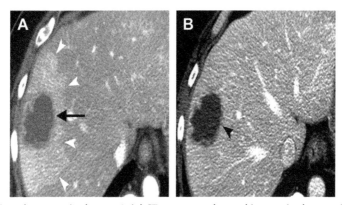

Fig. 16. Hepatic pyogenic abscess. Axial CT contrast-enhanced images in the arterial (*A*) and portal venous (*B*) phases show a complex cystic lesion (*arrow, A*) in the right hepatic lobe with thick irregularly enhancing wall (*black arrowhead, B*). The hyperenhancement on early postcontrast sequences (*white arrowheads, A*) represents vascular shunting from hyperemia.

microbubbles have unequivocally cleared, around 6 minutes after contrast has been injected. Reinjection of microbubble contrast can occur if needed for additional observations.[21]

There are a few contrast agents available and US Food and Drug Administration approved in the United States, including SonoVue/Lumason (sulfur hexafluoride lipid microspheres), octafluoropropane (perflutren with a lipid shell), and Sonazoid (perfluorobutane with a phospholipid shell). The microbubbles are 1 to 10 μm in size (equal to or smaller than red blood cells) and therefore macrovascular and microvascular structures can be visualized. The bubbles survive passage through the pulmonary circulation and recirculate, producing systemic ultrasonography enhancement. The highly echogenic microbubble gas core provides contrast and differentiates structures from background tissue.[36]

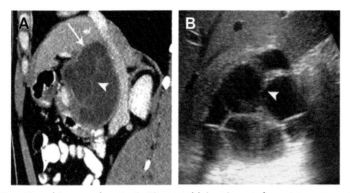

Fig. 17. Hepatic echinococcal cyst. A 19-year-old immigrant from Iraq presenting with abdominal pain. Sagittal contrast-enhanced CT (*A*) and sagittal ultrasonography images (*B*) show a complex cystic lesion (*arrow, A*) with numerous thickened internal septations (*arrowheads, A, B*). Echinococcal cysts commonly show a daughter cyst configuration. However, even in the absence of daughter cyst appearance this entity should be considered in the setting of a complex cystic lesion with an appropriate history.

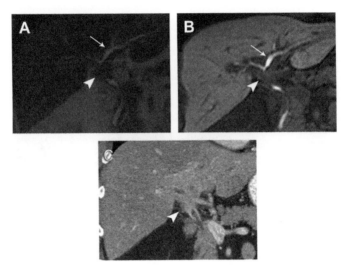

Fig. 18. Immunoglobulin (Ig) G4–related cholangiopathy mimicking hilar cholangiocarcinoma. Coronal MRCP (*A*) and T1 images with a HSCA in the hepatobiliary phase (*B*) show a severe stricture at the confluence of the right and left hepatic ducts extending into the common hepatic duct. On the hepatobiliary phase there is normal liver parenchymal enhancement, but hypointense soft tissue at the biliary hilum, and excreted contrast agent within the bile ducts (*arrow, A, B*). Coronal contrast-enhanced CT image in the portal venous phase (*C*) shows corresponding enhancing soft tissue causing the stricture seen by MRI. Cholangiocarcinoma would have a similar imaging appearance. IgG4-related cholangiopathy occurs within a spectrum of autoimmune conditions affecting multiple organ systems manifesting as tumorlike lymphoplasmacytic infiltration. This condition most often affects men, is associated with increased IgG4 levels, and shows response to treatment with steroids.

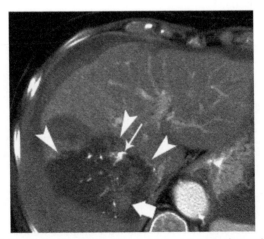

Fig. 19. Hepatic infarct. Axial portal venous phase contrast-enhanced CT image shows geographic hypointensity in the posterior right lobe (*arrowheads*). There are areas of linear hyperdense contrast material (*thin arrow*) compatible with material from recent endovascular embolization procedure. Internal regions of amorphous intermediate density (*thick arrow*) may represent areas of hemorrhage.

In centers with the necessary expertise, CEUS has become increasingly accepted as an alternative for diagnosing hepatic lesions that is equivalent to contrast-enhanced CT and MRI without the corresponding radiation. In addition to HCC screening, CEUS is most useful for incidental findings on routine ultrasonography, requiring a contrast study for further definition in patients who are unable to undergo contrast-enhanced CT or MRI (most commonly because of renal insufficiency) or when these studies are inconclusive. A downside of CEUS is that fat, being echogenic on ultrasonography, can attenuate the difference in appearance between the microbubbles and the liver tissue, making lesion characterization in fatty livers more challenging.[37] In experienced hands, CEUS has an estimated sensitivity of 95% and a specificity of 94% for diagnosing malignancy, which is similar (and possibly superior) to contrast-enhanced CT and MRI in the diagnosis of focal hepatic lesions.[38–40]

Although a promising technique, CEUS is not yet standard of care because it is only available in specialized centers of expertise and can be labor intensive. In contrast with non-CEUS, in which sonographers can independently perform the examination, many centers require a radiologist to also be in attendance for CEUS in order to direct the examination and monitor for adverse contrast reaction. CEUS should not be used for staging because it can only visualize a limited number of lesions per study[21] and the radiologist needs to have a road map of where to look in the liver. Therefore, in current practice, CEUS can be a useful tool to further characterize a known liver lesion.

Endoscopic Retrograde Cholangiopancreatography/Endoscopic Ultrasonography

There are some circumstances, mainly while working up a hilar or intrahepatic cholangiocarcinoma, in which there is no mass visualized on 4-phase CT or MRI/MRCP to account for the patient's jaundice. Under such circumstances, additional diagnostic testing may be warranted. Cholangiography, achieved via ERCP or percutaneous transhepatic biliary drain, may add additional information on the level of obstruction and biliary involvement, which are not seen on MRCP. Endoscopic ultrasonography occasionally shows a mass in the bile duct, not visible with cross-sectional imaging. However, these tests are usually performed for a therapeutic purpose or to obtain a biopsy rather than for diagnostic purposes.

SUMMARY

Contrast-enhanced CT and MRI (and in some centers CEUS) are the standard of care for diagnosing liver lesions, and high-quality imaging should be performed before performing a biopsy. With quick access to up-to-date standards such as the ACR Appropriateness Criteria, the medical community has guidance on which studies have been shown to be effective, efficient, and cost-effective for the evaluation of patients with liver masses. With this in mind, appropriate investigation and forethought are required before ordering a specific imaging test. In addition to gaining familiarity with national guidelines, the authors also encourage physicians to use the expertise of their radiology colleagues for specific guidance, because doing so can often guide the optimal imaging work-up and avoid unnecessary and wasteful imaging examinations, as well as inappropriate and avoidable biopsies. Importantly, history, physical examination, and laboratory investigations guide the treating clinicians and radiologists in the proper selection of an imaging study. The ability to accurately characterize lesions, even with the most modern imaging equipment, requires proper use and understanding of the technology and expert interpretation. When such expertise does not exist, strong consideration should be given to referring a patient to a center or physician that has experience in diagnosing and treating liver tumors.

REFERENCES

1. Matos A, Velloni F, Ramalho M, et al. Focal liver lesions: practical magnetic resonance imaging approach. World J Hepatol 2015;7(16):1987–2008.
2. Cogley JR, Miller FH. MR imaging of benign focal liver lesions. Radiol Clin North Am 2014;52:657–82.
3. Nault J, Bioulac-Sage P, Zucman-Rossi J. Hepatocellular benign tumors-from molecular classification to personalized clinical care. Gastroenterology 2013;144:888–902.
4. Fleischmann D, Kamaya A. Optimal vascular and parenchymal contrast enhancement: the current state of the art. Radiol Clin North Am 2009;47(1):13–26.
5. Coy D, Lin E, Kanne J. Body CT: the essentials. New York: McGraw-Hill Education; 2014.
6. Murakami T, Tsurusaki M. Hypervascular benign and malignant liver tumors that require differentiation from hepatocellular carcinoma: key points of imaging diagnosis. Liver Cancer 2014;3(2):85–96.
7. Donato H, França M, Candelária I, et al. Liver MRI: from basic protocol to advanced techniques. Eur J Radiol 2017;93:30–9.
8. Morana G, Grazioli L, Kirchin MA, et al. Solid hypervascular liver lesions: accurate identification of true benign lesions on enhanced dynamic and hepatobiliary phase magnetic resonance imaging after gadobenate dimeglumine administration. Invest Radiol 2011;46(4):225–39.
9. Ringe K, Husarik D, Sirlin C, et al. Gadoxetate disodium–enhanced MRI of the liver: part 1, protocol optimization and lesion appearance in the noncirrhotic liver. AJR Am J Roentgenol 2010;195:13–28.
10. Seale M, Catalano O, Saini S, et al. Hepatobiliary-specific MR contrast agents: role in imaging the liver and biliary tree. Radiographics 2009;29(6):1725–48.
11. Goodwin MD, Dobson JE, Sirlin CB, et al. Diagnostic challenges and pitfalls in MR imaging with hepatocyte-specific contrast agents. RadioGraphics 2011;31:1547–68.
12. Jhaveri K, Cleary S, Audet P, et al. Consensus statements from a multidisciplinary expert panel on the utilization and application of a liver-specific MRI contrast agent (gadoxetic acid). AJR Am J Roentgenol 2015;204(3):498–509.
13. National Lung Screening Trial Research Team. Reduced lung-cancer mortality with low-dose computed tomographic screening. N Engl J Med 2011;365:395–409.
14. Myers E, Moorman P, Gierisch J, et al. Benefits and harms of breast cancer screening: a systematic review. JAMA 2015;314:1615–34.
15. Mandel J, Church T, Bond J, et al. The effect of fecal occult-blood screening on the incidence of colorectal cancer. N Engl J Med 2000;343:1603–7.
16. Brechot C. Pathogenesis of hepatitis B virus-related hepatocellular carcinoma: old and new paradigms. Gastroenterology 2004;127:S56–61.
17. Marrero J, Kulik L, Sirlin C, et al. Diagnosis, staging, and management of hepatocellular carcinoma: 2018 practice guidance by the American Association for the Study of Liver Diseases. Hepatology 2018;68:723–50.
18. Zhang B, Yang B. Combined alpha fetoprotein testing and ultrasonography as a screening test for primary liver cancer. J Med Screen 1999;6:108–10.

19. Elsayes KM, Kielar AZ, Elmohr MM, et al. White paper of the Society of Abdominal Radiology hepatocellular carcinoma diagnosis disease-focused panel on LI-RADS v2018 for CT and MRI. Abdom Radiol (NY) 2018;43(10):2625–42.
20. CT/MRI LI-RADS v2018 CORE. In: American College of radiology. Available at: https://www.acr.org/Clinical-Resources/Reporting-and-Data-Systems/LI-RADS/CT-MRI-LI-RADS-v2018. Accessed December 22, 2018.
21. CEUS LI-RADS v2017 CORE. In: American College of radiology. Available at: https://www.acr.org/Clinical-Resources/Reporting-and-Data-Systems/LI-RADS/CEUS-LI-RADS-v2017. Accessed December 22, 2018.
22. Jones E, Chezmar J, Nelson R, et al. The frequency and significance of small (less than or equal to 15mm) hepatic lesions detected by CT. Am J Roentgenol 1992;158(3):535–9.
23. Schwartz L, Gandras E, Colangelo S, et al. Prevalence and importance of small hepatic lesions found at CT in patients with cancer. Radiology 1999;210(1):71–4.
24. Venturi A, Piscaglia F, Vidili G, et al. Diagnosis and management of hepatic focal nodular hyperplasia. J Ultrasound 2007;10(3):116–27.
25. Nault J, Couchy G, Balabaud C, et al. Molecular classification of hepatocellular adenoma associates with risk factors, bleeding, and malignant transformation. Gastroenterology 2017;152(4):880–94.
26. Chung K, Mayo-Smith W, Saini S, et al. Hepatocellular adenoma: MR imaging features with pathologic correlation. Am J Roentgenol 1995;165(2):303–8.
27. Blachar A, Federle M, Ferris J, et al. Radiologists' performance in the diagnosis of liver tumors with central scars by using specific CT criteria. Radiology 2002;223(2):532–9.
28. McLarney J, Rucker P, Bender G, et al. Fibrolamellar carcinoma of the liver: radiologic-pathologic correlation. Radiographics 1999;19(2):453–71.
29. Apisarnthanarak P, Pansri C, Maungsomboon K, et al. The CT appearances for differentiating of peripheral, mass-forming cholangiocarcinoma and liver metastases from colorectal adenocarcinoma. J Med Assoc Thai 2014;97(4):415–22.
30. Blodgett T, Meltzer C, Townsend D. PET-CT: form and function. Radiology 2007;242:360–85.
31. Banks K, Song W. Role of Positron Emission Tomography – Computed Tomography in gastrointestinal malignancies. Radiol Clin North Am 2013;51:799–831.
32. Lin E, Abass A. PET and PET/CT: a clinical guide. 2nd edition. New York: Thieme Medical Publishers; 2009.
33. Sacks A, Peller P, Surasi D, et al. Value of PET/CT in the management of primary hepatobiliary tumors, part 2. Am J Roentgenol 2011;197:260–5.
34. Kim J, Kim M, Lee T, et al. Clinical role of [18]FDG PET-CT in suspected and potentially operable cholangiocarcinoma: a prospective study compared with conventional imaging. Am J Gastroenterol 2008;103:1145–51.
35. Reinhard M, Strunk H, Gerhardt T, et al. Detection of Klatskin's tumour in extrahepatic bile duct strictures using delayed 18-F-FDG PET-CT: preliminary results for 22 patient studies. J Nucl Med 2005;46:1158–63.
36. Malhi H, Grant E, Duddalwar V. Contrast-enhanced ultrasound of the liver and kidney. Radiol Clin North Am 2014;52:1172–90.
37. Wilson S, Kim T, J H, et al. Enhancement pattern of focal liver masses: discordance between contrast-enhanced sonography and contrast-enhanced CT and MRI. Am J Roentgenol 2007;189(1):7–12.
38. Dietrich C, Kratzer W, Strobe D, et al. Assessment of metastatic liver disease in patients with primary extrahepatic tumors by contrast-enhanced sonography versus CT and MRI. World J Gastroenterol 2006;12(11):1699.

39. Guang Y, Xie L, Ding H, et al. Diagnostic value of focal liver lesions with SonoVue®-enhanced ultrasound compared with contrast-enhanced computed tomography and contrast-enhanced MRI: a meta-analysis. J Cancer Res Clin Oncol 2011;137(11):1595–605.
40. Seitz K, Bernatik T, Strobel D, et al. Contrast-enhanced ultrasound (CEUS) for the characterization of focal liver lesions in clinical practice (DEGUM Multicenter Trial): CEUS vs. MRI – a prospective comparison in 269 patients. Ultraschall Med 2010;31(5):492.

Nonsurgical Approaches to Treat Biliary Tract and Liver Tumors

Benjamin L. Green, MD, Michael G. House, MD*

KEYWORDS

- Cholangiocarcinoma • Hepatocellular carcinoma • Microwave ablation
- Radiofrequency ablation • Photodynamic therapy

KEY POINTS

- Most patients with primary hepatobiliary malignancies are not candidates for curative operative interventions.
- Nonoperative local therapies for patients with advanced hepatobiliary malignancies are advancing.
- Research into the outcomes of both monotherapy and combinational treatments suggests prolonged survival and reduced morbidity in patients with incurable disease.
- High-quality data regarding the superiority of any particular locoregional technique in controlling advanced hepatobiliary malignancies are lacking.

INTRODUCTION

The advent of percutaneous and endoscopic therapies has changed the management of hepatobiliary malignancies.[1,2] Although R0 surgical resection is the mainstay for therapy with curative intent, candidates for surgery are routinely excluded because of tumor location, stage, and patient-related comorbidity factors. Recent studies in endoscopic and percutaneous techniques for the local treatment of cholangiocarcinoma (CC) and hepatocellular carcinoma (HCC) are reviewed in this article. For perihilar cholangiocarcinoma (PHC), consideration is given to 3 endoscopic treatments: radiofrequency ablation (RFA), photodynamic therapy (PDT), and irreversible electroporation (IRE). The roles for percutaneous RFA, IRE, and microwave ablation (MWA) are discussed for HCC treatment. Multidisciplinary expertise in these techniques remains crucial to an institution's optimal practices for managing patients with HCC

Disclosures: The authors have nothing to disclose.
Department of Surgery, Indiana University School of Medicine-IU Health University Hospital, 545 Barnhill Drive, Emerson Hall 515, Indianapolis, IN 46202, USA
* Corresponding author.
E-mail address: michouse@iupui.edu

Surg Oncol Clin N Am 28 (2019) 573–586
https://doi.org/10.1016/j.soc.2019.06.013

and CC. Locoregional therapies for intrahepatic cholangiocarcinoma have been reviewed elsewhere.[3]

ENDOSCOPIC THERAPIES FOR CHOLANGIOCARCINOMA
Indications

Cholangiocarcinoma represents 2% of gastrointestinal malignancies. Distal cholangiocarcinoma and PHC arise distal and proximal to the insertion of the cystic duct, respectively. Together, they constitute more than half of all CCs, most being PHC.[4] Indications for operation with curative intent are technical resectability and lack of comorbid patient conditions. For distal cholangiocarcinoma, technical resectability is defined as the absence of locally advanced or metastatic disease.[5] For PHC, accepted criteria for resectability involve biliary, portal, and hepatic anatomic considerations after distant metastatic disease is excluded.[6] Postsurgical outcomes for PHC can be predicted from several established staging systems.[7]

Five-year survival rates for patients undergoing curative R0 operations for cholangiocarcinoma are 30% to 50%; however, only a minority of patients are considered surgical candidates.[8] When curative surgery is contraindicated, the standard of care is placement of a stent in the affected bile duct to relieve symptoms associated with obstructive jaundice. Stent placement has been shown to decrease secondary morbidity from obstructive jaundice, including pruritus, secondary biliary cirrhosis, and cholangitis. Self-expanding bare metal stents (SEMS) have superior patency durability compared with plastic stents.[9,10] However, stent placement is a temporizing treatment, and tumor progression can cause stent occlusion ultimately leading to major morbidity and mortality. Even for SEMS, the median stent patency time in the absence of locoregional therapy is 6 to 10 months.[10] PDT and RFA are endobiliary therapies that can occur simultaneously with stent placement or during stent maintenance (eg, replacement of an occluded stent). The utility of these interventions is being investigated for their potential to prolong stent patency and improve overall survival for patients with distal and perihilar cholangiocarcinoma.

Photodynamic Therapy

Protocols for PDT involve several steps. Before endoscopy, a photoactive compound is administered systemically, with cancer cells showing preferential uptake. Approximately 48 to 72 hours later, endoscopic cholangioscopy is performed to identify the diseased region of the bile duct. A diode laser system is typically used to irradiate the selected region of bile duct stricturing. Light of a certain wavelength is applied for several minutes. The subsequent cancer cell death occurs through multiple mechanisms, including creation of oxygen free radicals.[11] In addition, stenting of the bile duct stricture is maintained with percutaneous or endobiliary drainage tubes. Typically, multiple PDT sessions are required and often require biliary stent maintenance. Optimal time interval and number of PDT sessions have not been established. Outcomes after PDT and SEMS placement alone have been shown to be comparable.[12] Importantly, all patients must avoid direct sunlight exposure for a period of days to weeks after infusion with photoactive compounds because of the considerable risk of skin photoreaction. At present, areas under investigation include varying photoactive compounds and use of concurrent systemic chemotherapy.

Several experimental photoactive compounds are under investigation for patients with CC. A commonly used compound is porfimer sodium (Photofrin 2), activated by a laser at wavelength of 632 nm. Porfimer-based PDT has shown enhanced overall survival and prolonged stent patency times compared with stenting alone.[13] However, its estimated tumoricidal depth is limited to 4 mm of tissue penetration. Another common photoactive compound is hematoporphyrin (Photosan-3). Zoepf and colleagues[14] used hematoporphyrin-based PDT in a landmark randomized controlled trial (RCT) showing prolonged overall survival in patients compared with stenting alone. Notably, the cohort receiving PDT in this study had an increased rate of post–endoscopic retrograde cholangiopancreatography cholangitis. More recently, Yang and colleagues[15] prospectively compared a cohort receiving hematoporphyrin-based PDT plus plastic stenting with plastic stenting alone. The cohort receiving PDT had significantly longer mean survival compared with the group receiving biliary stenting only (13.8 months [6.2–16.5 months]vs 9.6 months [4.5–12.7 months]; $P<.001$).

Temoporfin (Foscan) is a compound used in PDT for oropharyngeal cancers with an estimated tumoricidal depth twice that of porfimer.[16] In a phase II prospective study, patients with unresectable PHC (n = 29) underwent temoporfin infusion followed by endobiliary exposure to light at a wavelength of 652 nm for 200 seconds. Compared with a matched historical group treated with porfimer-based PDT, time to tumor progression was significantly longer in the temoporfin group (6.5 vs 4.3 months; Mann-Whitney U test, $P<.01$). However, overall survival was not significantly different between the temoporfin group (15.4 months [10.7–20.0 months) and the porfimer group (9.3 months [6.5–12.1 months]; log rank test, $P = .72$). Complications of the temoporfin group included an increased rate of skin phototoxicity at the peripheral intravenous site of temoporfin infusion, an adverse event that the investigators claim can be avoided in the future by central venous administration.[17]

Combination Chemotherapy

Combination systemic chemotherapy and PDT have been shown to be tolerable. Recently, the PSC Nordic Study was a phase II RCT of temoporfin-based PDT and plastic stenting with or without chemotherapy (gemcitabine and capecitabine combination) in patients with locally advanced, recurrent, or metastatic PHC. Quality of life was the primary end point of this small study, and the two cohorts showed no differences.[18]

Although chemotherapy-PDT combination therapy may be feasible, the data on its efficacy compared with monotherapy are conflicting. Prior studies have been underpowered or used non–gemcitabine-based regimens.[19–21] Recently, 2 larger retrospective studies were performed. Gonzalez-Carmona and colleagues[22] compared 3 treatment groups in patients with unresectable PHC and distal cholangiocarcinoma, all of whom underwent biliary stenting: PDT (n = 34), chemotherapy (n = 26), and PDT plus chemotherapy (n = 36). Chemotherapy was mostly gemcitabine based. Photoactive compounds used for PDT were porfimer, hematoporphyrin, or temoporfin. Median overall survival was 20 months in the PDT plus chemotherapy group (95% confidence interval [CI], 16.38–23.62), compared with 15 months in the PDT group (95% CI, 10.02–19.98) and 10 months in the chemotherapy alone group (95% CI, 8.45–11.55). Despite the trend toward increased median overall survival, the difference between PDT plus chemotherapy and PDT groups was not statistically significant (log rank test, $P = .727$). Critics of this study have noted that cohorts had increased overall survival compared with previous prospective studies.[23]

Wentrup and colleagues[24] retrospectively compared patients with PHC after biliary stenting who received PDT (n = 35) or PDT plus chemotherapy (n = 33). Chemotherapy was mostly gemcitabine based; PDT was performed using porfimer. Mean overall survival from time of diagnosis for the PDT plus chemotherapy group was significantly increased at 520 days compared with 374 days in the PDT group

(Mann-Whitney U test, $P = .021$). Rates of cholangitis did not differ based on chemotherapy status. The discrepancy between overall survival rates observed in these two reports necessitates further studies to determine the utility of combination therapy in CC.

The most recent meta-analysis of PDT included 10 studies (n = 402) and showed survival benefit from PDT with stenting compared with stenting alone. The analysis included data from 2 RCTs, 5 prospective studies, and 3 retrospective studies using a variety of photoactive compounds and stent types. Most studies included patients treated with PDT using a percutaneous approach (P for χ^2 heterogeneity for all the pooled accuracy estimates was >.10). Overall, the group receiving PDT plus stenting had survival periods of 413 days (95%CI, 349.54–476.54), whereas stenting alone resulted in a survival period of 183 days (95%CI, 136.81–230.02); I^2 (inconsistency) = 85.1% (95%CI, 73.5%–90.2%); Egger (bias) = 5.09 (95%CI, 2.12–8.07), $P = .0043$. Odds ratio for postprocedure cholangitis was 0.57 (95%CI, 0.35–0.94). Approximately 10% of the patients receiving PDT sustained a self-resolving skin photosensitivity reaction. Subgroup analysis of the prospective studies also showed a significant overall survival advantage in patients receiving PDT.[25] These results are consistent with prior meta-analyses that have likewise shown a survival benefit for PDT.[26,27]

The PHOTOSTENT-02 trial was a multicenter phase III RCT that enrolled patients with biliary malignancy, including PHC, distal cholangiocarcinoma, intrahepatic CC, and gallbladder cancer. Cohorts underwent biliary stenting with (n = 46) or without (n = 46) porfimer-based PDT. Surprisingly, the addition of PDT resulted in a statistically significant decrease in overall survival of 6.2 months compared with 9.8 months for stenting alone (Cox proportional hazard model, hazard ratio [HR], 1.56; 95%CI, 1.00–2.43; $P = .048$). The trial was aborted once this effect was discovered. The cause of the poor outcomes in the PDT cohort has not been fully elucidated. The investigators noted that the cohort receiving PDT had a lower duration of salvage chemotherapy compared with the control group, but the effect did not fully explain the discrepancy in overall survival.[28] Although unfortunate in its outcome, understanding the results of the PHOTOSTENT-02 trial offers an important opportunity to learn the potential risks of this new technology as it is rapidly adopted into the therapeutic algorithm.

Although PDT is most commonly considered a first-line therapy for unresectable CC, several case series have explored alternative uses for PDT. One group successfully used PDT to downstage primary tumors previously considered unresectable. Seven patients who underwent resection following neoadjuvant PDT had similar outcomes compared with those predicted for patients undergoing initial R0 resection.[29] In addition, Shimizu and colleagues[30] reported a case in which PDT was used for local control of recurrence following surgical resection of the primary tumor.

Radiofrequency Ablation

Surgical and percutaneous approaches for RFA are well established for primary liver disorder. Recently, an endoscopic approach for RFA has been explored as novel therapy for PHC and distal cholangiocarcinoma. Briefly, endoscopy is performed and the common bile duct (CBD) is cannulated. Cholangiography is used to identify areas of malignant stricture. A catheter bearing electrodes is passed into the CBD and correct placement is fluoroscopically confirmed. The 2 commercially available RFA devices are Habib HPB-RF probe (Boston Scientific Corp., Marlborough, MA) and the ELRA RF catheter (Taewoong Medical, Gyeonggi-Do, South Korea). Ablation is performed at all sites of stricture for 2 minutes. In addition, a stent is placed across the treated area and the scope is withdrawn.[31–33] Use of RFA delivered via the percutaneous approach for distal cholangiocarcinoma and PHC has also been described.[34–37]

Several small phase I studies have shown that endoscopic RFA is safe and feasible in PHC and distal cholangiocarcinoma. In each study, postprocedure CBD diameter increased, and no major adverse events were related to the procedure.[38,39] Other case reports have described hepatic artery pseudoaneurysm[40] and hemobilia[41] following RFA. Excessive heating has been proposed as the cause of these complications. The newer ELRA RF catheter has a temperature probe that can theoretically avoid excessive heating, and a recent small prospective trial showed it to be safe and effective.[42]

A retrospective study by Cui and colleagues[43] investigated the effect of RFA on stent patency in malignant biliary obstruction from several tumor types. Subgroup analysis on the CC group showed no significant difference in overall survival when RFA was added to biliary stenting (6.7 months vs 4.5 months, respectively; log rank test, $P = .307$). However, stent patency time was significantly increased in the RFA group (n = 25) at 7.6 months compared with 4.3 months in the stenting-only group (n = 14; log rank test, $P = .009$).

Yang and colleagues[44] performed an RCT in patients with unresectable distal cholangiocarcinoma and PHC, with cohorts receiving either RFA with stenting (n = 32) or stenting only (n = 33). Compared with stenting only, the RFA cohort had statistically significant increases in both stent patency (6.8 months (95% CI, 3.6 – 8.2) versus 3.4 months (95% CI, 2.4–6.5); $P = .02$) and overall survival (13.2 ± 0.6 months [95% CI, 11.8–14.2] vs 8.3 ± 0.5 months [95% CI, 7.3–9.3]; $P<.001$). The most powerful predictive factor in determining overall survival by multivariable Cox regression analysis was RFA treatment status (HR, 0.182; 95% CI, 0.08–0.322; $P<.001$). Causes of death did not vary between groups significantly and were most commonly caused by tumor progression.

A meta-analysis by Sofi and colleagues[45] included 8 observational studies and 1 RCT of RFA in malignant biliary obstruction, most of which were CC. Overall survival was significantly increased in the RFA group (n = 504; HR = 1.395; 95%CI, 1.145–1.7; $P<.001$). Stent patency was significantly prolonged, with a pooled weighted mean difference of 50.6 days between RFA and control groups (95% CI, 32.83–68.48; Cochran Q test, $P = .002$; $I^2 = 79\%$). Surprisingly, subgroup analysis of patients with CC did not recapitulate these results. Treatment with RFA in CC resulted in a non–statistically significant increase of 42.7 days in stent patency compared with stenting alone (95% CI, 17.19–68.19; Cochran Q test, $P = .11$; $I^2 = 55\%$). The results from Yang and colleagues[44] were not included in this meta-analysis. Further prospective study is necessary to characterize the benefit of RFA in cholangiocarcinoma management.

Few studies have compared PDT with RFA, and none have shown superiority of either technique in the management of patients with cholangiocarcinoma. A retrospective analysis of patients with predominantly PHC treated with either porfimer-based PDT (n = 32) or RFA (n = 16) showed no difference in median overall survival (7.5 vs 9.6 months, respectively; $P = .799$). The RFA group received replacement stents at approximately half the rate of the PDT group, and experienced significantly higher rates of stent occlusion and cholangitis.[46] A second retrospective study of patients with PHC treated with porfimer-based PDT (n = 20) or RFA (n = 14) showed that RFA conferred a short-term advantage in decline in serum bilirubin level and the need for premature stent replacement; however, this study did not specifically assess overall survival.[47]

At present, no definitive long-term advantage follows PDT versus RFA in the treatment of unresectable PHC and distal cholangiocarcinoma. Surgical R0 resection represents the current upper limit of survival in this disease, but oncologic resection is available for only a minority of patients. Optimizing percutaneous and endoscopic techniques for PDT and RFA and exploring treatment combinations with systemic chemotherapy are imperative to improve outcomes in patients with CC. The low incidence of CC is a significant impediment to production of high-quality prospective studies. An algorithm has been proposed to guide the management of these patients.[48] Patient education must include the risks and benefits of both treatments, including skin photoreaction in PDT and potential vascular damage in RFA.

PERCUTANEOUS THERAPIES FOR HEPATOCELLULAR CARCINOMA
Indications

HCC is the most common primary liver cancer and is associated with a mortality exceeding 700,000 deaths per year worldwide.[49] Curative treatment of HCC includes both partial hepatectomy and transplant. However, most patients are not surgical candidates because of advanced tumor progression, size, vascular invasion, or presence of metastatic disease. Nonsurgical therapies for HCC are in widespread use, including systemic medical therapy and percutaneous techniques. Therapeutic algorithms for transplant, hepatectomy, percutaneous approaches, and systemic therapies have evolved from the Barcelona Clinic Liver Cancer (BCLC) guidelines.[50]

Percutaneous thermal ablation, like surgical ablation, controls disease by inducing coagulative necrosis of the selected region with a 5-mm to 10-mm margin, similar to an R0 surgical margin. Local ablative therapies have efficacy both as definitive treatment and as a bridge to transplant. These interventions can be performed safely on suboptimal surgical candidates with low morbidity. However, several challenges exist when performing local ablative therapies in HCC. First, the rich hepatic vascular supply is problematic for HCC located close to major vessels. Attempts at thermal ablation for these tumors often suffer from the heat-sink effect because local vascular blood flow decreases the temperature subtherapeutically within the treatment zone. Second, increased tumor size and difficult tumor locations can cause thermal heterogeneity within the tumor, leading to incomplete ablation. Particular care is taken when attempting ablations in proximity to sensitive anatomic structures such as the central biliary tree, gallbladder, and diaphragm. Third, different electromagnetic mechanisms of heat generation can produce varying efficacy of tumor ablation. Insufficient thermal treatment for any reason increases local recurrence rate of HCC.[50,51]

Percutaneous Radiofrequency Ablation

RFA is the most widely used thermal ablative technique for HCC. Under image guidance, electrodes are inserted directly into the tumor and electric current is passed through the tissue. Local desiccated tissue increases electrical impedance, and thermal energy passively diffuses through the ablation zone, inducing coagulative necrosis. Internal cooling systems using either saline or pulsed current prevent buildup of charred tissue around the electrode that would otherwise disrupt evenly circumferential heating. Average reported ablation zones vary but are approximately 3.0 cm in diameter for a single monopolar electrode. A critical final step of RFA is ablation of the percutaneous needle tract on electrode withdrawal, a technique that has significantly decreased needle tract recurrences.[52]

Several parameters of RFA are under investigation. Multielectrode systems have been developed for treating medium-sized tumors as large as 5.0 cm. In these multielectrode systems, energy delivery can be either alternated between electrodes or simultaneously administered for a faster treatment session.[52] Multipolar electrodes may expand the ablation zone of RFA. Cartier and colleagues[53] retrospectively compared traditional monopolar RFA (n = 158) with multipolar RFA (n = 56). Tumors less than 2.5 cm showed decreased residual tumor and recurrence with multipolar treatment. However, residual tumor and recurrence for tumors of 2.5 cm and greater were not significantly different with multipolar RFA. Although multipolar RFA is important in experimental studies, monopolar remains the more widely used RFA parameter.

The no-touch RFA protocol involves insertion of multiple electrodes within tissue surrounding the tumor. By avoiding direct contact with the tumor, the no-touch technique allows thermal ablation to be performed with higher intensity and decreased risk of tumor seeding of the probe tract. A multicenter retrospective study of HCC less than 5 cm in diameter (n = 362) observed that no-touch multibipolar RFA was more effective than monopolar RFA in the combined outcome of primary RFA failure and recurrence rates. However, 5-year overall survival rates were not statistically different between the two groups (monopolar 37.2% vs no-touch multibipolar 46.4%; P = .378).[54]

Casadei Gardini and colleagues[55] performed a meta-analysis on data pooled from 34 studies (n = 11,216) to determine factors predictive of improved outcomes in HCC treated with RFA. Strongest predictive factors for overall survival and recurrence-free survival following RFA treatment were Child-Pugh class A, albumin-bilirubin index of 1, and alpha fetoprotein level less than 20 ng/mL. In addition, survival was increased in the RFA treatment population with the presence of only 1 tumor nodule less than 2 cm. Thus, patient survival in RFA can be predicted reliably with small tumor size, low tumor number, and preserved hepatic function.

Several large studies have compared RFA with hepatectomy in the treatment of HCC. Xu and colleagues[56] performed a meta-analysis of 31 studies comparing RFA (n = 8252) with hepatectomy (n = 7851). Three RCTs and 28 observational studies were included. The hepatectomy group had significantly higher 3-year and 5-year survival rates (83.9% and 71.4%, respectively) compared with the RFA group (78.6% and 60.8%, respectively; P<.00001). Subgroup analysis showed that survival rates were similar between the two groups for tumors less than or equal to 2.0 cm. A second meta-analysis of 5 RCTs (n = 742) showed no difference in overall survival between hepatectomy and RFA at 1 and 3 years, but significantly increased survival in the hepatectomy group at 5 years (risk ratio, 1.91; 95% CI, 1.32, 2.79; P = .001).[57] These data align with those from the Surveillance, Epidemiology, and End Results (SEER) database comparing RFA and hepatectomy in patients stratified by age less than (n = 2784) or older than (n = 1912) 65 years. Patients older than 65 years with tumors less than 2.0 cm had similar survival to their propensity-matched group aged less than 65 years. However, age less than 65 years with tumors greater than 3.0 cm had significantly increased overall survival with hepatectomy compared with RFA.[58] A Cochran meta-analysis showed that although all-cause mortality was the same between RFA and hepatectomy, cancer-related mortality was higher in RFA compared with hepatectomy.[59]

Large-scale studies[56–59] are not able to incorporate the latest RFA techniques in the comparison with hepatectomy. Mohkam and colleagues[60] compared no-touch multibipolar RFA (n = 79) with hepatectomy (n = 62) in HCC 2.0 to 5.0 cm using inverse probability of treatment weighting. Morbidity was significantly lower for RFA, but local recurrence rates were higher than in hepatectomy at 1 year (7.4% vs 1.9%) and 3 years (27.8% vs 3.3%; P = .008). These data suggest that even advanced RFA technology carries inferior overall survival compared with hepatectomy. Further studies comparing outcomes in surgery versus RFA are warranted, especially as interventional technology continues to advance.

Transcatheter arterial chemoembolization (TACE) is a commonly used percutaneous nonablative treatment of HCC. Survival outcomes at 1 and 5 years in patients treated with TACE versus RFA monotherapy are comparable in HCCs less than 3.0 cm.[61] Combination TACE/RFA therapy is feasible, but so far the data on efficacy of cotreatment are primarily retrospective and conflicting. In a propensity-matching retrospective study (n = 92), Endo and colleagues[62] showed that 1-year, 3-year, and 5-year overall survival rates for TACE/RFA combination therapy (97.4%, 70.4%, and 60.4%, respectively) were significantly higher compared with a group receiving TACE monotherapy (92.7%, 55.7%, and 22.8%, respectively; $P = .045$). Another group found that TACE/RFA combination had better tumor response than TACE monotherapy, but it was no different than RFA monotherapy. TACE/RFA was also found to have a longer duration of hospital stay and more associated discomfort than RFA alone.[63]

Percutaneous Microwave Ablation

Thermal ablation using MWA occurs via a different physical mechanism from RFA. In MWA, an antenna generates high-frequency electromagnetic fields within the tumor. Rapid realignment of polar molecules throughout the tissue causes heat generation sufficient for tumor ablation. Local changes include desiccation and vaporization. Notably, MWA can successfully be performed within proximity to blood vessels and without a cooling system. Unlike RFA, electromagnetic fields generate and maintain ablative temperatures. Therefore, there is no potential for the heat-sink effect in tumors close to vessels, nor does charred local tissue impede propagation of heat conduction.[64]

Rates of recurrence in HCC treated with MWA versus RFA are variable. In a phase II RCT between RFA (n = 76) and MWA (n = 76) in HCCs less than 4 cm, no difference was found between local recurrence at 2 years (risk ratio 1.62; 95% CI, 0.66–3.94; $P = .27$). [65] In contrast, Liu and colleagues[66] retrospectively observed that 5-year recurrence-free survival was significantly higher in MWA (n = 126, 6.4%) compared with RFA (n = 436; 27.9%; $P<.001$) after performing propensity score matching for HCC within Milan criteria. Loriaud and colleagues[67] retrospectively analyzed 4-year progression rates of tumors less than 5 cm located near major vessels treated with 1 of 4 techniques: MWA, monopolar RFA, cluster RFA, and multibipolar RFA. Tumor progression was measured per nodule, n = 40 tumors for each group. Significantly lower 4-year tumor progression was observed in the multibipolar (16.3%) and cluster RFA (16.3%) compared with monopolar RFA (50.5%) and MWA (44.2%). Post hoc power analysis between MWA and RFA was 0.068.

Meta-analyses of trials comparing survival outcomes in MWA with those in RFA are based on low-quality data and generally show no difference between the techniques. Tan and colleagues[68] pooled data from 4 RCTs and 10 cohort studies, finding no significant difference in technically complete ablation or overall survival in MWA versus RFA. Another meta-analysis of 6 cohort studies and 3 RCTs also showed no difference in 1-year or 3-year overall survival between MWA and RFA. Complication rates of the two procedures are low and include subcapsular or intrahepatic hematoma.[69] Facciorusso and colleagues[70] analyzed data from 1 RCT and 6 retrospective studies (n = 774), finding no difference in 3-year overall survival.

Multiple studies have compared the effects of MWA/TACE combination therapy with monotherapy for HCCs of variable tumor size. For tumors less than or equal to 5.0 cm (n = 244), Chen and colleagues[71] performed retrospective analysis with propensity score matching and found that combination MWA/TACE therapy improved tumor response at 6 months posttreatment compared with TACE monotherapy. For intermediate HCC with 5 tumors or fewer less than 7.0 cm, a retrospective study (n = 150) showed significantly improved overall survival with MWA/TACE therapy compared with TACE monotherapy at 1, 3, and 5 years (93.1%, 79%, 67.7% vs 77.5%, 42.1%, 21%, respectively; P = .002).[72] For massive HCC, defined as tumor greater than or equal to 10.0 cm, MWA/TACE combination has been shown to significantly improve overall survival at 6, 12, and 18 months.[73] MWA and TACE likely represent an effective treatment combination for patients unable to receive operative management of HCC.

Percutaneous Irreversible Electroporation

IRE is a nonthermal ablation technique in HCC. In IRE, pulsed electric fields induce membrane nanopores. The resulting permeabilized cells undergo apoptosis but leave extracellular components relatively intact. The consequence is local ablation with minimal surrounding parenchymal damage. In addition, IRE relies on electric fields and is therefore not affected by the heat-sink effect. At present, the only commercially available IRE system is the NanoKnife (AngioDynamics, Latham, NY).[74] IRE has been shown to be safe and effective in ablation of liver tumors.[75] Several groups have analyzed comparisons in outcomes between IRE and thermal ablative techniques. Outcomes[76] and complication rates[77] seem to be similar based on retrospective data. With advantages in certain patient populations compared with thermal ablative techniques, IRE represents a technological advance with great potential for HCC. Further high-quality comparative studies are anticipated.

SUMMARY

Primary hepatobiliary cancer is a significant cause of morbidity and mortality worldwide. Surgery remains the most effective approach for prolonging survival in primary hepatobiliary malignancies. Inherently, removal of diseased tissue offers a biological advantage compared with other techniques that target tumor cells in situ. However, cancer is a systemic disease, and recurrences are frequent even after technically sufficient operations that accomplish complete tumor clearance. Furthermore, patient-related factors, including pulmonary, hepatic, renal, and nutritional function, must be sufficient to tolerate the physiologic challenges of a major abdominal surgery. Advanced disease presentation and underlying comorbidities force most patients into consideration for nonoperative therapy. Development of interventional techniques with lower morbidity is essential to prolong survival in a patient population inappropriate for operative management. Locoregional therapies may offer patients an opportunity for improved survival by controlling local disease progression. Understanding interventional techniques for local therapy along with anticipated outcomes is essential when counseling patients for nonoperative management of hepatobiliary cancer.

Endobiliary techniques have greatly reduced the morbidity of cholangitis in distal cholangiocarcinoma and PHC. Prolonging stent patency time can reduce comorbidity but also provides a window for administration of cytotoxic therapy. Multiple groups are experimenting with modifications to photoactive compounds in PDT, probe modifications in RFA, and combinations of concurrent chemotherapy with locoregional therapy. Optimizing these therapies by finding evidence of superiority of endoscopic parameters should be an important next step. However, the low incidence of CC makes it challenging to coordinate a sufficiently powered high-quality RCT comparing various techniques and treatment strategies. Interdisciplinary and institutional collaboration will be critical in this endeavor.

Percutaneous ablative therapies have been applied successfully to treat nonoperative HCC. Unlike CC, the anatomic variety found in HCC makes each technique valuable for different situations, such as vascular proximity and dangerous tumor locations. As various interventions evolve, certain ablative techniques may become less important in the therapeutic algorithm for primary liver cancer.[67] IRE represents a promising new nonthermal technology inducing cell death without violating the surrounding tissue stroma. The biological implications of this therapy need further characterization. The low morbidity associated with percutaneous and endoscopic interventional techniques makes combination therapies with systemic agents tolerable.

REFERENCES

1. Nault JC, Sutter O, Nahon PJ, et al. Percutaneous treatment of hepatocellular carcinoma: state of the art and innovations. J Hepatol 2018;68:783–97.
2. Labib PL, Davidson BR, Sharma RA, et al. Locoregional therapies in cholangiocarcinoma. Hepat Oncol 2017;4:99–109.
3. Mavros MN, Economopoulos KP, Alexiou VG, et al. Treatment and prognosis for patients with intrahepatic cholangiocarcinoma: systematic review and meta-analysis. JAMA Surg 2014;149:565–74.
4. Shaib Y, El-Serag HB. The epidemiology of cholangiocarcinoma. Semin Liver Dis 2004;24:115–25.
5. Goussous N, Patel ST, Cunningham SC. The management of bile duct cancer. In: Cameron JL, editor. Current surgical therapy. 12th edition. Toronto (Canada): Elsevier; 2017. p. 459.
6. Jarnigan WR, Fong Y, DeMatteo RP, et al. Staging, resectability, and outcome in 225 patients with hilar cholangiocarcinoma. Ann Surg 2001;234:507.
7. DeOliveira ML, Schulick RD, Nimura Y, et al. New staging system and a registry for perihilar cholangiocarcinoma. Hepatology 2011;53:1363–71.
8. DeOliveira ML, Cunningham SC, Cameron JL, et al. Cholangiocarcinoma: thirty-one-year experience with 564 patients at a single institution. Ann Surg 2007;245: 755–62.
9. Cassani LS, Chouhan J, Chan C, et al. Biliary decompression in perihilar cholangiocarcinoma improves survival: a single-center retrospective analysis. Dig Dis Sci 2019;64:561–9.
10. Sangchan A, Kongkasame W, Pugkhem A, et al. Efficacy of metal and plastic stents in unresectable complex hilar cholangiocarcinoma: a randomized controlled trial. Gastrointest Endosc 2012;76:93–9.
11. Abrahamse H, Hamblin MR. New photosensitizers for photodynamic therapy. J Biochem 2016;473:347–64.
12. Lee TY, Cheon YK, Shim CS, et al. Photodynamic therapy prolongs metal stent patency in patients with unresectable hilar cholangiocarcinoma. World J Gastroenterol 2012;18:5589–94.
13. Ortner ME, Caca K, Berr F, et al. Successful photodynamic therapy for nonresectable cholangiocarcinoma: a randomized prospective study. Gastroenterology 2003;125:1355–63.
14. Zoepf T, Jakobs R, Arnold JC, et al. Palliation of nonresectable bile duct cancer: improved survival after photodynamic therapy. Am J Gastroenterol 2005;100: 2426–30.
15. Yang J, Shen H, Jin H, et al. Treatment of unresectable extrahepatic cholangiocarcinoma using hematoporphyrin photodynamic therapy: a prospective study. Photodiagnosis Photodyn Ther 2016;16:110–8.

16. Wagner A, Kiesslich T, Neureiter D, et al. Photodynamic therapy for hilar bile duct cancer: clinical evidence for improved tumoricidal tissue penetration by temoporfin. Photochem Photobiol Sci 2013;12:1065–73.

17. Wagner A, Denzer UW, Neureiter D, et al. Temoporfin improves efficacy of photodynamic therapy in advanced biliary tract carcinoma: A multicenter prospective phase II study. Hepatology 2015;62:1456–65.

18. Hauge T, Hauge PW, Warloe T, et al. Randomised controlled trial of temoporfin photodynamic therapy plus chemotherapy in nonresectable biliary carcinoma—PCS Nordic study. Photodiagnosis Photodyn Ther 2016;13:330–3.

19. Park DH, Lee SS, Park SE, et al. Randomised phase II trial of photodynamic therapy plus oral fluoropyrimidine, S-1, versus photodynamic therapy alone for unresectable hilar cholangiocarcinoma. Eur J Cancer 2014;50:1259–68.

20. Knüppel M, Kubicka S, Vogel A, et al. Combination of conservative and interventional therapy strategies for intra- and extrahepatic cholangiocellular carcinoma: a retrospective survival analysis. Gastroenterol Res Pract 2012;2012:190708.

21. Fuks D, Bartoli E, Delcenserie R, et al. Biliary drainage, photodynamic therapy and chemotherapy for unresectable cholangiocarcinoma with jaundice. J Gastroenterol Hepatol 2009;24:1745–52.

22. Gonzalez-Carmona MA, Bolch M, Jansen C, et al. Combined photodynamic therapy with systemic chemotherapy for unresectable cholangiocarcinoma. Aliment Pharmacol Ther 2019;49:437–47.

23. Srinivasa S, Wigmore SJ. Editorial: shining a light on cholangiocarcinoma—a new dawn for photodynamic therapy? Aliment Pharmacol Ther 2019;49:952.

24. Wentrup R, Winkelmann N, Mitroshkin A, et al. Photodynamic therapy plus chemotherapy compared with photodynamic therapy alone in hilar nonresectable cholangiocarcinoma. Gut Liver 2016;10:470–5.

25. Moole H, Tathireddy H, Dharmapuri S, et al. Success of photodynamic therapy in palliating patients with nonresectable cholangiocarcinoma: A systematic review and meta-analysis. World J Gastroenterol 2017;23:1278–88.

26. Lu Y, Liu L, Wu JC, et al. Efficacy and safety of photodynamic therapy for unresectable cholangiocarcinoma: a meta-analysis. Clin Res Hepatol Gastroenterol 2015;39:718–24.

27. Leggett CL, Gorospe EC, Murad MH, et al. Photodynamic therapy for unresectable cholangiocarcinoma: a comparative effectiveness systematic review and meta-analyses. Photodiagnosis Photodyn Ther 2012;9:189–95.

28. Pereira SP, Jitlal M, Duggan M, et al. PHOTOSTENT-02: porfimer sodium photodynamic therapy plus stenting versus stenting alone in patients with locally advanced or metastatic biliary tract cancer. ESMO Open 2018;3:e000379.

29. Wagner A, Wiedmann M, Tannapfel A, et al. Neoadjuvant down-sizing of hilar cholangiocarcinoma with photodynamic therapy–long-term outcome of a phase ii pilot study. Int J Mol Sci 2015;16:26619–28.

30. Shimizu S, Nakazawa T, Hayashi K, et al. Photodynamic therapy using talaporfin sodium for the recurrence of cholangiocarcinoma after surgical resection. Intern Med 2015;54:2321–6.

31. Larghi A, Rimbaş M, Tringali A, et al. Endoscopic radiofrequency biliary ablation treatment: a comprehensive review. Dig Endosc 2019;31(3):245–55.

32. Auriemma F, De Luca L, Bianchetti M, et al. Radiofrequency and malignant biliary strictures: an update. World J Gastrointest Endosc 2019;11:95–102.

33. Wang F, Li Q, Zhang X, et al. Endoscopic radiofrequency ablation for malignant biliary strictures. Exp Ther Med 2016;11:2484–8.

34. Wu TT, Li WM, Li HC, et al. Percutaneous intraductal radiofrequency ablation for extrahepatic distal cholangiocarcinoma: a method for prolonging stent patency and achieving better functional status and quality of life. Cardiovasc Intervent Radiol 2017;40:260–9.

35. Wang Y, Cui W, Fan W, et al. Percutaneous intraductal radiofrequency ablation in the management of unresectable Bismuth types III and IV hilar cholangiocarcinoma. Oncotarget 2016;7:53911–20.

36. Cui W, Fan W, Lu M, et al. The safety and efficacy of percutaneous intraductal radiofrequency ablation in unresectable malignant biliary obstruction: A single-institution experience. BMC Cancer 2017;17:288.

37. Wang J, Zhao L, Zhou C, et al. Percutaneous intraductal radiofrequency ablation combined with biliary stent placement for nonresectable malignant biliary obstruction improves stent patency but not survival. Medicine 2016;95:e3329.

38. Laquière A, Boustière C, Leblanc S, et al. Safety and feasibility of endoscopic biliary radiofrequency ablation treatment of extrahepatic cholangiocarcinoma. Surg Endosc 2016;30:1242–8.

39. Sharaiha RZ, Sethi A, Weaver KR, et al. Impact of radiofrequency ablation on malignant biliary strictures: results of a collaborative registry. Dig Dis Sci 2015;60: 2164–9.

40. Topazian M, Levy MJ, Patel S, et al. Hepatic artery pseudoaneurysm formation following intraductal biliary radiofrequency ablation. Endoscopy 2013;45:E161–2.

41. Tal AO, Vermehren J, Friedrich-Rust M, et al. Intraductal endoscopic radiofrequency ablation for the treatment of hilar non-resectable malignant bile duct obstruction. World J Gastrointest Endosc 2014;6:13–9.

42. Lee YN, Jeong S, Choi HJ, et al. The safety of newly developed automatic temperature-controlled endobiliary radiofrequency ablation system for malignant biliary strictures: a prospective multicenter study. J Gastroenterol Hepatol 2019. [Epub ahead of print].

43. Cui W, Wang Y, Fan W, et al. Comparison of intraluminal radiofrequency ablation and stents vs. stents alone in the management of malignant biliary obstruction. Int J Hyperthermia 2017;33:853–61.

44. Yang J, Wang J, Zhou H, et al. Efficacy and safety of endoscopic radiofrequency ablation for unresectable extrahepatic cholangiocarcinoma: a randomized trial. Endoscopy 2018;50:751–60.

45. Sofi AA, Khan MA, Das A, et al. Radiofrequency ablation combined with biliary stent placement versus stent placement alone for malignant biliary strictures: a systematic review and meta-analysis. Gastrointest Endosc 2018;87:944–51.

46. Strand DS, Cosgrove ND, Patrie JT, et al. ERCP-directed radiofrequency ablation and photodynamic therapy are associated with comparable survival in the treatment of unresectable cholangiocarcinoma. Gastrointest Endosc 2014;80: 794–804.

47. Schmidt A, Bloechinger M, Weber A, et al. Short-term effects and adverse events of endoscopically applied radiofrequency ablation appear to be comparable with photodynamic therapy in hilar cholangiocarcinoma. United Eur Gastroenterol J 2016;4:570–9.

48. Buerlein RCD, Wang AY. Endoscopic retrograde cholangiopancreatography-guided ablation for cholangiocarcinoma. Gastrointest Endosc Clin N Am 2019; 29(2):351–67.

49. Bruix J, Reig M, Sherman M. Evidence-based diagnosis, staging, and treatment of patients with hepatocellular carcinoma. Gastroenterology 2016;150:835–53.

50. Lurje I, Czigany Z, Bednarsch J, et al. Treatment strategies for hepatocellular carcinoma - a multidisciplinary approach. Int J Mol Sci 2019;20:1465.
51. Kang TW, Lim HK, Cha DI. Percutaneous ablation for perivascular hepatocellular carcinoma: Refining the current status based on emerging evidence and future perspectives. World J Gastroenterol 2018;24:5331–7.
52. Lee DH, Lee JM. Recent advances in the image-guided tumor ablation of liver malignancies: radiofrequency ablation with multiple electrodes, real-time multi-modality fusion imaging, and new energy sources. Korean J Radiol 2018;19:545–59.
53. Cartier V, Boursier J, Lebigot J, et al. Radiofrequency ablation of hepatocellular carcinoma: mono or multipolar? J Gastroenterol Hepatol 2016;31:654–60.
54. Hocquelet A, Aubé C, Rode A, et al. Comparison of no-touch multi-bipolar vs. monopolar radiofrequency ablation for small HCC. J Hepatol 2017;66:67–74.
55. Casadei Gardini A, Marisi G, Canale M, et al. Radiofrequency ablation of hepatocellular carcinoma: a meta-analysis of overall survival and recurrence-free survival. Onco Targets Ther 2018;11:6555–67.
56. Xu Q, Kobayashi S, Ye X, et al. Comparison of hepatic resection and radiofrequency ablation for small hepatocellular carcinoma: a meta-analysis of 16,103 patients. Sci Rep 2014;4:7252.
57. Xu XL, Liu XD, Liang M, et al. Radiofrequency ablation versus hepatic resection for small hepatocellular carcinoma: systematic review of randomized controlled trials with meta-analysis and trial sequential analysis. Radiology 2018;287:461–72.
58. Jiang YQ, Wang ZX, Deng YN, et al. Efficacy of hepatic resection vs. radiofrequency ablation for patients with very-early-stage or early-stage hepatocellular carcinoma: a population-based study with stratification by age and tumor size. Front Oncol 2019;9:113.
59. Majumdar A, Roccarina D, Thorburn D, et al. Management of people with early- or very early-stage hepatocellular carcinoma: an attempted network meta-analysis. Cochrane Database Syst Rev 2017;(3):CD011650.
60. Mohkam K, Dumont PN, Manichon AF, et al. No-touch multibipolar radiofrequency ablation vs. surgical resection for solitary hepatocellular carcinoma ranging from 2 to 5 cm. J Hepatol 2018;68:1172–80.
61. Martin AN, Wilkins LR, Das D, et al. Efficacy of radiofrequency ablation versus transarterial chemoembolization for patients with solitary hepatocellular carcinoma ≤3 cm. Am Surg 2019;85:150–5.
62. Endo K, Kuroda H, Oikawa T, et al. Efficacy of combination therapy with transcatheter arterial chemoembolization and radiofrequency ablation for intermediate-stage hepatocellular carcinoma. Scand J Gastroenterol 2018;53:1575–83.
63. Kim W, Cho SK, Shin SW, et al. Combination therapy of transarterial chemoembolization (TACE) and radiofrequency ablation (RFA) for small hepatocellular carcinoma: comparison with TACE or RFA monotherapy. Abdom Radiol (NY) 2019;44(6):2283–92.
64. Meloni MF, Chiang J, Laeseke PF, et al. Microwave ablation in primary and secondary liver tumours: technical and clinical approaches. Int J Hyperthermia 2017;33:15–24.
65. Vietti Violi N, Duran R, Guiu B, et al. Efficacy of microwave ablation versus radiofrequency ablation for the treatment of hepatocellular carcinoma in patients with chronic liver disease: a randomised controlled phase 2 trial. Lancet Gastroenterol Hepatol 2018;3:317–25.

66. Liu W, Zheng Y, He W, et al. Microwave vs radiofrequency ablation for hepatocellular carcinoma within the Milan criteria: a propensity score analysis. Aliment Pharmacol Ther 2018;48:671–81.
67. Loriaud A, Denys A, Seror O, et al. Hepatocellular carcinoma abutting large vessels: comparison of four percutaneous ablation systems. Int J Hyperthermia 2018;34:1171–8.
68. Tan W, Deng Q, Lin S, et al. Comparison of microwave ablation and radiofrequency ablation for hepatocellular carcinoma: a systematic review and meta-analysis. Int J Hyperthermia 2019;36:264–72.
69. Luo W, Zhang Y, He G, et al. Effects of radiofrequency ablation versus other ablating techniques on hepatocellular carcinomas: a systematic review and meta-analysis. World J Surg Oncol 2017;15:126.
70. Facciorusso A, Di Maso M, Muscatiello N. Microwave ablation versus radiofrequency ablation for the treatment of hepatocellular carcinoma: A systematic review and meta-analysis. Int J Hyperthermia 2016;32:339–44.
71. Chen QF, Jia ZY, Yang ZQ, et al. Transarterial chemoembolization monotherapy versus combined transarterial chemoembolization-microwave ablation therapy for hepatocellular carcinoma tumors ≤5 cm: a propensity analysis at a single center. Cardiovasc Intervent Radiol 2017;40:1748–55.
72. Zhang R, Shen L, Zhao L, et al. Combined transarterial chemoembolization and microwave ablation versus transarterial chemoembolization in BCLC stage B hepatocellular carcinoma. Diagn Interv Radiol 2018;24:219–24.
73. Hu H, Chen GF, Yuan W, et al. Microwave ablation with chemoembolization for large hepatocellular carcinoma in patients with cirrhosis. Int J Hyperthermia 2018;34:1351–8.
74. Ruarus AH, Vroomen LGPH, Puijk RS, et al. Irreversible electroporation in hepatopancreaticobiliary tumours. Can Assoc Radiol J 2018;69:38–50.
75. Frühling P, Nilsson A, Duraj F, et al. Single-center nonrandomized clinical trial to assess the safety and efficacy of irreversible electroporation (IRE) ablation of liver tumors in humans: short to mid-term results. Eur J Surg Oncol 2017;43:751–7.
76. Bhutiani N, Philips P, Scoggins CR, et al. Evaluation of tolerability and efficacy of irreversible electroporation (IRE) in treatment of Child-Pugh B (7/8) hepatocellular carcinoma (HCC). HPB (Oxford) 2016;18:593–9.
77. Verloh N, Jensch I, Lürken L, et al. Similar complication rates for irreversible electroporation and thermal ablation in patients with hepatocellular tumors. Radiol Oncol 2019;53:116–22.

Intrahepatic Cholangiocarcinoma

Ramy El-Diwany, MPH[a], Timothy M. Pawlik, MD, MPH, PhD[b], Aslam Ejaz, MD, MPH[a,*]

KEYWORDS

- Intrahepatic cholangiocarcinoma • Hepatobiliary • Cholangiocarcionma

KEY POINTS

- Intrahepatic cholangiocarcinoma (ICC) occurs proximal to the segmental biliary ducts, and risk factors include chronic hepatitis and cirrhosis, biliary inflammatory diseases, and hepatobiliary flukes, although in most cases, no known risk factor is identified.
- ICCs generally present with vague abdominal pain and symptoms, unlike perihilar or extrahepatic tumors, which present more frequently with obstructive symptoms.
- Cholangiocarcinoma is a highly aggressive malignancy with long-term survival only observed in patients with R0 surgical resection.
- Nodal disease status is among the most important prognostic factors associated with a resection and requires a lymphadenectomy.
- Adjuvant chemotherapy can provide a significant survival benefit for patients with more advanced or aggressive tumors.
- Systemic, locoregional, and targeted therapies exist for patients with unresectable or metastatic disease.

INTRODUCTION

Cholangiocarcinoma (CCA) is the second most common primary liver malignancy after hepatocellular carcinoma[1] and arises from the epithelial cells of the intrahepatic and extrahepatic bile ducts.[2] CCA is classified based on the anatomic location of the tumor in relation to the biliary tree. CCA occurring in the periphery of the liver, proximal to the second-degree (segmental) bile ducts, is designated as intrahepatic cholangiocarcinoma (ICC, **Fig. 1**A). CCAs occurring more distal in the biliary tree, from the level of the confluence of the left and right hepatic ducts to the level of the insertion of the cystic duct into the common hepatic duct, are designated as perihilar cholangiocarcinoma (PCC, Klatskin tumor; **Fig. 1**B). CCA occurring below the level of the insertion of the cystic duct into the common bile duct down to the level of the ampulla of Vater is

The authors have nothing to disclose.
[a] Department of Surgery, Johns Hopkins University, 600 N. Wolfe St, Tower 110 Baltimore, MD 21287, USA; [b] Department of Surgery, The Ohio State University, 320 W. 10th Avenue, M-260 Starling Loving Hall, Columbus, OH 43210, USA
* Corresponding author. The Ohio State University, 320 W. 10th Avenue, M-260 Starling Loving Hall, Columbus, OH 43210.
E-mail address: aslam.ejaz@osumc.edu

A   B   C

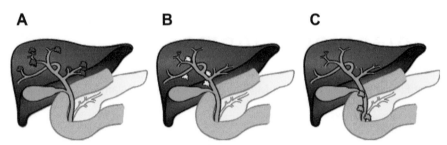

Fig. 1. Anatomic variants of cholangiocarcinoma. (*A*) Intrahepatic cholangiocarcinoma (ICC, red circles). (*B*) Perihilar cholangiocarcinoma (PSS, Klatskin tumor, yellow circles). (*C*) Extrahepatic cholangiocarcinoma (ECC, blue circles).

designated as extrahepatic cholangiocarcinoma (ECC, **Fig. 1**C). ICC and ECC account for approximately 25% each of all CCAs, with PCC accounting for the remaining 50% of CCAs.

ICC is an aggressive malignancy with 1- and 5-year overall survival rates of approximately 30% and 18%, respectively.[3] Complete surgical resection involving a formal liver resection and portal lymphadenectomy provides the best hope for long-term survival among patients with ICC.[4,5] Unfortunately, most patients with ICC are found to have locally advanced or metastatic disease at the time of diagnosis.[6] However, as newer and more effective chemotherapeutic and targeted agents become available, a multidisciplinary approach including surgical, systemic, locoregional, and radiotherapy is critical for the optimal treatment of patients with ICC.

EPIDEMIOLOGY/RISK FACTORS

Most ICCs arise de novo with no identifiable risk factor. The incidence of CCA, and in particular ICC, varies substantially across the globe. In the United States, the incidence of ICC has been increasing from 3.2 cases per 1,000,000 population between 1975 and 1979 to 8.5 cases per 1,000,000 population between 1995 and 1999. The peak age of diagnosis is in the seventh decade of life, with an approximately 50% higher prevalence in men.[1] A more recent analysis of ICCs from 1999 to 2013 supports that this trend is continuing across sex and racial/ethnic groups; there was an age-adjusted incident rate of 9.8 cases per 1,000,000 person-years from 2011 to 2013 compared with 14.5 cases per 1,000,000 person-years from 1999 to 2001 (*P*<.0001) in women, with a similar trend observed in men.[7]

In western countries, primary sclerosing cholangitis imparts the highest risk (hazard ratio [HR] 171.8, 95% confidence interval [CI] 57.1–517.4) for the development of ICC, with an overall estimated lifetime risk of 9% to 18% in this patient population.[8–10] Approximately 50% of the CCAs detected in PSC patients are detected in the first year of diagnosis of PSC, and they are almost exclusively identified in patients with dominant strictures.[8] Other risk factors for the development of ICC include infection with the hepatobiliary fluke worms *Opusthorchus viverrini* and *Clonorchis sinensis,* which are prevalent in Southeast Asia. In fact, endemic areas of these parasites have the highest prevalence of CCA globally (>100 cases per 100,000 population).[11]

Cirrhosis of any etiology is also strongly associated with the development of CCA (odds ratio [OR] 22.9). Given that viral hepatitis is a major etiology of cirrhosis, it was previously thought that associations between CCA and chronic viral hepatitis were exclusively related to liver cirrhosis. However, it has now been shown in multiple populations that chronic viral hepatitis itself imparts an increased risk for CCA, even without the presence of liver cirrhosis.[12–14] Similarly, nonalcoholic fatty liver disease and nonalcoholic steatohepatitis are also increasingly becoming substantial contributors to the liver disease burden in the United States.[15] Additional risk factors for the development of ICC include inflammatory bowel disease, drugs and toxins (Thorotrast), primary biliary cholangitis, cholelithiasis, bile duct adenoma, and biliary papillomatosis.

INTRAHEPATIC CHOLANGIOCARCINOMA TUMOR CLASSIFICATION
Morphologic Subtypes

ICCs are classified into 3 specific subtypes: mass-forming, periductal infiltrating, and intraductal growth. The mass-forming subtype is the most common, accounting for 60% to 80% of all ICCs.[16] This subtype of ICC classically appears as solid nodules distinct from hepatic parenchyma on imaging. Macroscopically, they appear as firm, pale, well-demarcated, solid tumors lacking a capsule and are usually polylobulated with no macroscopically detectable connection with the bile duct (**Fig. 2**A). Lymph node metastasis is more commonly observed in this subtype. The periductal infiltrating subtype is the second most common subtype, accounting for 15% to 35% of all ICCs (**Fig. 2**B).[16] Unlike the mass-forming subtype, periductal infiltrating ICC invades the parenchyma around portal structures and is often associated with stenosis of the involved ducts. This can lead to proximal obstructive biliary dilation and potentially cholangitis. Approximately 10% of ICCs are intraductal growth pattern (**Fig. 2**C), characterized by a papillary growth into the bile duct lumen and more often associated with advanced disease. Some controversy surrounding the relative prognosis of the intraductal growth pattern exists, with some sources suggesting better prognosis, while others report a similar prognosis as the mass-forming subtype.[17,18] Finally, the mixed mass-forming and periductal infiltrating subtype is believed to be the most aggressive subtype and accounts for approximately 25% of all ICCs.[16] This mixed subtype carries a significantly worse prognosis. The isolated mass-forming and isolated periductal-infiltrating subtypes (without hilar invasion) have a 5-year survival after surgery of 41.2% and 85.7%, respectively,[19] compared with no reported 5-year survivors with the mixed mass-forming and periductal-infiltrating subtype and a median overall survival of 8.3 months in these patients.[20]

Histology

ICCs are classically well- to moderately differentiated adenocarcinomas with a fibrotic core and foci of calcifications and necrosis. Infiltration often occurs through sinusoids

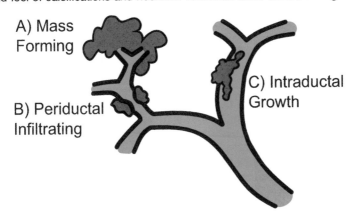

A) Mass Forming

B) Periductal Infiltrating

C) Intraductal Growth

Fig. 2. Macroscopic cholangiocarcinoma subtypes.

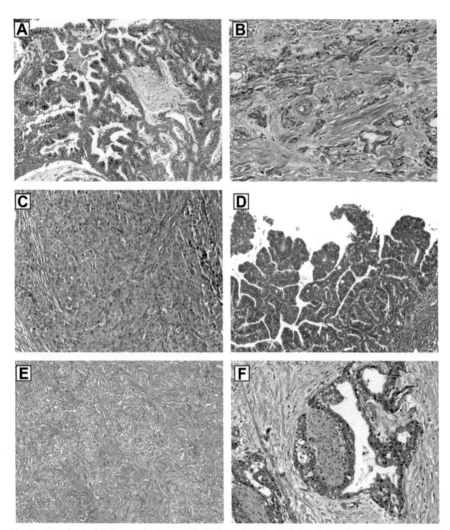

Fig. 3. Histology. (*A*) Large duct growth pattern (more common in perihilar cholangiocarcinoma). (*B*) Small duct growth pattern (more common in ICC). (*C*) Solid growth pattern (can mimic hepatocellular carcinoma on biopsy). (*D*) Intraductal papillary biliary neoplasm (a recognized precursor to cholangiocarcinoma). (*E*) Desmoplasia. (*F*) Perineural invasion. (*Courtesy of* M. Torbenson, MD, Rochester, Minnesota.)

coopting portal tracts and invading portal venules, lymphatics, and nerves at early stages. The large duct growth pattern (**Fig. 3**A) is more common in PCCs, and the small duct growth pattern (**Fig. 3**B) is more common in ICC. Solid growth patterns (**Fig. 3**C) can be observed with ICCs and can mimic HCCs on biopsy. Intraductal papillary biliary neoplasms (**Fig. 3**D) are rare recognized precursors to cholangiocarcinoma. Molecular and genetic analyses of CCA have revealed that the microenvironment of tumors is a key component of disease progression and pathogenesis consistent with previous observations that CCA is desmoplastic tumor (**Fig. 3**E).[21,22] Perineural invasion is frequently observed in CCA and portends a poor prognosis (**Fig. 3**F). Other rare histologic carcinoma variants include adenosquamous, squamous, mucinous, signet-ring cell, clear cell, and lymphoepithelioma-like carcinoma.[19] Although ICC is generally described as arising from cholangiocytes, there are some data that challenge this paradigm, suggesting that a more fluid constitution and reconstitution of the liver exist.[23,24]

CLINICAL EVALUATION
Presentation

By definition, ICC occurs proximal to the second-degree bile ducts, so symptoms of biliary obstruction (jaundice, pruritus, clay-colored stools, and dark urine) are much less common compared with extrahepatic and perihilar CCA. In a single-institution case series of 564 patients with operable CCA, only 16% of patients with ICC presented with jaundice, compared with 89% and 91% of perihilar and extrahepatic CCAs, respectively.[25] As a result, patients with ICC often present with nonspecific symptoms such as dull right upper quadrant pain, and possibly weight loss. As such, ICC is most commonly found as an incidental finding in patients with or without cirrhosis on cross-sectional imaging performed for other reasons. Given how vague and infrequent these symptoms are, diagnosis is frequently made in the late stages.

Diagnosis

The broad differential diagnosis for liver masses in patients without primary sclerosing cholangitis or cirrhosis includes metastasis, HCC, CCA, and benign liver lesions among others. A broad investigation of hepatic pathology and other malignancies should be conducted. Colon cancer risk and screening history, alcohol consumption history, viral hepatitis risk and serologies, autoimmune hepatitis serologies, iron studies (hemochromatosis), copper studies (Wilson disease), body mass index (BMI) (nonalcoholic steatohepatitis), travel history (liver flukes), and exposure to hepatotoxins (Thorotrast, aflatoxin) should be assessed. CA 19 to 9, CEA, and AFP should also be an early part of the investigation. In patients with PSC with or without ulcerative colitis, the development of CCA can be predicted with CA 19-9; a proposed cut-off level of 130 U/mL (normal <55 U/mL) carries a sensitivity and specificity of 78.6% and 98.5%, respectively and a negative predictive value of 99.4%.[26] However, CA-19 can be independently elevated by bacterial cholangitis or biliary dilation and may provide a false-negative result in those who are genetically devoid of the antigen (7% of people).[27]

Staging

There are 3 major staging systems for ICC including the American Joint Committee on Cancer (AJCC)/Union for International Cancer Control (UICC) tumor, node, metastasis (TNM) staging system, the Liver Cancer Study Group of Japan (LCSGJ),[28] and the National Cancer Center of Japan staging system.[29] The only major difference between these staging systems is related to the T staging, particularly with the relation to tumor size and the presence of vascular invasion.[30] Although previous iterations of the AJCC system were adaptations from the HCC staging system, the seventh edition had been to revised with more relevant T-stage distinction and stage survival correlation for ICC.[31] Additional analysis of the LCSGJ and NCCJ systems failed to stratify patients based on T stage and provided suboptimal survival correlation.[6,32,33] As a result, the eighth edition AJCC/UICC staging system subsequently reclassified T- and overall stage categories.

Imaging

Typically, ICCs are well defined or infiltrative liver lesions without a capsule. Classic computed tomography (CT) findings include global hypodensity and peripheral rim enhancement in both the arterial and portal venous phases.[34] However, this classic appearance on CT imaging is only observed in approximately 50% to 60% of cases.[34,35] Bile duct dilation peripheral to the mass is observed in approximately 50% of ICCs. In up to 20% of cases, there may be capsular contraction near the mass. If CT imaging is equivocal for ICC and there is still a high suspicion, additional studies such as magnetic resonance cholangiopancreatography (MRCP), endoscopic ultrasound (EUS) with fine needle aspiration (FNA), or endoscopic retrograde cholangiopancreatography (ERCP) with biopsy should be performed.

PREOPERATIVE MANAGEMENT

Preoperative management should include a comprehensive evaluation for metastatic or occult disease including CT of the chest, abdomen, and pelvis. High-quality imaging of the lesion is the mainstay in determining surgical technical resectability. Technical resectability is defined as the ability to achieve negative margins while preserving adequate liver function with the future liver remnant (FLR). As a result, macrovascular invasion and multifocal disease may preclude curative-intent surgical resection. Furthermore, peritoneal disease and distant lymph node metastasis deem a patient unresectable.

Postresection liver failure and complications are inversely related to the quantity and quality of liver parenchyma in the remnant liver.[36] Preoperative biliary drainage should be performed in the FLR if jaundice is present. In otherwise healthy individuals, 20% to 25% of FLR is the standard cut off, while 40% FLR is often required in individuals with underlying liver disease.[37-39] Portal venous embolization of the affected segments of the liver is often employed to induce hypertrophy in the FLR to increase functional capacity. Because of ethical considerations, true randomization of portal vein embolization (PVE) has not been assessed. However, studies have shown that in patients with marginal predicted FLR, PVE led to a significant increase in FLR volume and no significant difference in R0 resection and major complication rates when compared to patients with higher predicted FLRs who did not undergo PVE.[37]

In addition to technical resectability, physiologic resectability should be considered. This is an assessment of a patient's ability to tolerate a major liver resection. Assessment of a patient's physiologic status includes a comprehensive assessment of the patient's comorbidities and functional status. Patients with unresectable disease, either caused by technical considerations or a patient's physiologic status, should be considered for alternative modalities such as systemic (eg, chemotherapy or targeted therapy) or regional therapies such as transarterial chemoembolization, radioembolization, or external beam radiation.

OPERATIVE MANAGEMENT
Diagnostic Laparoscopy

The role of diagnostic laparoscopy in hepatobiliary malignancies remains mostly determined by surgeon preference. However, in patients with ICC, the authors recommend a diagnostic laparoscopy prior to definitive surgical resection because of the high incidence of occult metastatic disease; upwards of 30% of patients may harbor occult metastatic disease that was not visualized on preoperative cross-sectional staging imaging.[40] The sensitivity of a diagnostic laparoscopy may be aided by the use of intraoperative liver ultrasound to assess the extent of disease. The data suggest that approximately 1 in 3 patients with ICC may be spared a laparotomy with the utilization of diagnostic laparoscopy.[40-42]

Liver Resection

The surgical approach to patients with ICC involves hepatic resection with negative margins and a portal lymphadenectomy. With advances in preoperative evaluation, intraoperative surgical techniques, and perioperative management, morbidity and mortality from liver resection have greatly improved over the past several decades. Still, overall morbidity rates are high and quoted between 6% and 43%, with mortality rates quoted between 1% and 5% at high-volume specialized centers. The most common causes of morbidity in liver resection for ICC are superficial wound infection (13.1%), abscess (7.5%), sepsis (6.3%), and biliary leak (4%).[25] Curative-intent surgical resection (R0 resection) is achieved in 46% to 98% of cases and varies dramatically by institution.[5,20,25,37,43] This is likely multifactorial and due to surgeon and hospital experience, pathologic evaluation, and patient selection.

Vascular Resection

Major vascular involvement is a common finding of ICC. In an international multicenter trial of 1089 patients with histologically confirmed ICCs who underwent curative-intent resection, vascular invasion was noted to be an independently poor prognostic factor. This study also examined the impact of macroscopic and microscopic vascular invasion on overall survival and found a median overall survival of 39 versus 21 months, respectively; patients without any vascular invasion had the longest median overall survival at 45 months.[44] Despite this, vascular resection may be necessary to achieve negative margins. Major vascular resection may be performed safely without an increase in perioperative morbidity or mortality.[45] As such, the need for major vascular resection should not preclude surgical resection if negative margins can be obtained.

Lymphadenectomy

In addition to an R0 resection, lymph node status is among the most important long-term prognostic factors for patients with ICC.[16,19,20,25,46,47] Thus, evaluation of the draining lymph node through the completion of a portal lymphadenectomy is imperative. As such, National Comprehensive Cancer Network (NCCN) guidelines recommend retrieval of at least 6 lymph nodes. A formal lymphadenectomy of the celiac axis should be performed and includes dissection along the gastrohepatic ligament, hepatoduodenal ligament, and retropancreatic lymph nodes.

Minimally Invasive Resection

The use of a minimally invasive approach for liver lesions has been increasingly used in recent years. Previous retrospective studies have found that patients undergoing minimally invasive liver resection had a shorter length of stay and a lower incidence of complications compared with patients undergoing an open liver resection.[48-50] A study of Medicare patients undergoing liver and pancreatic resections found that patients undergoing a minimally invasive resection had lower complication and readmission rates and shorter length of stay.[48] Despite these purported benefits, an investigation of the Nationwide Inpatient Sample database found that over 95% of resections were performed using a traditional open approach. As such, a minimally invasive approach may be considered in the well-selected patient by surgeons with technical expertise in this area.

Transplantation

There are mixed data supporting the use of orthotopic liver transplant (OLT) with respect to ICCs. The earliest data for the use of OLT for ICCs is a 54-patient study from 1981 to 1994 where 20 patients with either unresectable disease or cirrhosis underwent OLT and were compared with 34 patients who underwent hepatectomy for ICC during the same time interval.[51] Although the study reiterated the impact of tumor number, margin positivity, and metastatic disease on survival, it failed to show any clinically significant difference between survival in patients managed with OLT versus hepatectomy. It is important to note that these patients did not receive neoadjuvant systemic therapy and that the overall survival was low in both groups. A more contemporary 2011 study showed a 33% disease recurrence-free survival after OLT compared to 0% without OLT among patients who received varying chemotherapy and locoregional therapies.[52–54] Ongoing studies are examining algorithmic risk-based approaches to neoadjuvant chemotherapy, locoregional chemotherapy, and adjuvant chemotherapy in conjunction with OLT for patients with ICC.

ADJUVANT CHEMOTHERAPY AND RADIATION

Prospective or randomized clinical investigation of standardized adjuvant chemotherapy in patients with R0 resection is limited. Combination therapy with gemcitabine and cisplatin may provide some survival benefit based on prospective controlled trials of unresected biliary tract cancers. Among patients with resected tumors, the recent BILCAP trial evaluated the use of adjuvant capecitabine among patients with invasive gallbladder cancer and cholangiocarcinoma. In this study, patients were randomized to receive 6 months of capecitabine versus observation following R0 resection. Overall survival was found to be higher in the capecitabine group, although significance was not achieved in the intention-to-treat analysis. In the per protocol analysis of capecitabine (n = 210) and observation (n = 220), the overall survival was 53 months versus 36 months (P=.028), respectively, suggesting that there is a survival advantage associated with the use of adjuvant capecitabine following R0 resection for ICC.[55]

In a retrospective analysis involving 1154 patients undergoing curative-intent hepatectomy for ICC across 14 institutions, adjuvant therapy was associated with better survival in patients with N1 disease and in patients with T2-T4 tumors.[56] Approximately 50% of these patients received gemcitabine-based therapy. These data suggest that adjuvant chemotherapy can provide a significant survival benefit for patients with more advanced or aggressive tumors, particularly those with nodal disease. Further studies are needed to clarify the role of standardized adjuvant chemotherapy in ICC, particularly in high-risk patients with nodal disease and locally advanced tumors.

UNRESECTABLE/METASTATIC DISEASE
Systemic Therapy

Patients with metastatic or unresectable ICC are often treated with systemic chemotherapy. The ABC-02 trial found that patients with advanced biliary cancer and treated with combination gemcitabine/cisplatin chemotherapy had a significant survival advantage compared with patients treated with gemcitabine alone.[57] Other reported regimens include other combination gemticatbine- or fluorouracil-based chemotherapies.

Locoregional Therapy

Because of the late diagnosis of the majority of these tumors, approximately 70% of ICCs are deemed unresectable at diagnosis. Accordingly, great interest exists in the use of regional therapies with the goal of either downstaging or improving survival in patients with unresectable ICC. Transarterial regional therapies involve the delivery of drugs or radiation through the hepatic arterial system supplying the affected tissue. This technique relies on the fact that healthy liver parenchyma obtains most of its blood supply through portal venous branches, while liver malignancies tend to derive most of their blood supply through the hepatic arterial system. Three major varieties of locoregional therapy exist including conventional transcatheter arterial chemoembolization (cTACE), drug-eluting beads (DEB)-TACE, and Yttrium-90 radioembolization (Y90-RE).

Conventional transcatheter arterial chemoembolization
In this approach, contrast-lipid emulsion (typically Lipiodol or Ethiodol) is delivered into the tumor-supplying branch of the hepatic artery. Centrally located tumors should have bilateral hepatic artery angiographic evaluation, as there is a high possibility that these tumors are supplied by bilateral arteries. After localization of the blood supply, a chemotherapeutic agent is delivered. Typically doxorubicin, cisplatin, and mitomycin-C are used, although the use of gemcitabine has also been described.[58–60] Following the administration of this chemotherapy, embolic occlusion is typically achieved with gelfoam, polyvinyl-alcohol (PVA), or triacryl gelatin (TG) microspheres to devascularize the tumor and prevent washout of the chemotherapy payload. cTACE has been shown to increase overall survival in unresectable ICC as well as in postoperative patients with poor prognosis.[59,61] Its efficacy is best observed in patients receiving multimodal treatment including systemic chemotherapy.[60] cTACE is typically well tolerated, although a mild-to-moderate postembolization syndrome can be seen, which includes abdominal pain, nausea, fever, and transaminase elevation.[60]

Drug-eluting beads
In this method, PVA or superabsorbant beads are typically loaded with doxorubicin or irnoctecan, although the technology is amenable to loading with a range of agents. Delivery of these agents through the beads allows for an even higher sustained intratumoral chemotherapeutic concentration. Small prospective studies have shown an overall survival benefit for drug-eluting beads in unresectable disease. As with cTACE, the technique is often used in conjunction with systemic chemotherapy, and significant variation exists among regimens used.

Yttrium-90 radioembolization
This method utilizes small (approximately 30 μm) glass- or resin-based embolic particles loaded with the radionucleotide Y90 that are intra-arterially delivered. The Y90 emits β-radiation with a target dose of 120 Gy, which is significantly higher than what can be achieved with external beam radiation. Furthermore, liver tissue is extremely sensitive to radiation, and rarely can tumoricidal doses be administered before toxicities preclude ongoing treatment. Similar to other forms of locoregional therapy, studies of Y-90-RE are mostly focused in patients with unresectable disease and/or in conjunction with systemic chemotherapy. In this context, over 80% of patients have partial response or stable disease at 3 months, and in several instances, downstaging to resectable disease was achieved.[62] An area of active investigation is the use of systemic chemotherapy as a means of radiosensitization prior to Y90 delivery as a means of increasing the therapeutic index. Early trials suggest that over 170 Gy of Y90 can be safely delivered with capecitabine radiosensitization.[63]

FUTURE DIRECTIONS

Recent advances have been made regarding the molecular and genetic makeup of ICC. This improved understanding allows for the identification of potentially targetable mutations. In the MOSCATO-01 trial, 68% of patients with ICC were found to have an actionable molecular target.[64] Used as a second-line therapy, the overall response rate was found to be 33%, and the disease control rate was 88%. Compared with a match group of patients who did not receive a molecular targeted agent, these patients had a lower risk of death. A deeper understanding of the role of these targeted agents as well as other newer modalities, such as immune checkpoint inhibitors, is needed to further evaluate their role in the treatment of ICC.

SUMMARY

ICC is an aggressive primary hepatic malignancy occurring in the periphery of the liver, proximal to the second-degree (segmental) bile ducts. High-quality cross-sectional imaging is necessary to determine the extent of disease and resectability. The mainstay of treatment for ICC remains curative-intent liver resection with a portal lymphadenectomy. The use of systemic therapy in the neoadjuvant and adjuvant settings can be utilized to improve survival. In addition, systemic and locoregional therapies provide effective options for patients with unresectable disease, and in some cases downstage previously unresectable patients. Molecular profiling of these tumors may be helpful to identify targeted agents useful in the treatment of this aggressive disease.

REFERENCES

1. Khan SA, Toledano MB, Taylor-Robinson SD. Epidemiology, risk factors, and pathogenesis of cholangiocarcinoma. HPB (Oxford) 2008;10(2):77–82.
2. Rahnemai-Azar AA, Weisbrod A, Dillhoff M, et al. Intrahepatic cholangiocarcinoma: molecular markers for diagnosis and prognosis. Surg Oncol 2017;26(2): 125–37.
3. Brown KM, Parmar AD, Geller DA. Intrahepatic cholangiocarcinoma. Surg Oncol Clin N Am 2014;23(2):231–46.
4. Lang H, Sotiropoulos GC, Sgourakis G, et al. Operations for intrahepatic cholangiocarcinoma: single-institution experience of 158 patients. J Am Coll Surg 2009; 208(2):218–28.
5. Jonas S, Thelen A, Benckert C, et al. Extended liver resection for intrahepatic cholangiocarcinoma: a comparison of the prognostic accuracy of the fifth and sixth editions of the TNM classification. Ann Surg 2009;249(2):303–9.
6. Nathan H, Aloia TA, Vauthey J-N, et al. A proposed staging system for intrahepatic cholangiocarcinoma. Ann Surg Oncol 2009;16(1):14–22.
7. Van Dyke AL, Shiels MS, Jones GS, et al. Biliary tract cancer incidence and trends in the United States by demographic group, 1999-2013. Cancer 2019. https://doi.org/10.1002/cncr.31942.
8. Chapman MH, Webster GJM, Bannoo S, et al. Cholangiocarcinoma and dominant strictures in patients with primary sclerosing cholangitis: a 25-year single-centre experience. Eur J Gastroenterol Hepatol 2012;24(9):1051–8.
9. Claessen MMH, Vleggaar FP, Tytgat KMAJ, et al. High lifetime risk of cancer in primary sclerosing cholangitis. J Hepatol 2009;50(1):158–64.
10. Bergquist A, Ekbom A, Olsson R, et al. Hepatic and extrahepatic malignancies in primary sclerosing cholangitis. J Hepatol 2002;36(3):321–7.

11. Kaewpitoon N, Kaewpitoon S-J, Pengsaa P, et al. Opisthorchis viverrini: the carcinogenic human liver fluke. World J Gastroenterol 2008;14(5):666–74.
12. Wang Z, Sheng Y-Y, Dong Q-Z, et al. Hepatitis B virus and hepatitis C virus play different prognostic roles in intrahepatic cholangiocarcinoma: a meta-analysis. World J Gastroenterol 2016;22(10):3038–51.
13. Jeong S, Luo G, Wang Z-H, et al. Impact of viral hepatitis B status on outcomes of intrahepatic cholangiocarcinoma: a meta-analysis. Hepatol Int 2018;12(4):330–8.
14. Tao L-Y, He X-D, Xiu D-R. Hepatitis B virus is associated with the clinical features and survival rate of patients with intrahepatic cholangiocarcinoma. Clin Res Hepatol Gastroenterol 2016;40(6):682–7.
15. Wongjarupong N, Assavapongpaiboon B, Susantitaphong P, et al. Non-alcoholic fatty liver disease as a risk factor for cholangiocarcinoma: a systematic review and meta-analysis. BMC Gastroenterol 2017;17(1):149.
16. Lendvai G, Szekerczés T, Illyés I, et al. Cholangiocarcinoma: classification, histopathology and molecular carcinogenesis. Pathol Oncol Res 2018. https://doi.org/10.1007/s12253-018-0491-8.
17. Suh KS, Roh HR, Koh YT, et al. Clinicopathologic features of the intraductal growth type of peripheral cholangiocarcinoma. Hepatology 2000;31(1):12–7.
18. Bagante F, Weiss M, Alexandrescu S, et al. Long-term outcomes of patients with intraductal growth sub-type of intrahepatic cholangiocarcinoma. HPB (Oxford) 2018;20(12):1189–97.
19. Vijgen S, Terris B, Rubbia-Brandt L. Pathology of intrahepatic cholangiocarcinoma. Hepatobiliary Surg Nutr 2017;6(1):22–34.
20. Yeh C-N, Yeh T-S, Chen T-C, et al. Gross pathological classification of peripheral cholangiocarcinoma determines the efficacy of hepatectomy. J Gastroenterol 2013;48(5):647–59.
21. Kajiyama K, Maeda T, Takenaka K, et al. The significance of stromal desmoplasia in intrahepatic cholangiocarcinoma: a special reference of "scirrhous-type" and "nonscirrhous-type" growth. Am J Surg Pathol 1999;23(8):892–902.
22. DeClerck YA. Desmoplasia: a response or a niche? Cancer Discov 2012;2(9):772–4.
23. Sekiya S, Suzuki A. Intrahepatic cholangiocarcinoma can arise from Notch-mediated conversion of hepatocytes. J Clin Invest 2012;122(11):3914–8.
24. Fan B, Malato Y, Calvisi DF, et al. Cholangiocarcinomas can originate from hepatocytes in mice. J Clin Invest 2012;122(8):2911–5.
25. DeOliveira ML, Cunningham SC, Cameron JL, et al. Cholangiocarcinoma: thirty-one-year experience with 564 patients at a single institution. Ann Surg 2007;245(5):755–62.
26. Levy C, Lymp J, Angulo P, et al. The value of serum CA 19-9 in predicting cholangiocarcinomas in patients with primary sclerosing cholangitis. Dig Dis Sci 2005;50(9):1734–40.
27. Steinberg W. The clinical utility of the CA 19-9 tumor-associated antigen. Am J Gastroenterol 1990;85(4):350–5.
28. Yamasaki S. Intrahepatic cholangiocarcinoma: macroscopic type and stage classification. J Hepatobiliary Pancreat Surg 2003;10(4):288–91.
29. Okabayashi T, Yamamoto J, Kosuge T, et al. A new staging system for mass-forming intrahepatic cholangiocarcinoma: analysis of preoperative and postoperative variables. Cancer 2001;92(9):2374–83.
30. Blechacz B, Komuta M, Roskams T, et al. Clinical diagnosis and staging of cholangiocarcinoma. Nat Rev Gastroenterol Hepatol 2011;8(9):512–22.

31. Farges O, Fuks D, Le Treut Y-P, et al. AJCC 7th edition of TNM staging accurately discriminates outcomes of patients with resectable intrahepatic cholangiocarcinoma: by the AFC-IHCC-2009 study group. Cancer 2011;117(10):2170–7.

32. Sotiropoulos GC, Miyazaki M, Konstadoulakis MM, et al. Multicentric evaluation of a clinical and prognostic scoring system predictive of survival after resection of intrahepatic cholangiocarcinomas. Liver Int 2010;30(7):996–1002.

33. Uenishi T, Yamazaki O, Yamamoto T, et al. Serosal invasion in TNM staging of mass-forming intrahepatic cholangiocarcinoma. J Hepatobiliary Pancreat Surg 2005;12(6):479–83.

34. Valls C, Gumà A, Puig I, et al. Intrahepatic peripheral cholangiocarcinoma: CT evaluation. Abdom Imaging 2000;25(5):490–6.

35. Iavarone M, Piscaglia F, Vavassori S, et al. Contrast enhanced CT-scan to diagnose intrahepatic cholangiocarcinoma in patients with cirrhosis. J Hepatol 2013;58(6):1188–93.

36. van den Broek MAJ, Olde Damink SWM, Dejong CHC, et al. Liver failure after partial hepatic resection: definition, pathophysiology, risk factors and treatment. Liver Int 2008;28(6):767–80.

37. Abdalla EK, Barnett CC, Doherty D, et al. Extended hepatectomy in patients with hepatobiliary malignancies with and without preoperative portal vein embolization. Arch Surg 2002;137(6):675–80 [discussion: 680–1].

38. Vauthey JN, Chaoui A, Do KA, et al. Standardized measurement of the future liver remnant prior to extended liver resection: methodology and clinical associations. Surgery 2000;127(5):512–9.

39. Kubota K, Makuuchi M, Kusaka K, et al. Measurement of liver volume and hepatic functional reserve as a guide to decision-making in resectional surgery for hepatic tumors. Hepatology 1997;26(5):1176–81.

40. Weber SM, Jarnagin WR, Klimstra D, et al. Intrahepatic cholangiocarcinoma: resectability, recurrence pattern, and outcomes. J Am Coll Surg 2001;193(4): 384–91.

41. Davidson JT, Jin LX, Krasnick B, et al. Staging laparoscopy among three subtypes of extra-hepatic biliary malignancy: a 15-year experience from 10 institutions. J Surg Oncol 2019;119(3):288–94.

42. Tian Y, Liu L, Yeolkar NV, et al. Diagnostic role of staging laparoscopy in a subset of biliary cancers: a meta-analysis. ANZ J Surg 2017;87(1–2):22–7.

43. Tang Z, Yang Y, Zhao Z, et al. The clinicopathological factors associated with prognosis of patients with resectable perihilar cholangiocarcinoma: a systematic review and meta-analysis. Medicine (Baltimore) 2018;97(34):e11999.

44. Hu L-S, Weiss M, Popescu I, et al. Impact of microvascular invasion on clinical outcomes after curative-intent resection for intrahepatic cholangiocarcinoma. J Surg Oncol 2019;119(1):21–9.

45. Reames BN, Ejaz A, Koerkamp BG, et al. Impact of major vascular resection on outcomes and survival in patients with intrahepatic cholangiocarcinoma: a multi-institutional analysis. J Surg Oncol 2017;116(2):133–9.

46. Yoh T, Hatano E, Seo S, et al. Long-term survival of recurrent intrahepatic cholangiocarcinoma: the impact and selection of repeat surgery. World J Surg 2018; 42(6):1848–56.

47. Ruys AT, Busch OR, Rauws EA, et al. Prognostic impact of preoperative imaging parameters on resectability of hilar cholangiocarcinoma. HPB Surg 2013;2013: 657309.

48. Ejaz A, Sachs T, He J, et al. A comparison of open and minimally invasive surgery for hepatic and pancreatic resections using the Nationwide Inpatient Sample. Surgery 2014;156(3):538–47.
49. Morino M, Morra I, Rosso E, et al. Laparoscopic vs open hepatic resection: a comparative study. Surg Endosc 2003;17(12):1914–8.
50. Kaneko H, Takagi S, Otsuka Y, et al. Laparoscopic liver resection of hepatocellular carcinoma. Am J Surg 2005;189(2):190–4.
51. Casavilla FA, Marsh JW, Iwatsuki S, et al. Hepatic resection and transplantation for peripheral cholangiocarcinoma. J Am Coll Surg 1997;185(5):429–36.
52. Hong JC, Jones CM, Duffy JP, et al. Comparative analysis of resection and liver transplantation for intrahepatic and hilar cholangiocarcinoma: a 24-year experience in a single center. Arch Surg 2011;146(6):683–9.
53. Ghali P, Marotta PJ, Yoshida EM, et al. Liver transplantation for incidental cholangiocarcinoma: analysis of the Canadian experience. Liver Transpl 2005;11(11):1412–6.
54. Sapisochin G, Facciuto M, Rubbia-Brandt L, et al. Liver transplantation for "very early" intrahepatic cholangiocarcinoma: international retrospective study supporting a prospective assessment. Hepatology 2016;64(4):1178–88.
55. Bridgewater JA, Fox R, Primrose JN. Exploratory analyses of the BILCAP study. J Clin Oncol 2018;36(15_suppl):e16132.
56. Reames BN, Bagante F, Ejaz A, et al. Impact of adjuvant chemotherapy on survival in patients with intrahepatic cholangiocarcinoma: a multi-institutional analysis. HPB (Oxford) 2017;19(10):901–9.
57. Valle J, Wasan H, Palmer DH, et al. Cisplatin plus gemcitabine versus gemcitabine for biliary tract cancer. N Engl J Med 2010;362(14):1273–81.
58. Yang G-W, Zhao Q, Qian S, et al. Percutaneous microwave ablation combined with simultaneous transarterial chemoembolization for the treatment of advanced intrahepatic cholangiocarcinoma. Onco Targets Ther 2015;8:1245–50.
59. Shen WF, Zhong W, Liu Q, et al. Adjuvant transcatheter arterial chemoembolization for intrahepatic cholangiocarcinoma after curative surgery: retrospective control study. World J Surg 2011;35(9):2083–91.
60. Kiefer MV, Albert M, McNally M, et al. Chemoembolization of intrahepatic cholangiocarcinoma with cisplatinum, doxorubicin, mitomycin C, ethiodol, and polyvinyl alcohol: a 2-center study. Cancer 2011;117(7):1498–505.
61. Hyder O, Marsh JW, Salem R, et al. Intra-arterial therapy for advanced intrahepatic cholangiocarcinoma: a multi-institutional analysis. Ann Surg Oncol 2013;20(12):3779–86.
62. Al-Adra DP, Gill RS, Axford SJ, et al. Treatment of unresectable intrahepatic cholangiocarcinoma with yttrium-90 radioembolization: a systematic review and pooled analysis. Eur J Surg Oncol 2015;41(1):120–7.
63. Hickey R, Mulcahy MF, Lewandowski RJ, et al. Chemoradiation of hepatic malignancies: prospective, phase 1 study of full-dose capecitabine with escalating doses of yttrium-90 radioembolization. Int J Radiat Oncol Biol Phys 2014;88(5):1025–31.
64. Verlingue L, Malka D, Allorant A, et al. Precision medicine for patients with advanced biliary tract cancers: an effective strategy within the prospective MOSCATO-01 trial. Eur J Cancer 2017;87:122–30.

Surgical Considerations of Hilar Cholangiocarcinoma

Blaire Anderson, MD[a], M.B. Majella Doyle, MD, MBA[b],*

KEYWORDS

- Hilar cholangiocarcinoma • Hepatic resection • Liver transplantation
- Vascular resection

KEY POINTS

- The goal of successful oncologic outcome is achieved with margin negative resection including the extrahepatic bile duct with concomitant ipsilateral liver resection with caudate.
- Vascular resection and reconstruction of the portal vein should not be a contraindication to resection for cure. Arterial resection should be performed only in select patients at experienced centers.
- A functional liver remnant of 40% or greater is advised, which can be facilitated by portal vein embolization with biliary decompression of the future liver remnant improving regenerative capacity. Prohibitive mortality has been reported with Associating Liver Partition and Portal Vein Ligation for hilar cholangiocarcinoma.
- Liver transplant after neoadjuvant protocol is appropriate for a subset of carefully selected patients who have nonmetastatic locally advanced lesions that are not amenable to resection.

INTRODUCTION

Cholangiocarcinoma is a rare tumor of the bile duct epithelium, accounting for only 3% of gastrointestinal malignancies.[1] It can be divided into intrahepatic, hilar (at the confluence of the right and left hepatic duct), and extrahepatic cholangiocarcinoma. Hilar cholangiocarcinoma (HC) is the most common and will be the focus of this discussion. Resection and transplantation are the main modalities of curative treatment, whereas patients with inoperable tumors are best served with palliative chemoradiation. The consensus of a multidisciplinary committee including surgeons, medical and radiation oncologists, gastroenterologists, radiologists, and pathologists should drive treatment.

Disclosure Statement: The authors have nothing to disclose.
[a] Division of Transplantation Surgery, Department of Surgery, University of Nebraska Medical Center, 983285 Nebraska Medical Center, Omaha, NE 68198, USA; [b] Section of Abdominal Organ Transplant, Department of Surgery, Washington University School of Medicine, Washington University, 660 South Euclid Avenue, Campus Box 8109, St Louis, MO 63110, USA
* Corresponding author.
E-mail address: doylem@wustl.edu

Surg Oncol Clin N Am 28 (2019) 601–617
https://doi.org/10.1016/j.soc.2019.06.003
1055-3207/19/© 2019 Elsevier Inc. All rights reserved.

surgonc.theclinics.com

DIAGNOSIS

HC almost always presents with obstructive jaundice, unless only the left or right duct is intimately involved. Tea colored urine, clay colored stools, anorexia, weight loss, vague abdominal pain, and pruritis are common complaints. Physical examination is often nonrevealing other than clinical jaundice and possibly hepatomegaly. If the mass extends to the level of the cystic duct, a distended, palpable gallbladder may be appreciated. An obstructive pattern is found on laboratory values. Tumor markers including carcinoembryonic antigen (CEA) and carbohydrate antigen 19-9 (CA 19-9) should be evaluated and may be elevated; however, this is nonspecific for cholangio-carcinoma and can be increased in the setting of biliary obstruction from other causes. None the less, baseline values should be established and when extremely high can be predictive of metastatic disease.

Abdominal cross-sectional imaging, including high-quality pancreas protocol computed tomography (CT) or MRI/magnetic resonance cholangiopancreatography, should be performed to evaluate for metastatic disease and determine local resectability. These studies should ideally be performed before biliary decompression with stent placement. A CT of the chest completes the staging workup. Imaging will reveal local, regional, and distant extent of disease. Specifically, one should assess for metastatic disease, ductal involvement, vascular involvement, and extent of hepatic atrophy. PET scan has limited sensitivity in biliary cancers; however, it may have some utility in the setting of equivocal CT or MRI findings.[2–5] Routine use of PET scan is not recommended, as it rarely changes surgical management.

Direct cholangiography (endoscopic retrograde cholangiopancreatography [ERCP] or percutaneous transhepatic cholangiography [PTC]) provide biliary tree anatomic information, tissue for histology, and biliary drainage when required. ERCP with biliary brushings is routinely used in the diagnostic workup of biliary strictures. Overall, cytology has low sensitivity for diagnosis of ductal cancers due to the desmoplastic nature of these tumors, limiting the ability to obtain adequate tissue for analysis. Despite a specificity of 100%, cytology alone has a sensitivity as low as 5% to 40%.[6,7] The addition of fluorescent in situ hybridization (FISH), a means of identifying chromosomal abnormalities, namely polysomy or amplification, can improve sensitivity upward of 84%, maintaining a high specificity of 97%.[8] Adjunctive techniques including direct cholangioscopy and endoscopic ultrasound (EUS) with fine-needle aspiration (FNA) or biopsy may increase diagnostic yield further.

Brooks and colleagues[9] reviewed the workup of consecutive biliary strictures, evaluating the performance of FISH, cholangioscopic biopsy, and EUS-FNA. FISH polysomy/9p21 was 99% specific and 56% sensitive for diagnosis. The use of EUS-FNA for distal strictures and cholangioscopic biopsy for proximal strictures increased sensitivity from 33% to 93% and 48% to 76% in cytology-negative strictures.[10]

Immunoglobulin G4 (IgG4)-related sclerosing cholangitis mimics HC. Serum IgG4 levels should be assessed in cases of biliary stricture with diagnostic uncertainty to rule out this diagnosis. Biopsy findings of infiltrates of IgG4 plasma cells and severe interstitial fibrosis although pathognomonic are not present in all cases due to limitations of bile duct tissue sampling.[10] Of note, resection can be performed based on malignant-appearing stricture in the absence of tissue diagnosis in carefully selected cases. This results in benign final diagnosis approximately 10% of the time.[11,12]

FUTURE LIVER REMNANT

When evaluating for resectability the capacity to leave adequate hepatic parenchyma is essential. A future liver remnant (FLR) of at least 20% is advised when underlying liver is otherwise healthy.[13] Major and liver-related complications, hepatic dysfunction or insufficiency, longer hospital stays, and 90-day mortality are increased when FLR is less than 20%.[14] In addition, long duration of chemotherapy and FLR less than 30% are independent risk factors for hepatic insufficiency.[15] Because neoadjuvant treatment is not currently standard of care before resection, these patients should not have significant hepatic injury from chemotherapy; however, of note, the functional capacity of cholestatic liver is not equivalent to normal liver, as cholestasis impairs regenerative capacity.

Portal vein embolization (PVE) can be used to increase the FLR by a hemodynamic change and redistribution of growth factors leading to hypertrophy, thus improving the safety of major hepatic resections. Japanese surgeons, who have the most extensive experience of PVE in the setting of HC, generally suggest PVE if FLR is less than 40%.[16,17] A 2008 meta-analysis of 1140 patients showed an average increase of 8% to 27% after PVE/with this technique.[18] Importantly, the degree of hypertrophy indicates outcome. Kinetic growth rate has been brought forward as an early marker of regenerative capacity. Shindoh and colleagues[15] compared kinetic growth rate, standardized FLR volume, and degree of hypertrophy as predictive factors of overall and liver-specific postoperative morbidity and mortality, establishing cutoffs of 30%, 8%, and 2% per week, respectively. Because patients have variable hypertrophic response to PVE development of a composite score, using several volumetric parameters could more accurately predict postoperative liver failure.

Alternatively, Associating Liver Partition and Portal Vein Ligation (ALPPS) is an operative procedure used to induce rapid FLR hypertrophy by staged hepatectomy, facilitating extended resections. In the first stage, ligation of the portal vein branch and in situ splitting of liver parenchyma is undertaken. After a 1- to 2-week waiting period, the second stage involves division of the hepatic arterial supply, bile duct, and systemic venous outflow, with removal of intended liver. Most of the ALPPS publications include heterogenous cohorts of varying hepatic and biliary pathologies with 2-staged extended resection in the small-for-size setting.[19,20] Unparalleled liver hypertrophy with upward of 74% volume increase at a mean of 9 days after stage one has been reported.[19] A recent case-control analysis from 2 high-volume centers specifically assessed ALPPS for HC. Olthof and colleagues[21] reported significantly higher mortality rate, 48% for ALPPS compared with 28% for extended resection without ALPPS. Given inferior outcomes compared with PVE with subsequent resection, PVE should remain the gold standard to augment FLR in resectable HC.

BILIARY DECOMPRESSION

There are advocates and critics of routine biliary drainage with indications and even the means of decompression still debated. Biliary obstruction has been associated with increased postoperative mortality, and decompression has resulted in decreased risk of postoperative liver failure and mortality.[22–25] This is likely secondary to impaired hepatic regeneration in cholestatic liver, with drainage improving functional regenerative capacity.[26] As such, decompression provides relief of jaundice and improved liver function, at the risk of increased infectious complications, seeding of malignancy, and delay in treatment.[25,27,28]

Biliary decompression is clearly indicated when the patient is cholangitic, when treatment includes preoperative antineoplastic therapy or PVE, in cases of hyperbilirubinemia-induced malnutrition, and in hepatic or renal insufficiency.[13] Outside of these indications it perhaps should be reserved for small FLR cases, as complications may outweigh benefits in subgroups with sufficient FLR.[29–31] The

FLR should be prioritized for drainage, as this optimizes regenerative capacity. It is not advised to drain the atrophic liver lobe given the risk of persistent biliary infection. A preoperative bilirubin of less than 2 mg/dL is ideal. This can be achieved with ERCP, percutaneous transhepatic cholangiogram, and endoscopic nasobiliary drainage with proponents for each.

LAPAROSCOPY AND INTRAOPERATIVE ULTRASOUND

Staging laparoscopy before resection is controversial; there is no consensus in the literature as to its role. It has been reported that up to 47% of HC cases are found to be unresectable at the time of laparotomy.[32,33] The primary utility of staging laparoscopy is to screen these patients avoiding unnecessary major surgery. Staging laparoscopy is most useful in identifying those with liver and peritoneal metastasis; unfortunately, HC is more commonly locally invasive, and carcinomatosis is the reason for unresectability in only one-third of cases.[32] Coelen and colleagues,[34] in a recent systematic review and meta-analysis including 12 studies with 832 patients with HC, reported wide variability in yield of staging laparoscopy, from 6% to 45% with a pooled yield of 24%. Of note, in subgroup analysis the yield and sensitivity were lower for studies after 2010, likely attributable to improved preoperative imaging detecting metastatic disease and unresectability before going to the operating room.

The addition of intraoperative ultrasound has improved diagnostic yield in hepatobiliary malignancies with the advantage of the ability to assess involvement of biliary and vascular structures.[35,36] Russolillo and colleagues[37] analyzed the role of laparoscopic ultrasound during staging for proximal biliary cancers, including gallbladder, HC, and borderline resectable intrahepatic cholangiocarcinoma. Their series of 100 patients, 35 with HC, showed that laparoscopic ultrasound increased overall yield from 18% to 24% and accuracy from 60% to 80%. Interestingly, there was no advantage in the HC group with an overall yield and accuracy of 15% and 56%, respectively. Biliary drainage limits evaluation of portal structures secondary to stent artifact and associated inflammatory processes. In keeping, drainage procedure was found to be predictive of negative yield.

HEPATIC RESECTION

As surgeons continue to push the limits technically, the definition of resectable disease is in constant evolution (**Table 1**).[13] The goal is to remove the diseased bile ducts and restore biliary continuity with the ability to leave adequate hepatic parenchyma. Metastatic disease obviously precludes both resection and transplantation, in which case palliative chemoradiation therapy may be an option. Partial hepatectomy with en bloc resection of the extrahepatic bile duct, portal lymphadenectomy, and Roux-en-Y hepaticojejunostomy is required for most hilar tumors. Extrahepatic bile duct resection alone is associated with worse outcomes, given propensity for submucosal longitudinal extension of malignant cells along the biliary tract, but may be appropriate in select patients.[38–40] The Bismuth-Corlette classification was the original description of anatomic location of HC along the biliary tree (**Table 2**).[41] More recently, Blumgart and colleagues[42] have incorporated vascular invasion and lobar atrophy into the Memorial Sloan-Kettering preoperative T-stage criteria for HC (**Table 3**).

Generally right-sided lesions require right hepatic resections and left-sided lesions require left hepatic resections. The right hepatic artery is more commonly involved than the left, as it courses in close proximity to the biliary confluence. The right hepatic

Table 1
Criteria for unresectability of hilar cholangiocarcinoma

Patient Factors	Tumor Factors	
	Local	**Distant**
• Multiple medical comorbidities, unable to tolerate major operation • Underlying liver disease (cirrhosis with portal hypertension, primary sclerosing cholangitis)	• Extension of tumor to bilateral segmental ducts • Unilateral hepatic atrophy with either contralateral segmental duct involvement *or* vascular inflow involvement • Extension of tumor to unilateral segmental ducts with contralateral vascular inflow involvement	• Lymph node involvement beyond the hepatoduodenal ligament (N2 disease: periaortic, pericaval, superior mesenteric artery, and/or celiac artery lymph nodes) • Metastatic disease

Adapted from Mansour JC, Aloia TA, Crane CH, et al. Hilar cholangiocarcinoma: expert consensus statement. HPB (Oxford). 2015;17:691-699; and Jarnagin WR, Fong Y, DeMatteo RP, et al. Staging, resectability, and outcome in 225 patients with hilar cholangiocarcinoma. Ann Surg 2001; 234:507-17; with permission.

duct is short and anatomically variable, thus left-sided resections are more complex. The choice of hemi-hepatectomy or extended hepatectomy seems to be center specific with no difference in margin-negative resection or survival reported in the literature.[43–45]

Table 2
Summary of the Bismuth-Corlette classification of hilar cholangiocarcinoma

Classification	Description	Operative Approach
I	At the level of the cystic duct but below the bifurcation of the right and left hepatic ducts	Extrahepatic bile duct resection from the hepatic hilus to the pancreas with cholecystectomy, lymphadenectomy, right hepatic resection, caudate lobectomy, and biliary reconstruction (Hepatic resection may not be required in select cases)
II	At the bifurcation of right and left hepatic ducts	
IIIa	At the duct bifurcation with extension into the right hepatic duct	Extrahepatic bile duct resection from the hepatic hilus to the pancreas with cholecystectomy, lymphadenectomy, right hepatic resection, caudate lobectomy, and biliary reconstruction
IIIb	At the duct bifurcation with extension into the left hepatic duct	Extrahepatic bile duct resection from the hepatic hilus to the pancreas with cholecystectomy, lymphadenectomy, left hepatic resection, caudate lobectomy, and biliary reconstruction
IV	Extension into both right and left hepatic ducts or multicentric disease	Neoadjuvant chemoradiotherapy and liver transplantation

Adapted from Bismuth H, Corlette MB. Intrahepatic chlangioenteric anastomosis in carcinoma of the hilus of the liver. Surg Gynecol Obstet 1975;140:170-8; with permission.

Table 3
Summary of the Memorial Sloan-Kettering T-stage criteria for hilar cholangiocarcinoma

Stage	Criteria	Operative Approach
T1	Involvement of the biliary confluence ± unilateral extension to second-order biliary radicles	Extrahepatic bile duct resection from the hepatic hilus to the pancreas with cholecystectomy, lymphadenectomy, ipsilateral hepatic resection, caudate lobectomy, and biliary reconstruction
T2	Involvement of the biliary confluence ± unilateral extension to second-order biliary radicles *and* ipsilateral portal vein involvement ± ipsilateral hepatic lobe atrophy	
T3	Involvement of the biliary confluence ± bilateral extension to second-order biliary radicles; *or* "unilateral extension to second-order biliary radicles with contralateral portal vein involvement; *or* unilateral extension to second-order biliary radicles with contralateral hepatic lobe atrophy; *or* main or bilateral portal venous involvement"	Neoadjuvant chemoradiotherapy and liver transplantation

Adapted from Jarnagin WR, Fong Y, DeMatteo RP, et al. Staging, resectability, and outcome in 225 patients with hilar cholangiocarcinoma. Ann Surg 2001; 234:507-17; with permission.

Surgical approach is commonly as follows:

- First, exploration is undertaken to rule out distant metastatic disease of the peritoneum and liver as well as distant lymph nodes beyond the porta. Retropancreatic nodes should be assessed by performing a Kocher maneuver. Suspicious nodes outside of the hepatoduodenal ligament represent distant metastatic disease and unresectability. Intraoperative ultrasound is used both to rule out intrahepatic metastases to the contralateral liver and to aid in confirming local resectability by examining the extent of tumor and proximity to critical structures.
- If resectable, the next step is portal lymphadenectomy, which concurrently exposes hilar structures. Adenectomy of the cystic, pericholedochal, periportal and retroportal, hepatic artery, hilar, and superior pancreaticoduodenal nodes yield prognostic value with complete extirpation of lymph nodes having no effect on survival.[46]
- Early division of the distal bile duct allows for frozen-section margin evaluation. Typically, reresection is undertaken when frozen section reveals invasive disease or high-grade dysplasia. If tumor invades the proximal bile duct margin reexcision is warranted with possible pancreaticoduodenectomy. Achieving an R0 margin with reresection is associated with improved long-term survival and outcomes similar to those with primary R0 resection, thus every attempt should be made to clear surgical margins when possible.[47,48]
- Division of ipsilateral hepatic artery and portal vein completes the portal portion.
- This is followed by parenchymal transection, of which the authors favor low central venous pressure with intermittent Pringle maneuver and use an ultrasonic dissector with an energy-sealing device.
- Division of the proximal bile duct is generally completed during parenchymal transection.
- The hepatic vein is divided where it enters the inferior vena cava.
- Finally, the bile duct is reconstructed with a Roux-en-Y hepaticojejunostomy.

Perioperative morbidity and mortality following resection of HC are much higher than those reported for other elective operations. At high-volume centers morbidity ranges between 30% and 60% and mortality from 5% to 10%.[1,32,43–45,49,50] A better understanding of FLR requirements in cholestatic liver and utilization of PVE has led to decreased incidence of hepatic insufficiency. However, biliary compilations including bile leak, biloma, and intraabdominal abscess are still frequent. With resection, 5-year survival rates of 20% to 43% have been reported, with surgical margin status and lymph node involvement being the most significant independent prognostic factors.[1,32,43–45,49,50]

CAUDATE

Pathologically the caudate lobe is involved in 40% of cases.[51] There is literature to support resection of the caudate for HC in an effort to decrease local recurrence rates. Resecting the caudate leads to increased margin-negative (R0) resections with no difference in morbidity or mortality.[52,53] Favorable survival was demonstrated when comparing American and Japanese cohorts with 8% and 89% caudate resections, respectively.[54] A recent multiinstitutional analysis of the US extrahepatic biliary malignancy consortium also demonstrated a reduction in margin positivity with caudate resection; this was not, however, associated with any difference in recurrence free or overall survival when compared with patients who did not have a caudate resection.[55] In the authors' opinion the caudate lobe should be resected routinely.

VASCULAR RESECTION

Vascular involvement by tumor is common, given the close proximity of the bile duct bifurcation to vascular inflow to the liver. Traditionally vascular invasion was a strong relative contraindication to surgical resection, as the risk involved with surgery outweighed the benefit. With improvements in microsurgical techniques and experience with liver transplantation, resection and reconstruction of both the portal vein and hepatic artery have become acceptable when necessary to extirpate all disease. Abutment of tumor on imaging often does not reflect tumor invasion. Thus, the ability to resect vascular structures improves radical resection options, increasing the number of patients for whom surgical exploration is possible, providing the opportunity to significantly prolong survival.

Portal vein resection has become an established practice for many hepatopancreatobiliary malignancies. Although technical complexity may increase perioperative morbidity and mortality, several high-volume centers have reported acceptable results.[1,44,50,56,57] Neuhaus and colleagues[45] endorse the "no-touch" technique of routine hilar en bloc resection. This involves extended hepatic resection of segments 4 to 8 with regional lymphadenectomy and resection of the extrahepatic bile ducts, portal vein bifurcation, and right hepatic artery. In a study of 100 patients, 50 in each group, they report 1-, 3-, and 5-year survival rates of 87%, 70%, and 58% with hilar en bloc resection, compared with 79%, 40%, and 29%, respectively for conventional major hepatectomy ($P = .021$). de Jong and colleagues[1] published the results of an international multiinstitutional database including 305 resections for HC, of which 51 underwent portal vein resection. Both 30-day (5% vs 12%, $P = .11$) and 90-day (15% vs 18%, $P = .65$) mortality were higher in the portal vein resection group but were not statistically different. Interestingly, 5-year survival rate for 32 patients who had disease that grossly involved the main portal vein and necessitated portal vein resection was comparable to the 19 patients who underwent the "no-touch" technique of routine portal vein resection ($P = .32$).

Hepatic arterial resection is being integrated into aggressive resection practices at select centers. Overall it is controversial, with operative mortality upward of 56% reported without long-term survivors.[58,59] The complexity of these cases sometimes requires alternative liver inflow via the gastroduodenal or left hepatic artery or the use of interposition grafts.[60,61] Portal venous arterialization has been described but is associated with the potential for significant portal hypertension and biliary complications and thus is ill advised.[62,63] The largest series of combined arterial and portal venous resection and reconstruction comes from Japan and reports the results of 50 consecutive cases. Negative margins were achieved in 66% of cases with only one perioperative mortality. Results were significantly better than early reports with 1-, 3-, and 5-year survivals of 79%, 36%, and 30%.[64]

A meta-analysis of 24 studies examined the benefit of vascular resection in the treatment of HC. Portal vein resection was achievable with no impact on postoperative mortality. Increased morbidity and mortality and no proven survival benefit with hepatic arterial resection was reported. Of note, overall, vascular resection did not improve margin negative rates and had no impact on long-term survival, which were often worse (5-year survival 25% vs 39%, $P = .004$).[65] It is not surprising that no survival benefit is conferred, as those undergoing vascular resection have higher rates of locally advanced disease (T3 and T4) with biologically more aggressive tumors. In fact, near equivalent survival is outstanding, as in the past these patients would have been deemed unresectable with limited treatment options.

Ultimately, the goal of successful oncologic outcome is achieved with R0 resection with or without vascular resection, as obtaining negative margins is the most important factor in achieving prolonged survival (**Fig. 1**). In summary, portal vein resection should not be standard practice for all HCs; however, requirement for en bloc vascular resection and reconstruction of the portal vein should not be a contraindication to resection for cure. Arterial resection should be performed only in select patients at experienced centers.

TRANSPLANT

Transplant, a therapeutic option that obviates the concerns with achieving negative surgical margins, is thought to be appropriate for a subset of patients who have nonmetastatic, locally advanced HC that is not amenable to resection.[13] Unfortunately, initial reports of transplant for cholangiocarcinoma had very poor outcomes. Locoregional dissemination was common with tumor recurrence of 53% to 84% and dismal long-term survival, thus liver transplant was deemed inappropriate for this indication.[66–70] Over time, the addition of neoadjuvant therapy to control progression and potentially downstage tumors, along with more careful patient selection yielded improved early results.[71–73]

The goal of patient selection is to identify those who are least likely to develop metastatic disease and most likely to respond to neoadjuvant chemoradiotherapy, as these are the patients with the highest probability of long-term survival after liver transplant. It is commonly agreed on that transplant eligibility requires a malignant appearing stricture and at least one of the following[13,51,74]:

1. Endoluminal biopsy or cytology that is positive or highly suspicious for malignancy including polysomy by FISH,
2. A mass lesion on imaging at the site of the malignant appearing stricture, or
3. CA 19-9 greater than 100 U/mL.

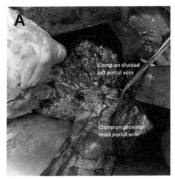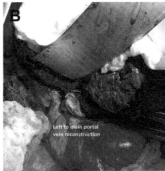

Fig. 1. Portal vein resection during extended right hepatectomy for cholangiocarcinoma. (*A*) Clamp on left portal vein and the main portal vein. (*B*) Anastomosis of left proximal main portal vein.

For HC, neoadjuvant treatment and transplant on protocol is contraindicated for the following[13,51,74]:

1. Primary tumors greater than 3 cm in radial diameter,
2. Any nodal or distant metastatic disease,
3. Attempted resection or transperitoneal tumor biopsy,
4. Previous chemoradiation that precludes full-dose neoadjuvant therapy, or
5. History of malignancy within 5 years.

The most common multimodality protocol is that from the Mayo Clinic, which includes high-dose radiation and chemotherapy followed by operative staging with regional hepatic lymph node sampling, and finally, liver transplant.[72] Suspicious regional lymphadenopathy should be further assessed with endoscopic ultrasound or laparoscopic FNA, as positive results would preclude patients form transplant protocols. Patients being considered for liver transplantation should not undergo transperitoneal biopsy due to the extremely high rate of peritoneal seeding with dissemination at the time of operative staging.[75] Therefore, as stated intraluminal brushings with cytology or direct visualization cholangioscopy and biopsy are preferred for diagnostic purposes, with EUS providing opportunity to evaluate and sample regional nodes. Following the completion of neoadjuvant therapy, patients undergo a staging procedure, laparoscopy or laparotomy, with biopsy of any suspicious lesions as well as regional hepatic lymph nodes. Only patients with negative staging are eligible for transplant.

Darwish Murad and colleagues[76] reported their 10-year experience of 199 patients treated under neoadjuvant transplant protocol, of which 137 eventually underwent transplant. Predictors of drop-out pretransplant were CA 19-9 greater than 500 U/mL, mass greater than 3 cm, malignant brushings or biopsy, and model for end-stage liver disease greater than 20. Posttransplant 1-, 2-, and 5-year survival of 91%, 85%, and 71%, respectively were reported, similar to survival for other liver transplant indications. At median follow-up of 23 months, 20% of patients had developed recurrent disease.

Radiation effects on portal structures have been of concern as vascular endothelial cells, particularly arteries, are very radiosensitive. Increased late portal venous, 22%, and hepatic arterial, 21%, complications have been reported; however, can be mitigated by early percutaneous transhepatic portal angioplasty and stent placement as well as the use of donor iliac arterial conduit to the infrarenal aorta.[77]

A multicenter retrospective study of 304 patients who underwent either resection or transplant for HC was recently published. Transplant was associated with improved outcome over resection with 5-year overall survival of 64% versus 18% (P<.001). This held true in subgroup analysis including only resection patients with tumors less than 3 cm and node-negative disease (transplant candidates) and when eliminating those transplant patients with unconfirmed pathologic diagnosis and primary sclerosing cholangitis, who overall have lower risk of recurrence posttransplant. Intention to treat analysis also showed survival benefit of transplant over resection. This led investigators to conclude that resection for HC that meets criteria for transplant (less than 3 cm and N0 disease) is associated with significantly decreased survival when compared with transplant protocols.[78]

Results are mixed however. Croome and colleagues[79] similarly demonstrated that overall and progression-free survival were better in patients undergoing multimodality transplant protocol compared with resection alone (5-year overall survival 59% vs 36%, P = .003; 5-year progression-free survival 54% vs 29%, P<.001). Intention-to-treat analysis was accordant; however, when R0 resection was achieved with negative nodes, no difference in survival was found regardless of surgical treatment (P = .41). This result supported resection for clearly resectable cases, as evidence did not demonstrate improved outcomes with transplant.

Treatment effects of neoadjuvant therapy must be acknowledged. In their series, Rea and colleagues[80] found that 16 out of 38 explanted livers had no evidence of residual carcinoma; 9 of these had unequivocal pathologic confirmation before neoadjuvant therapy and transplant. Rate of perineural invasion (33% vs 78%, P<.001) and lymph node positivity (19% vs 38%, P = .004) have been reported as much lower after neoadjuvant transplant protocols compared with resection alone, possibly reflecting treatment effect of radiation and chemotherapy and contributing to overall improved outcomes.[78] The role of neoadjuvant chemoradiotherapy before resection is in evolution.

With changes in allocation policies and redistribution of organs, it is unclear how exception points and transplantation for malignancy will be affected. If an organ does not become available before progression of disease outside of transplant protocol, the opportunity for surgery is lost. Thus, perhaps it is still advisable to resect tumors if R0 resection is obtainable. In the authors' practice they continue to resect HCs that are resectable and reserve transplant for patients with nonmetastatic locally advanced lesions that are unresectable. When resectability is in question and the patient meets transplant criteria, enrolling them in protocol is the best option, given very poor outcomes with margin positive resections.

SUMMARY

Cholangiocarcinoma is an aggressive malignancy of the extrahepatic bile ducts with hilar lesions being most common. Patients present with obstructive jaundice and intrahepatic bile duct dilation. Cross-sectional imaging reveals local, regional, and distant extent of disease, with direct cholangiography providing tissue for diagnosis. The consensus of a multidisciplinary committee dictates treatment with resection and transplantation options for curative treatment and palliative chemoradiotherapy the treatment of choice for those with inoperable tumors or metastatic disease. The goal of surgery is to remove the tumor with negative surgical margins, which almost always requires concomitant hepatic resection. Resection necessitates the ability to leave an adequate FLR that may be achieved by PVE. Biliary decompression may be required and the FLR should be drained preferentially. Resection and reconstruction of the portal vein should not be a contraindication to resection for cure. Arterial resection should be performed only in select patients at experienced centers. Liver transplant after neoadjuvant protocol is appropriate for a subset of carefully selected patients who have nonmetastatic locally advanced lesions that are not amenable to resection.

REFERENCES

1. de Jong MC, Marques H, Clary BM, et al. The impact of portal vein resection on outcomes for hilar cholangiocarcinoma: a multi-institutional analysis of 305 cases. Cancer 2012;118:4737–47. Available at: https://onlinelibrary.wiley.com/doi/epdf/10.1002/cncr.27492.
2. Li J, Kuehl H, Grabellus F, et al. Preoperative assessment of hilar cholangiocarcinoma by dual-modality PET/CT. J Surg Oncol 2008;98:438–43. Available at: https://onlinelibrary.wiley.com/doi/epdf/10.1002/jso.21136.
3. Corvera CU, Blumgart LH, Akhurst T, et al. 18F-fluorodeoxyglucose positron emission tomography influences management decisions in patients with biliary cancer. J Am Coll Surg 2008;206:57–65. Available at: https://www.sciencedirect.com/science/article/pii/S1072751507011623?via%3Dihub.
4. Anderson CD, Rice MH, Pinson CW, et al. Fluorodeoxyglucose PET imaging in the evaluation of gallbladder carcinoma and cholangiocarcinoma. J Gastrointest Surg 2004;8:90–7. Available at: https://www.sciencedirect.com/science/article/abs/pii/S1091255X03002282.
5. Ruys AT, Bennink RJ, van Westreenen HL, et al. FDG-positron emission tomography/computed tomography and standardized uptake value in the primary diagnosis and staging of hilar cholangiocarcinoma. HPB (Oxford) 2011;13:256–62. Available at: https://www.ncbi.nlm.nih.gov/pmc/articles/PMC3081626/pdf/hpb0013-0256.pdf.
6. Renshaw AA, Madge R, Jiroutek M, et al. Bile duct brushing cytology: statistical analysis of proposed diagnostic criteria. Am J Clin Pathol 1998;110:635–40. Available at: https://www.ncbi.nlm.nih.gov/pubmed/9802349.
7. de Bellis M, Sherman S, Fogel EL, et al. Tissue sampling at ERCP in suspected malignant biliary strictures (Part 1). Gastrointest Endosc 2002;56:552–61. Available at: https://www.sciencedirect.com/science/article/pii/S0016510702704422?via%3Dihub.
8. Gonda TA, Glick MP, Sethi A, et al. Polysomy and p16 deletion by fluorescence in situ hybridization in the diagnosis of indeterminate biliary strictures. Gastrointest Endosc 2012;75:74–9. Available at: https://www.sciencedirect.com/science/article/pii/S0016510711021043?via%3Dihub.
9. Brooks C, Gausman V, Kokoy-Mondragon C, et al. Role of fluorescent in situ hybridization, cholangioscopic biopsies, and EUS-FNA in the evaluation of biliary strictures. Dig Dis Sci 2018;63:636–44. Available at: https://link.springer.com/article/10.1007%2Fs10620-018-4906-x.
10. Tabata T, Kamisawa T, Hara S, et al. Differentiating immunoglobulin G4-related sclerosing cholangitis from hilar cholangiocarcinoma. Gut Liver 2013;7:234–8. Available at: https://www.ncbi.nlm.nih.gov/pmc/articles/PMC3607779/pdf/gnl-7-234.pdf.
11. Wetter LA, Ring EJ, Pellegrini CA, et al. Differential diagnosis of sclerosing cholangiocarcinomas of the common hepatic duct (Klatskin tumors). Am J Surg 1991;161:57–62 [discussion: 62–3]. Available at: https://www.sciencedirect.com/science/article/pii/000296109190361G?via%3Dihub.

12. Juntermanns B, Kaiser GM, Reis H, et al. Klatskin-mimicking lesions: still a diag-nostical and therapeutical dilemma? Hepatogastroenterology 2011;58:265–9. Available at: https://www.ncbi.nlm.nih.gov/pubmed/21661379.

13. Mansour JC, Aloia TA, Crane CH, et al. Hilar cholangiocarcinoma: expert consensus statement. HPB (Oxford) 2015;17:691–9. Available at: https://www.ncbi.nlm.nih.gov/pmc/articles/PMC4527854/.

14. Ribero D, Abdalla EK, Madoff DC, et al. Portal vein embolization before major hepatectomy and its effects on regeneration, resectability and outcome. Br J Surg 2007;94:1386–94. Available at: https://onlinelibrary.wiley.com/doi/full/10.1002/bjs.5836.

15. Shindoh J, Truty MJ, Aloia TA, et al. Kinetic growth rate after portal vein emboli-zation predicts posthepatectomy outcomes: toward zero liver-related mortality in patients with colorectal liver metastases and small future liver remnant. J Am Coll Surg 2013;216:201–9. Available at: https://www.ncbi.nlm.nih.gov/pmc/arti-cles/PMC3632508/pdf/nihms427772.pdf.

16. Higuchi R, Yamamoto M. Indications for portal vein embolization in perihilar chol-angiocarcinoma. J Hepatobiliary Pancreat Sci 2014;21:542–9. Available at: https://onlinelibrary.wiley.com/doi/epdf/10.1002/jhbp.77.

17. Glantzounis GK, Tokidis E, Basourakos SP, et al. The role of portal vein emboliza-tion in the surgical management of primary hepatobiliary cancers. A systematic review. Eur J Surg Oncol 2017;43:32–41. Available at: https://reader.elsevier.com/reader/sd/pii/S0748798316301779?token=ADCD3FE8C4E539ACFE862389 6959782E4C9ADF75FF0AEB923E3FD800EEA4C7114CA6AF7A2503DBC0C275 F10835F22025.

18. Abulkhir A, Limongelli P, Healey AJ, et al. Preoperative portal vein embolization for major liver resection: a meta-analysis. Ann Surg 2008;247:49–57. Available at: https://journals.lww.com/annalsofsurgery/fulltext/2008/01000/Preoperative_Portal_Vein_Embolization_for_Major.10.aspx.

19. Schnitzbauer AA, Lang SA, Goessmann H, et al. Right portal vein ligation com-bined with in situ splitting induces rapid left lateral liver lobe hypertrophy enabling 2-staged extended right hepatic resection in small-for-size settings. Ann Surg 2012;255:405–14. Available at: https://journals.lww.com/annalsofsurgery/fulltext/2012/03000/Right_Portal_Vein_Ligation_Combined_With_In_Situ.1.aspx.

20. Schadde E, Ardiles V, Robles-Campos R, et al. Early survival and safety of ALPPS: first report of the International ALPPS registry. Ann Surg 2014;260:829–36 [discussion : 836–8]. https://www.zora.uzh.ch/id/eprint/104291/1/00000658-201411000-00016.pdf.

21. Olthof PB, Wiggers JK, Groot Koerkamp B, et al. Postoperative liver failure risk score: identifying patients with resectable perihilar cholangiocarcinoma who can benefit from portal vein embolization. J Am Coll Surg 2017;225:387–94. Avail-able at: https://www.sciencedirect.com/science/article/pii/S1072751517305665?via%3Dihub.

22. Blamey SL, Fearon KC, Gilmour WH, et al. Prediction of risk in biliary surgery. Br J Surg 1983;70:535–8. https://onlinelibrary.wiley.com/doi/abs/10.1002/bjs.1800700910.

23. Belghiti J, Hiramatsu K, Benoist S, et al. Seven hundred forty-seven hepatec-tomies in the 1990s: an update to evaluate the actual risk of liver resection. J Am Coll Surg 2000;19:38–46. Available at: https://www.sciencedirect.com/sci-ence/article/pii/S1072751500002611?via%3Dihub.

24. Dixon JM, Armstrong CP, Duffy SW, et al. Factors affecting morbidity and mortality after surgery for obstructive jaundice: a review of 373 patients. Gut 1983;24:

845–52. Available at: https://www.ncbi.nlm.nih.gov/pmc/articles/PMC1420091/pdf/gut00406-0087.pdf.

25. Iacono C, Ruzzenente A, Campagnaro T, et al. Role of preoperative biliary drainage in jaundiced patients who are candidates for pancreatodudodenectomy or hepatic resection: highlights and drawbacks. Ann Surg 2013;257:191–204. Available at: https://insights.ovid.com/pubmed?pmid=23013805.

26. Yokoyama Y, Nagino M, Nimura Y. Mechanism of impaired hepatic regeneration in cholestatic liver. J Hepatobiliary Pancreat Surg 2007;14:159–66. Available at: https://onlinelibrary.wiley.com/doi/epdf/10.1007/s00534-006-1125-1.

27. Laurent A, Tayar C, Cherqui D. Cholangiocarcinoma: preoperative biliary drainage (con). HPB (Oxford) 2008;10:126–9. Available at: https://www.ncbi.nlm.nih.gov/pmc/articles/PMC2504392/pdf/MHPB10-126.pdf.

28. Nimura Y. Preoperative biliary drainage before resection for cholangiocarcinoma (pro). HPB (Oxford) 2008;10:130–3. Available at: https://www.ncbi.nlm.nih.gov/pmc/articles/PMC2504393/pdf/MHPB10-130.pdf.

29. Wiggers JK, Groot Koerkamp B, Cieslak KP, et al. Postoperative mortality after liver resection for perihilar cholangiocarcinoma: development of a risk score and importance of biliary drainage of the future liver remnant. J Am Coll Surg 2016;223:321–31. Available at: https://www.ncbi.nlm.nih.gov/pmc/articles/PMC4961586/pdf/nihms776337.pdf.

30. Farges O, Regimbeau JM, Fuks D, et al. Multicentre European study of preoperative biliary drainage for hilar cholangiocarcinoma. Br J Surg 2013;100:274–83. Available at: https://onlinelibrary.wiley.com/doi/epdf/10.1002/bjs.8950.

31. Kennedy TJ, Yopp A, Qin Y, et al. Role of preoperative biliary drainage of liver remnant prior to extended liver resection for hilar cholangiocarcinoma. HPB (Oxford) 2009;11:445–51. Available at: https://www.ncbi.nlm.nih.gov/pmc/articles/PMC2742615/pdf/hpb0011-0445.pdf.

32. Matsuo K, Rocha FG, Ito K, et al. The Blumgart preoperative staging system for hilar cholangiocarcinoma: analysis of resectability and outcomes in 380 patients. J Am Coll Surg 2012;215:343–55. Available at: https://www.sciencedirect.com/science/article/pii/S1072751512004140?via%3Dihub.

33. Ruys AT, Busch OR, Gouma DJ, et al. Staging laparoscopy for hilar cholangiocarcinoma: is it still worthwhile? Ann Surg Oncol 2011;18:2647–53. Available at: https://www.ncbi.nlm.nih.gov/pmc/articles/PMC3162633/pdf/10434_2011_Article_1576.pdf.

34. Coelen RJS, Ruys AT, Besselink MGH, et al. Diagnostic accuracy of staging laparoscopy for detecting metastasized or locally advanced perihilar cholangiocarcinoma: a systematic review and meta-analysis. Surg Endosc 2016;30:4163–73. Available at: https://www.ncbi.nlm.nih.gov/pmc/articles/PMC5009158/pdf/464_2016_Article_4788.pdf.

35. Callery MP, Strasberg SM, Doherty GM, et al. Staging laparoscopy with laparoscopic ultrasonography: optimizing resectability in hepatobiliary and pancreatic malignancy. J Am Coll Surg 1997;185:33–9. Available at: https://www.sciencedirect.com/science/article/pii/S107275150100878X.

36. Minnard EA, Conlon KC, Dougherty EC, al at. Laparoscopic ultrasound enhances standard laparoscopy in the staging of pancreatic cancer. Ann Surg 1998;228:182–7. Available at: https://www.ncbi.nlm.nih.gov/pmc/articles/PMC1191458/pdf/annsurg00006-0054.pdf.

37. Russolillo N, D'Eletto M, Langella S, et al. Role of laparoscopic ultrasound during diagnostic laparoscopy for proximal biliary cancers: a single series of 100 patients. Surg Endosc 2016;30:1212–8. Available at: https://link.springer.com/content/pdf/10.1007%2Fs00464-015-4333-4.pdf.

38. Lim JH, Choi GH, Choi SH, et al. Liver resection for Bismuth type I and type II hilar cholangiocarcinoma. World J Surg 2013;37:829–37. Available at: https://link.springer.com/article/10.1007%2Fs00268-013-1909-9.

39. Miyazaki M, Ito H, Nakagawa K, et al. Aggressive surgical approaches to hilar cholangiocarcinoma: hepatic or local resection? Surgery 1998;123:131–6. Available at: https://www.sciencedirect.com/science/article/pii/S0039606098702491?via%3Dihub.

40. Ito F, Agni R, Rettammel RJ, et al. Resection of hilar cholangiocarcinoma concomitant liver resection decreases hepatic recurrence. Ann Surg 2008;248:273–9. Available at: https://insights.ovid.com/pubmed?pmid=18650638.

41. Bismuth H, Corlette MB. Intrahepatic chlangioenteric anastomosis in carcinoma of the hilus of the liver. Surg Gynecol Obstet 1975;140:170–8. Available at: https://www.ncbi.nlm.nih.gov/pubmed/1079096.

42. Burke EC, Jarnagin WR, Hochwald SN, et al. Hilar cholangiocarcinoma: patterns of spread, the importance of hepatic resection for curative operation, and a pre-surgical clinical staging system. Ann Surg 1998;228:385–94. Available at: https://www.ncbi.nlm.nih.gov/pmc/articles/PMC1191497/.

43. Nagino M, Ebata T, Yokoyama Y, et al. Evolution of surgical treatment for perihilar cholangiocarcinoma: a single-center 34-year review of 574 consecutive resections. Ann Surg 2013;258:129–40. Available at: https://insights.ovid.com/pubmed?pmid=23059502.

44. Hemming AW, Mekeel K, Khanna A, et al. Portal vein resection in management of hilar cholangiocarcinoma. J Am Coll Surg 2011;212:604–13. Available at: https://www.sciencedirect.com/science/article/pii/S1072751510012913?via%3Dihub.

45. Neuhaus P, Thelen A, Jonas S, et al. Oncological superiority of hilar en bloc resection for the treatment of hilar cholangiocarcinoma. Ann Surg Oncol 2012;19:1602–8. Available at: https://link.springer.com/content/pdf/10.1245%2Fs10434-011-2077-5.pdf.

46. Ito K, Ito H, Allen PJ, et al. Adequate lymph node assessment for extrahepatic bile duct adenocarcrcinoma. Ann Surg 2010;251:675–81. Available at: https://insights.ovid.com/pubmed?pmid=20224368.

47. Ribero D, Amisano M, Lo Tesoriere R, et al. Additional resection of an intraoperative margin-positive proximal bile duct improves survival in patients with hilar cholangiocarcinoma. Ann Surg 2011;254:776–81 [discussion: 781–3]. Available at: https://insights.ovid.com/pubmed?pmid=22042470.

48. Zhang XF, Squires MH III, Bagante F, et al. The impact of intraoperative re-resection of a positive bile duct margin on clinical outcomes for hilar cholangiocarcinoma. Ann Surg Oncol 2018;25:1140–9. Available at: https://link.springer.com/content/pdf/10.1245%2Fs10434-018-6382-0.pdf.

49. Nuzzo G, Giuliante F, Ardito F, et al. Improvement in perioperative and long-term outcome after surgical treatment of hilar cholangiocarcinoma: results of an Italian multicenter analysis of 440 patients. Arch Surg 2012;147:26–34. Available at: https://jamanetwork.com/journals/jamasurgery/fullarticle/1107306.

50. Igami I, Nishio H, Ebata T, et al. Surgical treatment of hilar cholangiocarcinoma in the "new era": the Nagoya University experience. J Hepatobiliary Pancreat Sci 2010;17:449–54. Available at: https://onlinelibrary.wiley.com/doi/epdf/10.1007/s00534-009-0209-0.

51. Zaydfudim VM, Rosen CB, Nagorney DM. Hilar cholangiocarcinoma. Surg Oncol Clin N Am 2014;23:247–63. Available at: https://www.sciencedirect.com/science/article/pii/S1055320713001099?via%3Dihub.

52. Dinant S, Gerhards MF, Busch ORC, et al. The importance of complete excision of the caudate lobe in resection of hilar cholangiocarcinoma. HPB (Oxford) 2005;7: 263–7. Available at: https://www.ncbi.nlm.nih.gov/pmc/articles/PMC2043102/pdf/MHPB07-263.pdf.

53. Cheng QB, Yi B, Wang JH, et al. Resection with total caudate lobectomy confers survival benefit in hilar cholangiocarcinoma of Bismuth type III and IV. Eur J Surg Oncol 2012;38:1197–203. Available at: https://www.sciencedirect.com/science/article/pii/S0748798312012085?via%3Dihub.

54. Tsao JI, Nimura Y, Kamiya J, et al. Management of hilar cholangiocarcinoma: comparison of an American and a Japanese experience. Ann Surg 2000;232: 166–74. Available at: https://www.ncbi.nlm.nih.gov/pmc/articles/PMC1421125/pdf/20000800s00003p166.pdf.

55. Bhutiani N, Scoggins CR, McMasters KM, et al. The impact of caudate lobe resection on margin status and outcomes in patients with hilar cholangiocarcinoma: a multi-institutional analysis from the US Extrahepatic Biliary Malignancy Consortium. Surgery 2018;163:726–31. Available at: https://www.sciencedirect.com/science/article/pii/S0039606017307626?via%3Dihub.

56. Hoffman K, Luible S, Goeppert B, et al. Impact of portal vein resection on oncologic long-term outcome in patients with hilar cholangiocarcinoma. Surgery 2015; 158:1252–60. Available at: https://www.sciencedirect.com/science/article/pii/S003960601500361X?via%3Dihub.

57. Ebata T, Nagino M, Kamiya J, et al. Hepatectomy with portal vein resection for hilar cholangiocarcinoma: audit of 52 consecutive cases. Ann Surg 2003;238: 720–7. Available at: https://www.ncbi.nlm.nih.gov/pmc/articles/PMC1356151/pdf/20031100s00013p720.pdf.

58. Miyazaki M, Kato A, Ito H, et al. Combined vascular resection in operative resection for hilar cholangiocarcinoma: does it work or not? Surgery 2007;141:581–8. Available at: https://www.sciencedirect.com/science/article/pii/S0039606006007367?via%3Dihub.

59. Gerhards MF, van Gulik TM, de Wit LT, et al. Evaluation of morbidity and mortality after resection for hilar cholangiocarcinoma: a single center experience. Surgery 2000;127:395–404. Available at: https://www.sciencedirect.com/science/article/pii/S0039606000312132?via%3Dihub.

60. de Santibanes E, Ardiles V, Alvarez FA, et al. Hepatic artery reconstruction first for the treatment of hilar cholangiocarcinoma bismuth type IIIB with contralateral arterial invasion: a novel technical strategy. HPB (Oxford) 2012;14:67–70. Available at: https://www.ncbi.nlm.nih.gov/pmc/articles/PMC3252994/pdf/hpb0014-0067.pdf.

61. Kondo S, Hirano S, Ambo Y, et al. Arterioportal shunting as an alternative to microvascular reconstruction after hepatic artery resection. Br J Surg 2004;91: 248–51. Available at: https://onlinelibrary.wiley.com/doi/full/10.1002/bjs.4428.

62. Bhangui P, Salloum C, Lim C, et al. Portal vein arterialization: a salvage procedure for a totally de-arterialized liver. The Paul Brousse Hospital experience. HPB (Oxford) 2014;16(8):723–38. Available at: https://www.ncbi.nlm.nih.gov/pmc/articles/PMC4113254/pdf/hpb0016-0723.pdf.

63. Chen Y, Liu Z, Duan W, et al. Modified arterioportal shunting in radical resection of hilar cholangiocarcinoma. Hepatogastroenterology 2014;61:9–11. Available at: https://www.ncbi.nlm.nih.gov/pubmed/24895784.

64. Nagino M, Nimura Y, Nishio H, et al. Hepatectomy with simultaneous resection of the portal vein and hepatic artery for advanced perihilar cholangiocarcinoma: an

audit of 50 consecutive cases. Ann Surg 2010;252:115–23. Available at: https://insights.ovid.com/pubmed?pmid=20531001.

65. Abbas S, Sandroussi C. Systematic review and meta-analysis of the role of vascular resection in the treatment of hilar cholangiocarcinoma. HPB (Oxford) 2013;15:492–503. Available at: https://www.ncbi.nlm.nih.gov/pmc/articles/PMC3692018/pdf/hpb0015-0492.pdf.

66. Meyer CG, Penn I, James L. Liver transplantation for cholangiocarcinoma: results in 207 patients. Transplantation 2000;69:1633–7. Available at: https://journals.lww.com/transplantjournal/Fulltext/2000/04270/LIVER_TRANSPLANTATION_FOR_CHOLAN-GIOCARCINOMA_.19.aspx.

67. Iwatsuki S, Todo S, Marsh JW, et al. Treatment of hilar cholangiocarcinoma (Klatskin tumors) with hepatic resection or transplantation. J Am Coll Surg 1998;187:358–64. Available at: https://www.ncbi.nlm.nih.gov/pmc/articles/PMC2991118/pdf/nihms249869.pdf.

68. Robles R, Figueras J, Turrion VS, et al. Spanish experience in liver transplantation for hilar and peripheral cholangiocarcinoma. Ann Surg 2004;239:265–71. Available at: https://www.ncbi.nlm.nih.gov/pmc/articles/PMC1356221/pdf/20040200s00019p265.pdf.

69. Ghali P, Marotta PJ, Toshida EM, et al. Liver transplantation for incidental cholangiocarcinoma: analysis of the Canadian experience. Liver Transpl 2005;11:1412–6. Available at: https://aasldpubs.onlinelibrary.wiley.com/doi/epdf/10.1002/lt.20512.

70. Brandsaeter B, Isoniemi H, Broome U, et al. Liver transplantation for primary sclerosing cholangitis; predictors and consequences of hepatobiliary malignancy. J Hepatol 2004;40:815–22. Available at: https://www.sciencedirect.com/science/article/pii/S0168827804000078?via%3Dihub.

71. Sudan D, DeRoover A, Chinnakotla S, et al. Radiochemotherapy and transplantation allow long-term survival for nonresectable hilar cholangiocarcinoma. Am J Transplant 2002;2:774–9. Available at: https://onlinelibrary.wiley.com/doi/epdf/10.1034/j.1600-6143.2002.20812.x.

72. De Vreede I, Steers JL, Burch PA, et al. Prolonged disease-free survival after orthotopic liver transplantation plus adjuvant chemoirradiation for cholangiocarcinoma. Liver Transpl 2000;6:309–16. Available at: https://aasldpubs.onlinelibrary.wiley.com/doi/epdf/10.1053/lv.2000.6143.

73. Heimbach JK, Gores GJ, Haddock MG, et al. Liver transplantation for unresectable perihilar cholangiocarcinoma. Semin Liver Dis 2004;24:201–7. Available at: https://www.thieme-connect.com/products/ejournals/abstract/10.1055/s-2004-828896.

74. Gores GJ, Gish RG, Sudan D, et al. Model for end-stage liver disease (MELD) exception for cholangiocarcinoma or biliary dysplasia. Liver Transpl 2006;12:S95–7. Available at: https://aasldpubs.onlinelibrary.wiley.com/doi/epdf/10.1002/lt.20965.

75. Heimbach JK, Sanchez W, Rosen CB, et al. Trans-peritoneal fine needle aspiration biopsy of hilar cholangiocarcinoma is associated with disease dissemination. HPB (Oxford) 2011;13:356–60. Available at: https://www.sciencedirect.com/science/article/pii/S1365182X15304391?via%3Dihub.

76. Darwish Murad S, Kim WR, Therneau T, et al. Predictors of pretransplant dropout and posttransplant recurrence in patients with perihilar cholangiocarcinoma. Hepatology 2012;56:972–81. Available at: https://www.ncbi.nlm.nih.gov/pmc/articles/PMC3830980/pdf/nihms507185.pdf.

77. Mantel HT, Rosen CB, Heimbach JK, et al. Vascular complications after orthotopic liver transplantation after neoadjuvant therapy for hilar cholangiocarcinoma.

Liver Transpl 2007;12:1372–81. Available at: https://aasldpubs.onlinelibrary.wiley.com/doi/epdf/10.1002/lt.21107.

78. Ethun CG, Lopez-Aguiar AG, Anderson DJ, et al. Transplantation versus resection for hilar cholangiocarcinoma: an argument for shifting treatment paradigms for resectable disease. Ann Surg 2018;267:797–805. Available at: https://insights.ovid.com/pubmed?pmid=29064885.

79. Croome KP, Rosen CB, Heimback JK, et al. Is liver transplantation appropriate for patients with potentially resectable de novo hilar cholangiocarcinoma? J Am Coll Surg 2015;221:130–9. Available at: https://www.sciencedirect.com/science/article/pii/S1072751515001829?via%3Dihub.

80. Rea DJ, Heimbach JK, Rosen CB, et al. Liver transplantation with neoadjuvant chemoradiation is more effective than resection for hilar cholangiocarcinoma. Ann Surg 2005;242:451–61. Available at: https://www.ncbi.nlm.nih.gov/pmc/articles/PMC1357753/pdf/20050900s00016p451.pdf.

Gallbladder Cancer
Managing the Incidental Diagnosis

Leonid Cherkassky, MD, Michael D'Angelica, MD*

KEYWORDS

- Incidental gallbladder cancer management • Operative strategy for reresection
- Recurrence patterns • Prognostic factors • Neoadjuvant chemotherapy

KEY POINTS

- Incidental gallbladder carcinoma is diagnosed on pathologic assessment following chole-cystectomy for presumed benign disease.
- Standard management includes reresection to remove sites at risk for harboring residual disease with the ultimate goal of cure, or at least prolonged survival.
- The goal of curative intent reresection is achieving negative resection (R0) margin status and optimal staging while limiting morbidity.
- Gallbladder cancer is characterized by an early and frequently distant recurrence pattern that is the most common cause of surgical failure.
- Patients identified as high-risk for eventual distant recurrence (eg, node-positive disease, advanced tumor stage, residual disease, and poorly differentiated histology) may benefit from neoadjuvant chemotherapy before reresection.

INTRODUCTION

Incidental gallbladder carcinoma (IGBC) is diagnosed on pathologic assessment following cholecystectomy for presumed benign disease. Traditional management includes resection of the gallbladder liver bed and regional lymph nodes to remove residual disease (RD) with the ultimate goal of cure, or at least prolonged survival. The surgeon must exclude those patients who are already metastatic to spare the morbidity of an operation for those who cannot benefit. Cross-sectional imaging revealing metastatic disease excludes surgery and is best treated with systemic therapy.

Although on the surface this decision-making seems simple enough, it does not take into account a recurrence pattern characterized by frequent and early distant recurrence with only 35% 5-year survival rate. Although there is a lack of level 1 evidence

Disclosure Statement: The authors have no disclosures.
Department of Surgery, Memorial Sloan-Kettering Cancer Center, 1275 York Avenue, New York, NY, 10065 USA
* Corresponding author.
E-mail address: dangelim@mskcc.org

Surg Oncol Clin N Am 28 (2019) 619–630
https://doi.org/10.1016/j.soc.2019.06.005
1055-3207/19/© 2019 Elsevier Inc. All rights reserved.

supporting neoadjuvant chemotherapy for patients diagnosed with IGBC, the overall poor prognosis suggests considering at least the selective use of neoadjuvant systemic therapy for patients at high risk of recurrence in order to optimally select those patients most likely to benefit from surgery.

After a decision to proceed to the operating room is made, additional considerations regarding operative strategy are whether to perform staging laparoscopy (SL), the extent of liver and bile duct resection, the extent of lymphadenectomy, and whether to resect port sites. This article summarizes the management of IGBC. The authors aim to summarize the staging techniques used and the debates that concern operative decision-making, and to understand the underlying natural history of gallbladder cancer in order to counsel patients with the ultimate goal of optimizing the benefits of surgery and limiting surgical morbidity.

RERESECTION IS THE STANDARD APPROACH TO MANAGING INCIDENTAL GALLBLADDER CARCINOMA

Historically, gallbladder cancer presented at advanced stages with symptomatic large tumors and jaundice with dismal outcomes: median overall survival (OS) of 5 months and 5 years ranging from 5% to 17%, depending on resectability.[1,2] Outcomes have significantly improved since then, reflecting adoption by surgeons of curative-intent extended cholecystectomy and increasing rates of detection at earlier stages of disease. More modern series using curative-intent resection report 5-year survivals of 60% to 80% for tumor stage (T)-2 tumors[3–6] and 21% to 28% for T3 to T4 tumors.[7]

Because simple cholecystectomy is not an oncologically adequate operation except for the earliest stage (T1a), reresection is generally indicated for IGBC. For T1b tumors (invasion into the muscle layer) and higher, transection along the muscular wall-cystic plate plane is a substandard cancer operation that risks leaving RD within the liver and regional lymph nodes. Therefore, the rationale for reresection is to remove tissue at risk for gross and/or microscopic RD left behind at the initial cholecystectomy, which is found in 45% to 60% of patients.[8–10] When compared with nonoperative management, reresection is associated with significantly improved oncologic outcomes. A French cohort study demonstrated 5-year OS rates of 41% for reresection when compared with 15% for those subjects treated nonoperatively.[9] When stratified by T stage, 5-year OS for reresected T2 subjects reached 62% and for T3 19% (vs 0% for simple cholecystectomy only). Multiple other multicenter and single institution cohort studies in Japan, Europe, and the United States also observed an association with a survival advantage for reresection (**Table 1**).[7,11–14]

One other question that affects the justification for reresection is whether violating the subserosal plane at the time of simple cholecystectomy risks tumor spillage that offsets the association of reresection with a survival advantage. This break in the principle of en bloc resection is of particular concern in the case of gallbladder cancer given its predisposition to port site,[15,16] biopsy tract, and peritoneal seeding.[13] Despite this theoretic risk, the authors' experience is of similar outcomes for reresected IGBC patients compared with primarily resected patients when matched for stage. In fact, those patients presenting with IGBC are more likely to undergo curative-intent resection (32% vs 14%), likely because of presentation at earlier stages of disease and a lower likelihood of involvement of biliary and vascular structures.[7] Based on the experience of 2 high-volume US centers, those patients who undergo reresection reach median OS of 26 to 35 months and 5-year OS rates of 38% to 49%.[7,17]

Table 1
Selected series of reresection for incidentally diagnosed gallbladder cancer

Reference, Year	Number of Subjects	Procedure	5-y OS (%)	Comments
Shirai et al,[6] 1992, Japan single-institution	10 35	EC (reresection) SC	90[a] 41	T2 subjects summarized, low number of T3 or T4 subjects
Fong et al,[7] 2000, MSKCC	37 16	EC SC	61[a] 19	16 subjects either refused or were not offered reresection (comparison made for only T2 tumors)
Ouchi et al,[13] 2002, multicenter Japan	153 (T2), 30 (T3) 48 (T2), 10 (T3)	EC SC	70% for T2, 20%[a] for T3	P<.05 for T3, P = .051 for T2, no difference for T1 or T4
Foster et al,[11] 2007, Roswell	13 25	EC SC	62[a] 16	T2 and T3 subjects
Shih et al,[17] 2007, Hopkins	29 5	EC SC	49[a] 0	T3 subjects
Goetze & Paolucci,[12] 2010, multicenter German	231 393	EC SC	41[a] 25	—
Fuks et al,[9] 2011, multicenter French	148 70	EC SC	41[a] 15	—

Abbreviations: EC, extended cholecystectomy; MSKCC, Memorial Sloan-Kettering Cancer Center; SC, simple cholecystectomy.
[a] P<.05.
Data from Refs.[7,11–14]

Reresection is typically performed only for *American Joint Committee on Cancer* (AJCC) T1b to T3 tumors.[18] T1a (confined to the mucosa and not invading the muscularis layer) cancers are considered cured by cholecystectomy alone.[6] T4 tumors are considered unresectable due to main portal vein or hepatic artery invasion or invasion of 2 or more extrahepatic organs, do not benefit from resection, and are staged in the IV category.[17] Reresection for T1b cancers is somewhat controversial. Although some series report 95% to 100% 5-year OS rates for all T1 stage subjects who undergo simple cholecystectomy alone,[13,14] these studies are limited by a low number of T1b subjects. A Surveillance, Epidemiology, and End Results (SEER) database study that included larger numbers (300 T1a subjects and 536 T1b subjects) found that extended cholecystectomy is associated with improved disease-specific survival (DSS) and OS for extended cholecystectomy in T1b but not T1a subjects.[19] Furthermore, RD can be present in up to 35% (5 out of 14 subjects in the authors' series) of subjects staged T1b following simple cholecystectomy,[20] further supporting reresection for T1b subjects.

STAGING EVALUATION: IMAGING

Gallbladder cancer frequently metastasizes to the liver, lungs, intraabdominal lymph nodes, and peritoneum. Therefore, these patients must be accurately staged to spare patients a nontherapeutic laparotomy and resection. Cross-sectional imaging and SL both contribute as effective staging tools to select patients for reresection. The authors' center typically obtains a contrast-enhanced computed tomography (CT) scan of the chest, abdomen, and pelvis to evaluate for locally unresectable and/or metastatic disease. Clear evidence of nonregional nodal (outside of the porta hepatis, including aortocaval pancreatic or retropancreatic, celiac, and superior mesenteric arterial nodes) or visceral metastatic disease is best treated with chemotherapy because resection is associated with universal and rapid recurrence. Suspicion of remaining gross disease following initial cholecystectomy may indicate additional imaging (MRI liver protocol or a multiphase CT study) to assess for proper hepatic artery or main portal vein involvement that would signify locally advanced disease and preclude resection.

As for the utility of PET imaging, a retrospective study from the authors' institution in which both CT-MRI and PET imaging were available in 100 subjects,[21] PET definitively changed management in very few (5%) subjects. However, it did confirm suspicious CT findings for an additional 12 subjects, and was especially helpful in confirming distant nodal disease suggested by CT. Given that it might also be harmful to patients (3% of subjects had PET findings that led to invasive procedures that did not affect management) and because performance was significantly lower in subjects with IGBC, the authors do not routinely perform PET imaging but do use it selectively for clarification when there are findings concerning for distant disease on CT-MRI. The explanation for decreased utility in the case of the incidental diagnosis may be because these tumors are commonly diagnosed at earlier stages, these patients have already passed a test of laparoscopic exploration, and because the postoperative gallbladder bed is PET-avid from postoperative inflammation.[22] To the contrary, a previous study at the authors' institution analyzing gallbladder cancer cases from an earlier time period found a higher incidence of altered management (23%),[23] and so the authors have come to appreciate that improvement of CT and MR imaging over the years has likely diminished the added value of PET. Retrospective series from other institutions demonstrate yields up to 25%,[24] although no information on other imaging is provided to ascertain the added value of PET.

STAGING EVALUATION: LAPAROSCOPY

Even with the most sensitive imaging available, aborted resection rates in the literature range from 24% to 46%.[8,10,25] In the series previously reported in which subjects (including all those with cases of gallbladder cancer) received both CT-MRI and PET,[21] 27 of 100 cases resulted in an aborted resection. Most metastatic disease found at surgery was peritoneal (identified in 13 cases), which is commonly detected by laparoscopy and for which imaging has low sensitivity. Overall, however, only 6 subjects were spared nontherapeutic laparotomy by incorporating SL. Therefore, SL can spare nontherapeutic laparotomies and has demonstrated the highest yields and accuracies specifically for gallbladder cancer when compared with other hepatobiliary malignancies (yields 23%–48% and accuracies 58%–94%).[26–28]

Although these results suggest a low threshold for the use of laparoscopy in gallbladder cancer overall, in the authors' experience, the utility significantly decreases in the case of IGBC. This is not surprising because these patients have already undergone laparoscopic exploration at the time of initial cholecystectomy and because the presentation is typically at earlier stages. In the authors' series, out of 136 consecutive subjects with IGBC submitted to exploration for reresection,[29] SL was performed in 46 cases. Ten of these subjects had distant disease that was identified by SL in only 2 subjects (yield 4.3%, accuracy 20%). The authors, therefore, selectively perform laparoscopy for those patients at highest risk for disseminated disease as identified in the authors' analysis: positive margin at initial cholecystectomy, poorly differentiated tumor, T3 disease, or imaging studies suggesting RD. Other high-risk factors associated with higher risk of occult metastatic disease that may indicate SL are node-positive disease (typically found in cystic duct lymph node if removed) and occurrence of bile spillage at initial cholecystectomy, which risks peritoneal dissemination.[30,31]

OPERATIVE STRATEGY

The overarching goal of reresection is to resect RD at local and regional sites, attaining a negative resection (R0) margin with curative intent. Secondary goals are to obtain locoregional control and accurately stage the patient for prognostic purposes. This article reviews, in turn, the operative strategy for liver, bile duct, and lymph node resection, and discusses how to limit operative morbidity and optimize curative intent, locoregional control, and staging information. Given these goals, the authors' approach for IGBC is a limited hepatectomy, portal lymphadenectomy, with or without bile duct resection and reconstruction depending on suspected involvement of the common duct.

MANAGEMENT OF PORT SITES

Given the predisposition to peritoneal implantation, tumor cell contamination at the time of initial laparoscopic simple cholecystectomy risks port-site contamination. The authors' experience demonstrates that routine port-site resection has little benefit but significant risk of morbidity. At the time the most recent analysis of this issue was published,[32] port sites were resected in most patients with IGBC (61%). The rate of positive port-site disease on pathologic assessment was 19%, although it is much less common in a French series (2%).[33] Despite the high positive rate, in almost all patients, port-site disease represented generalized peritoneal spread; 10 of 13 positive patients had either peritoneal disease at the time of excision or developed peritoneal disease subsequently. Thus, the authors believe that port-site resection does not benefit oncologic outcomes, including peritoneal recurrence. Furthermore, because it requires removal of a cylinder of tissue down to peritoneum, it can be disfiguring and is associated with an incisional hernia rate of at least 8%.[33] The authors, therefore, do not recommend routine port-site excision.

EXTENT OF RESECTION: LYMPH NODES

Intraoperative staging includes palpation of the celiac, superior mesenteric artery, and retropancreatic regions to exclude nodal disease in these regions, which are equivalent to distant metastasis and should lead to an aborted resection. As for regional lymphadenectomy, its role in locoregional control is secondary to its importance in staging the patient. Node-positive disease is a marker of poor prognosis and risk for distant recurrence. In early-stage disease, nodal status is the most relevant predictor of outcomes.[3]

Retrospective studies demonstrate that adequate staging is associated with improved OS. In keeping with the principle of lymph node dissection as a staging tool, this association is likely due to stage migration rather than true therapeutic benefit. The population staged as no cancer in lymph nodes (N0) likely contains inaccurately staged node-positive patients. In assessing the SEER database, a group from Howard University demonstrated an association with OS for those patients who had 1 to 4 lymph nodes (LNs) and 5 or more nodes excised.[34] In the series by Ito and colleagues,[35] a lymph node yield of 3 or more was associated with improved recurrence-free survival (RFS) and DSS, with an optimal yield identified as at least 6 nodes. These data are reflected in the AJCC 8th edition staging criteria, which recommends harvest of at least 6 nodes.[18]

Reality, however, dictates that optimal nodal staging quality is achieved in only a minority of patients because the median lymph node yield was 3 in the authors' series. Techniques to increase lymph node counts may be considered; however, (1) extrahepatic bile duct resection is not associated with increased yield and (2) lymph nodes along the visceral vessels could be harvested but positive nodes in the aortocaval, superior mesenteric artery, and celiac chains entail a prognosis similar to that of metastasis stage (M)-1 disease.[36]

To balance accurate staging and added morbidity, the authors perform a portal lymphadenectomy to include the hepatoduodenal ligament and common hepatic artery nodes. This corresponds to the pattern of nodal spread as defined by a Japanese group that used intralymphatic injection of indigo carmine to map the drainage pattern of gallbladder lymphatics.[37] These studies note a lymphatic path around the bile ducts, through the cystic node, into the pericholedochal lymph nodes, and then into the retroportal and peripancreatic nodes, indicating that the cystic and pericholedochal LNs are the most common sites of initial tumor spread.[38]

EXTENT OF RESECTION: LIVER AND BILE DUCT RESECTION

The extent of liver resection at the authors' center is based on disease extent and proximity to major inflow pedicles at exploration, with the goal being to achieve an R0 resection. Liver resection is typically a liver wedge resection to include the gallbladder fossa or an anatomic 4B plus 5 segmentectomy, whereas major hepatectomy is limited to large or poorly placed tumors that involve the right inflow structures. Major hepatectomy, if not necessary to achieve negative margins, only adds morbidity. Similarly, bile duct resection is done selectively only when it is necessary to achieve a negative margin and additional cystic duct resection is not adequate. This approach reflects the authors' experience comparing patients undergoing major liver and extended bile duct resection (commonly performed in the authors' early experiences) to those patients with a more limited hepatic resection (either 4B/5 segmentectomy or extending resection as a wedge to include the gallbladder fossa). The performance of a major hepatectomy or a common bile duct (CBD) excision was not associated with other clinicopathologic variables or long-term survival[39]; instead, the variables that were associated with outcomes were those reflecting tumor biology: T stage, N stage, differentiation, and CBD involvement. Routine major liver resection and extrahepatic bile duct resection were associated with increased morbidity, with a high (33%) incidence of grade 3 or 4 events typical of bilioenteric anastomoses to a normal nondilated bile duct. The 5% mortality all occurred in patients who underwent combined major hepatectomy and bile duct excision as a result of intraabdominal sepsis with multiorgan failure or liver failure. In conclusion, major resections should be limited to fit patients with localized but poorly placed tumors involving major inflow structures. Similarly, bile duct resection is only performed when necessary to clear locally invasive tumors or adherent nodal disease.

GALLBLADDER CANCER IS ASSOCIATED WITH FREQUENT AND DISTANT RECURRENCE

Although traditional management for IGBC is upfront reresection with the goal of achieving cure, gallbladder carcinoma is characterized by a high risk of distant recurrence which is the major cause of surgical failure. Recurrence occurs early with a median time to recurrence of 11 months and almost all patients who recur do so within 2 years; 62% within 12 months and 88% within 24 months. Almost all recurrences include distant sites (85%). Salvage is exceedingly rare and, therefore, the OS of 21 months closely mirrors the timing of recurrence.[20,40] Such early and distant recurrence likely reflects a high frequency of occult micrometastatic disease at the time of initial diagnosis and should frame patient expectations as to the benefits of reresection. Furthermore, patients who are preoperatively defined to be at particularly high risk of early, distant recurrence should be considered for upfront systemic therapy (see later discussion).

As these data are reviewed, it should be mentioned that IGBC is a unique situation that provides supplemental pathologic assessment staging information before reresection. This includes T staging and may include N staging based on the cholecystectomy specimen. Furthermore, a positive gallbladder or cystic duct margin indicates possible RD, which, although a justification for reresection, also serves as a marker of poor prognosis.

FACTORS ASSOCIATED WITH POOR ONCOLOGIC OUTCOMES

T and N stage prognosticate outcome, and advanced T stage and node-positive disease, are associated with poor oncologic outcomes. A French cohort study of IGBC demonstrated that 5-year OS is associated with T stage at diagnosis: 100% (T1), 62% (T2), 19% (T3), and 0% (T4) subjects were alive at 5 years.[9] So, although reresection was associated with improvement in OS in T3 subjects within this cohort, there are only few T3 long-term survivors, and a sizable fraction (44%) of subjects died within 1 year. Multiple other retrospective studies, including single-center studies and national database analyses, have similarly identified an association between T stage and oncologic outcomes.[7,35,39,41,42]

Another high-risk population is patients with node-positive disease. In a series published from the authors' institution, 5-year DSS for node-positive subjects was 17% (compared with 51% for node negative), and N stage was associated with worse DSS on multivariate analysis.[39] Consistent with the typical pattern of early recurrence, the time to event was approximately 1 year for most subjects. Other series similarly support an association with poor prognosis for node-positive disease.[20,35,43] It is important to recognize that node-positive disease must be discussed in the context of the nodes sampled at the time of curative-intent resection: those along the cystic duct, CBD, hepatic artery, and portal vein, as compared with nodes along visceral vessels (periaortic, pericaval, superior mesenteric artery, and celiac artery), which are representative of distant metastases.[18]

Other clinicopathological factors prognostic of survival include (1) histologic grade of differentiation (poorly differentiated tumors having 18 to 31 months median DSS[20,35,39,43]); (2) lymphovascular invasion[20]; (3) total lymph node count of 6 or more, which adequately stages patients[35]; (4) CBD involvement[39]; (5) jaundice[7]; and (6) port site,[15,16] biopsy tract, and peritoneal seeding.[13] A retrospective Canadian study also found that bile spillage at index cholecystectomy was associated with peritoneal carcinomatosis and worse disease-free survival (DFS).[44]

RESIDUAL DISEASE ASSOCIATES WITH POOR OUTCOMES

As previously discussed, justification for reresection following a diagnosis of IGBC is performed with the goal of removing RD and achieving R0 margin status. Ironically however, even while reresection is associated with better outcomes, RD found at the time of curative-intent resection or on pathologic assessment is also a marker of poor prognosis.[9,20] Butte and colleagues[20] studied 135 subjects with IGBC: 61% of subjects with RD had an associated DFS of 11 months and a DSS of 25 months as compared with 93 months and not reached for those without RD. Furthermore, RD remained an independent predictor of outcomes in multivariate analysis. Also, for those subjects who underwent R0 resection, local RD within the gallbladder fossa was associated with similarly poor outcomes as regional (regional nodes or involvement of bile duct or cystic duct stump) and distant (peritoneum, port sites, liver metastases) RD. That local disease seems to be the clinical equivalent of regional and metastatic disease may be explained by initially inadequate staging, the possibility that local gallbladder fossa disease actually represented metastatic microscopic disease, and that even the metastatic subjects included in the analysis did not have gross metastatic disease (and all underwent curative-intent R0 resection).

The authors also note that RD may be known following simple cholecystectomy (before proceeding to reresection) either by cross-sectional imaging or in the case of a positive cholecystectomy margin; however, in many cases, it is only known following reresection. If known before reresection, this information could theoretically be used to counsel patients and make treatment decisions.

HEPATIC SIDE TUMORS AS A MARKER OF POOR PROGNOSIS

As part of the AJCC 8th edition staging criteria, T2 gallbladder cancers are now further stratified based on location at the hepatic or peritoneal side.[18] These staging criteria come from a study of 437 subjects conducted at 4 centers in the United States, Chile, Italy, and Japan, which found an independent association for hepatic side tumor location and worse OS following curative-intent resection, specifically, and only for T2 stage disease (5-year OS for hepatic side was 42.6% vs 64.7%). Tumors are classified as peritoneal side when tumor infiltrates subserosa only at the free serosal side and as hepatic when at least part of the tumor infiltrates subserosal tissue in the part of the gallbladder wall attached to the liver. This prognostic difference might be explained by a dense network of lymphatics and larger vessels on the hepatic side of the gallbladder,[45] allowing for a more direct drainage route to nodes and intrahepatic portal veins.[46] The hypothesis that this anatomic difference facilitates spread is supported by association of hepatic side with distant node and intrahepatic recurrence, as well as positive correlation with node-positive disease, vascular invasion, and microscopic disease in the adjacent liver. The limitations of these results are that surgeons cannot stratify patients based on preoperative imaging, thereby limiting utility, and conclusions are based on 1 study without validation as of yet.

CHEMOTHERAPY FOR GALLBLADDER CANCER HAS LIMITED EFFICACY

Currently available evidence indicates that systemic chemotherapy is relatively ineffective for gallbladder cancer. In the advanced biliary cancers (ABC)-02 trial comparing gemcitabine-cisplatin with gemcitabine alone for metastatic and locally advanced disease,[47] although doublet therapy improved progression-free survival (PFS) and OS, response rates were only 26%, PFS 8 months, and OS less than a year. Extrapolating these results to gallbladder cancer specifically (only 36% of the subjects) is not possible. The authors' experience further supports limited efficacy in treating locally advanced or node-positive patients; treatment with what was most often a gem or platinum doublet resulted in a response rate of only 23%.[48]

In the adjuvant setting, the 2 randomized controlled trials performed thus far are both negative. In the multicenter UK capecitabine compared with observation in resected biliary tract cancer (BILCAP) trial, in which 18% of the subjects had gallbladder carcinoma, the adjuvant capecitabine group demonstrated a clinically significant but not statistically significant benefit of 7 months RFS and 15 months OS.[49] The multicenter French study comparing gemcitabine and oxaliplatin with observation also did not find any benefit for RFS or OS.[50] These studies included all biliary cancers and cannot specifically be extrapolated to gallbladder cancer.

ALTERING THE TREATMENT SEQUENCE IN INCIDENTAL GALLBLADDER CARCINOMA

Given that gallbladder cancer is characterized by a high risk of distant failure, a systemic therapy-first approach may be considered with the theoretic benefits of (1) early treatment of micrometastatic disease and (2) optimizing patient selection for curative-intent resection. Patients who progress at distant sites during systemic treatment can be spared the morbidity and mortality of surgery. Although there is no level 1 evidence that supports a benefit to upfront chemotherapy for gallbladder cancer, the authors consider and often use this strategy for patients who are at high risk of distant recurrence in order to optimally balance surgical morbidity with chemotherapy toxicity. The predictors of poor prognosis that identify these high-risk patients were previously discussed and the authors are often able to identify these patients before reresection, especially with the benefit of staging and pathologic information provided by the initial cholecystectomy specimen and cross-sectional imaging. Thus, T3, node-positive, or poor differentiation as identified on cholecystectomy specimen; or suggestion of RD, either by margin positivity or detection on imaging, may justify a test of time and systemic therapy to optimally select patients for surgery. Those patients who progress during the 3 months of upfront chemotherapy are likely those who already had metastatic but radiologically occult disease at the time of diagnosis and can be spared the morbidity of an operation. This strategy should be used carefully. As previously discussed, systemic therapy is fairly ineffective for gallbladder cancer and indiscriminate use for patients at low risk for early distant recurrence theoretically risks local progression and an impaired functional status for an otherwise fit surgical candidate. A true test of the neoadjuvant strategy awaits validation with a randomized trial, 1 of which is in the planning stages and in which the authors' institution is participating.

FINAL THOUGHTS AND PRACTICAL CONSIDERATIONS

Cross-sectional imaging to exclude distant disease is a necessary first step and, if positive, indicates treatment with systemic chemotherapy. PET scans may be used to supplement staging, especially in the case of suspicious regional or distant nodal disease noted on standard cross-sectional imaging. The surgical oncologist should carefully review the cholecystectomy operative report and consider a discussion with the operating surgeon to clarify any missed details, such as bile spillage that places the patient at increased risk for peritoneal recurrence or evidence of peritoneal disease that was misinterpreted within the context of presumed benign disease. Pathologic analysis should be rereviewed by an experienced pathologist.

Next, risk factors for poor prognosis should be identified to facilitate patient counseling and clinical decision-making. IGBC provides a unique situation in which pathologic assessment of the cholecystectomy specimen can contribute to identifying patients at higher risk for the early distant recurrence that characterizes gallbladder cancer. Node-positivity, T3 disease, poor differentiation, or RD, as suggested by a positive margin or imaging, identify patients with poor prognosis. These patients may benefit from upfront chemotherapy. However, systemic therapy in the neoadjuvant setting must not be applied indiscriminately because there is no level 1 evidence for its efficacy.

After the decision for curative-intent reresection is made, the authors perform laparoscopic staging in those patients at high risk for previously unidentified peritoneal disease: T3, positive margin, and poorly differentiated tumors. Resection is performed to remove sites at risk for RD, achieve an R0 resection, and optimally stage the patient while limiting morbidity and mortality. This typically includes a wedge resection of the gallbladder fossa or a more formal resection of segments 4b/5 and portal lymphadenectomy with major hepatectomy and extrahepatic bile duct resection performed only when necessary in order to achieve negative margins.

REFERENCES

1. Cubertafond P, Gainant A, Cucchiaro G. Surgical treatment of 724 carcinomas of the gallbladder. Results of the French Surgical Association Survey. Ann Surg 1994;219:275–80.
2. Piehler JM, Crichlow RW. Primary carcinoma of the gallbladder. Surg Gynecol Obstet 1978;147:929–42.
3. Bartlett DL, Fong Y, Fortner JG, et al. Long-term results after resection for gallbladder cancer. Implications for staging and management. Ann Surg 1996;224: 639–46.
4. de Aretxabala XA, Roa IS, Burgos LA, et al. Curative resection in potentially resectable tumours of the gallbladder. Eur J Surg 1997;163:419–26.
5. Matsumoto Y, Fujii H, Aoyama H, et al. Surgical treatment of primary carcinoma of the gallbladder based on the histologic analysis of 48 surgical specimens. Am J Surg 1992;163:239–45.
6. Shirai Y, Yoshida K, Tsukada K, et al. Radical surgery for gallbladder carcinoma. Long-term results. Ann Surg 1992;216:565–8.
7. Fong Y, Jarnagin W, Blumgart LH. Gallbladder cancer: comparison of patients presenting initially for definitive operation with those presenting after prior noncurative intervention. Ann Surg 2000;232:557–69.
8. Pawlik TM, Gleisner AL, Vigano L, et al. Incidence of finding residual disease for incidental gallbladder carcinoma: implications for re-resection. J Gastrointest Surg 2007;11:1478–86 [discussion: 1486–7].
9. Fuks D, Regimbeau JM, Le Treut YP, et al. Incidental gallbladder cancer by the AFC-GBC-2009 Study Group. World J Surg 2011;35:1887–97.
10. Butte JM, Waugh E, Meneses M, et al. Incidental gallbladder cancer: analysis of surgical findings and survival. J Surg Oncol 2010;102:620–5.
11. Foster JM, Hoshi H, Gibbs JF, et al. Gallbladder cancer: defining the indications for primary radical resection and radical re-resection. Ann Surg Oncol 2007;14: 833–40.
12. Goetze TO, Paolucci V. Adequate extent in radical re-resection of incidental gallbladder carcinoma: analysis of the German Registry. Surg Endosc 2010;24: 2156–64.
13. Ouchi K, Mikuni J, Kakugawa Y, et al. Laparoscopic cholecystectomy for gallbladder carcinoma: results of a Japanese survey of 498 patients. J Hepatobiliary Pancreat Surg 2002;9:256–60.
14. Shirai Y, Yoshida K, Tsukada K, et al. Inapparent carcinoma of the gallbladder. An appraisal of a radical second operation after simple cholecystectomy. Ann Surg 1992;215:326–31.

15. Fong Y, Brennan MF, Turnbull A, et al. Gallbladder cancer discovered during laparoscopic surgery. Potential for iatrogenic tumor dissemination. Arch Surg 1993;128:1054–6.
16. Drouard F, Delamarre J, Capron JP. Cutaneous seeding of gallbladder cancer after laparoscopic cholecystectomy. N Engl J Med 1991;325:1316.
17. Shih SP, Schulick RD, Cameron JL, et al. Gallbladder cancer: the role of laparoscopy and radical resection. Ann Surg 2007;245:893–901.
18. Chun YS, Pawlik TM, Vauthey JN. 8th Edition of the AJCC Cancer Staging Manual: Pancreas and Hepatobiliary Cancers. Ann Surg Oncol 2018;25:845–7.
19. Hari DM, Howard JH, Leung AM, et al. A 21-year analysis of stage I gallbladder carcinoma: is cholecystectomy alone adequate? HPB (Oxford) 2013;15:40–8.
20. Butte JM, Kingham TP, Gonen M, et al. Residual disease predicts outcomes after definitive resection for incidental gallbladder cancer. J Am Coll Surg 2014;219:416–29.
21. Leung U, Pandit-Taskar N, Corvera CU, et al. Impact of pre-operative positron emission tomography in gallbladder cancer. HPB (Oxford) 2014;16:1023–30.
22. Shukla PJ, Barreto SG, Arya S, et al. Does PET-CT scan have a role prior to radical re-resection for incidental gallbladder cancer? HPB (Oxford) 2008;10:439–45.
23. Corvera CU, Blumgart LH, Akhurst T, et al. 18F-fluorodeoxyglucose positron emission tomography influences management decisions in patients with biliary cancer. J Am Coll Surg 2008;206:57–65.
24. Butte JM, Redondo F, Waugh E, et al. The role of PET-CT in patients with incidental gallbladder cancer. HPB (Oxford) 2009;11:585–91.
25. Duffy A, Capanu M, Abou-Alfa GK, et al. Gallbladder cancer (GBC): 10-year experience at Memorial Sloan-Kettering Cancer Centre (MSKCC). J Surg Oncol 2008;98:485–9.
26. Agrawal S, Sonawane RN, Behari A, et al. Laparoscopic staging in gallbladder cancer. Dig Surg 2005;22:440–5.
27. D'Angelica M, Fong Y, Weber S, et al. The role of staging laparoscopy in hepatobiliary malignancy: prospective analysis of 401 cases. Ann Surg Oncol 2003;10:183–9.
28. Weber SM, DeMatteo RP, Fong Y, et al. Staging laparoscopy in patients with extrahepatic biliary carcinoma. Analysis of 100 patients. Ann Surg 2002;235:392–9.
29. Butte JM, Gonen M, Allen PJ, et al. The role of laparoscopic staging in patients with incidental gallbladder cancer. HPB (Oxford) 2011;13:463–72.
30. Shibata K, Uchida H, Iwaki K, et al. Lymphatic invasion: an important prognostic factor for stages T1b-T3 gallbladder cancer and an indication for additional radical resection of incidental gallbladder cancer. World J Surg 2009;33:1035–41.
31. Park JS, Yoon DS, Kim KS, et al. Actual recurrence patterns and risk factors influencing recurrence after curative resection with stage II gallbladder carcinoma. J Gastrointest Surg 2007;11:631–7.
32. Maker AV, Butte JM, Oxenberg J, et al. Is port site resection necessary in the surgical management of gallbladder cancer? Ann Surg Oncol 2012;19:409–17.
33. Fuks D, Regimbeau JM, Pessaux P, et al. Is port-site resection necessary in the surgical management of gallbladder cancer? J Visc Surg 2013;150:277–84.
34. Downing SR, Cadogan KA, Ortega G, et al. Early-stage gallbladder cancer in the Surveillance, Epidemiology, and End Results database: effect of extended surgical resection. Arch Surg 2011;146:734–8.

35. Ito H, Ito K, D'Angelica M, et al. Accurate staging for gallbladder cancer: implications for surgical therapy and pathological assessment. Ann Surg 2011;254: 320–5.
36. Kondo S, Nimura Y, Hayakawa N, et al. Regional and para-aortic lymphadenectomy in radical surgery for advanced gallbladder carcinoma. Br J Surg 2000;87: 418–22.
37. Shirai Y, Yoshida K, Tsukada K, et al. Identification of the regional lymphatic system of the gallbladder by vital staining. Br J Surg 1992;79:659–62.
38. Tsukada K, Kurosaki I, Uchida K, et al. Lymph node spread from carcinoma of the gallbladder. Cancer 1997;80:661–7.
39. D'Angelica M, Dalal KM, DeMatteo RP, et al. Analysis of the extent of resection for adenocarcinoma of the gallbladder. Ann Surg Oncol 2009;16:806–16.
40. Jarnagin WR, Ruo L, Little SA, et al. Patterns of initial disease recurrence after resection of gallbladder carcinoma and hilar cholangiocarcinoma: implications for adjuvant therapeutic strategies. Cancer 2003;98:1689–700.
41. Tran TB, Nissen NN. Surgery for gallbladder cancer in the US: a need for greater lymph node clearance. J Gastrointest Oncol 2015;6:452–8.
42. Wang L, Dong P, Zhang Y, et al. Prognostic validation of the updated 8th edition Tumor-Node-Metastasis classification by the Union for International Cancer Control: Survival analyses of 307 patients with surgically treated gallbladder carcinoma. Oncol Lett 2018;16:4427–33.
43. Shindoh J, de Aretxabala X, Aloia TA, et al. Tumor location is a strong predictor of tumor progression and survival in T2 gallbladder cancer: an international multicenter study. Ann Surg 2015;261:733–9.
44. Horkoff MJ, Ahmed Z, Xu Y, et al. Adverse outcomes after bile spillage in incidental gallbladder cancers: a population-based study. Ann Surg 2019. [Epub ahead of print].
45. Nagahashi M, Shirai Y, Wakai T, et al. Perimuscular connective tissue contains more and larger lymphatic vessels than the shallower layers in human gallbladders. World J Gastroenterol 2007;13:4480–3.
46. Fahim RB, Mc DJ, Richards JC, et al. Carcinoma of the gallbladder: a study of its modes of spread. Ann Surg 1962;156:114–24.
47. Valle J, Wasan H, Palmer DH, et al. Cisplatin plus gemcitabine versus gemcitabine for biliary tract cancer. N Engl J Med 2010;362:1273–81.
48. Creasy JM, Goldman DA, Dudeja V, et al. Systemic chemotherapy combined with resection for locally advanced gallbladder carcinoma: surgical and survival outcomes. J Am Coll Surg 2017;224:906–16.
49. Primrose JN, Fox RP, Palmer DH, et al. Capecitabine compared with observation in resected biliary tract cancer (BILCAP): a randomised, controlled, multicentre, phase 3 study. Lancet Oncol 2019;20:663–73.
50. Edeline J, Benabdelghani M, Bertaut A, et al. Gemcitabine and oxaliplatin chemotherapy or surveillance in resected biliary tract cancer (PRODIGE 12-ACCORD 18-UNICANCER GI): a randomized phase III study. J Clin Oncol 2019;37:658–67.

Approaches and Outcomes to Distal Cholangiocarcinoma

Rachel M. Lee, MD, MSPH[a], Shishir K. Maithel, MD[b],*

KEYWORDS

- Distal cholangiocarcinoma • Extrahepatic cholangiocarcinoma • Adjuvant therapy
- Risk factors • Surgery

KEY POINTS

- Distal cholangiocarcinoma arises in the common bile duct distal to the insertion of the cystic duct and proximal to the ampulla of Vater and accounts for approximately 20% to 40% of all cholangiocarcinomas.
- The vast majority of distal cholangiocarcinomas arise de novo; however, risk factors include consumption of liver flukes, primary sclerosing cholangitis, hepatitis B and C, biliary enteric drainage, and choledochal cyst disease.
- Distal cholangiocarcinoma presents similarly and is often confused with pancreatic ductal adenocarcinoma. MRI is the gold-standard imaging modality for diagnosis and staging. Endoscopic brushings are often used for tissue diagnosis; however, the sensitivity of brushings and endoscopic biopsy are poor. Endoscopic retrograde cholangiopancreatography has the added therapeutic benefit of stent placement for obstructive lesions.
- Surgical management with pancreatoduodenectomy is the mainstay of treatment of resectable disease, and the only potential for cure.
- Optimal adjuvant therapy in resectable disease remains unknown; however, retrospective analyses have seen improved outcomes with the use of adjuvant chemoradiation, and the recently published BILCAP trial provided the first randomized controlled evidence that chemotherapy with capecitabine has overall survival benefit in the adjuvant setting. More study of neoadjuvant therapy is needed.

INTRODUCTION

Cholangiocarcinoma is the second most common primary liver cancer, accounting for approximately 10% to 15% of primary liver malignancies. Incidence varies greatly across the world, likely because of differences in the prevalence of risk factors; the highest incidence rates are seen in Southeast Asia, where liver flukes are common.[1,2]

Disclosure Statement: No financial or material disclosures.
[a] Division of Surgical Oncology, Department of Surgery, Winship Cancer Institute, Emory University School of Medicine, 1365B Clifton Road, 4th Floor, Atlanta, GA 30322, USA; [b] Division of Surgical Oncology, Department of Surgery, Emory Liver and Pancreas Center, Winship Cancer Institute, Emory University School of Medicine, 1365B Clifton Road, 4th Floor, Atlanta, GA 30322, USA
* Corresponding author.
E-mail address: smaithe@emory.edu

There are approximately 8000 cases of cholangiocarcinoma diagnosed in the United States every year.[3]

Relevant Anatomy/Pathophysiology

Cholangiocarcinoma is an epithelial cell malignancy subdivided into 3 types based on anatomic location. Intrahepatic cholangiocarcinoma arises proximal to the second-order bile ducts. It accounts for approximately 10% to 20% of all cholangiocarcinomas, although the incidence, and this percentage, is rapidly increasing.[1,4,5] Perihilar cholangiocarcinoma arises between the second-order bile ducts and the insertion of the cystic duct into the common bile duct and is the most common type, accounting for approximately 50% of all cholangiocarcinomas. Distal cholangiocarcinoma arises in the common bile duct distal to the insertion of the cystic duct and proximal to the ampulla of Vater. Distal cholangiocarcinomas account for approximately 20% to 40% of all cholangiocarcinomas.[4,5] In addition to location, cholangiocarcinomas are characterized by growth pattern as either mass forming, periductal infiltrating, or intraductal. Although any growth pattern may occur at any location, intrahepatic cholangiocarcinomas are commonly mass forming, whereas perihilar tumors are commonly periductal infiltrating. Intraductal growth pattern is the least common and may occur at any location.[6,7]

The vast majority of cases of cholangiocarcinoma arise de novo, with no identifiable risk factors.[5] Risk factors for cholangiocarcinoma include

- *Clonorchis sinensis* and *Opistorchis viverrini* flukes infect the liver after consumption of freshwater fish and induce chronic inflammation in small intrahepatic ducts and gallbladder.[1,5,8]
- Primary sclerosing cholangitis (PSC) causes diffuse inflammation and fibrosis of the intrahepatic and extrahepatic bile ducts. Patients with PSC have approximately a 5% to 10% incidence of cholangiocarcinoma, with a particular predilection for perihilar tumors.[5,9–11]
- Hepatitis B and C and cirrhosis have more recently been recognized as risk factors for cholangiocarcinoma, specifically intrahepatic cholangiocarcinoma; hepatitis C has been studied in the United States and Europe, where infection is more prevalent, and hepatitis B in Asia, where it is endemic.[12–17]
- Biliary-enteric drainage, including choledochoduodenostomy, transduodenal sphincteroplasty, and biliary reconstruction with hepaticojejunostomy, typically performed for benign diseases, including choledocholithiasis and benign biliary stricture, have been associated with cholangiocarcinoma rates between 1.9% for patients after hepaticojejunostomy and 5.8% and 7.9% for patients with transduodenal sphincteroplasty and choledochoduodenostomy, respectively. The pathophysiology of this increased risk is thought to be reflux of enteric contents into the distal bile duct, causing increasing rates of chronic relapsing cholangitis, leading to biliary epithelial hyperplasia, atypia, and ultimately malignant transformation. Cholangiocarcinoma onset typically occurs between 1 and 2 decades after the given procedure.[18–20]
- Choledochal cyst disease, with type I (solitary extrahepatic) and type IV (intrahepatic and extrahepatic dilation involving the ductal confluence) cysts having the highest risk of malignant transformation, has up to a 30% incidence of cholangiocarcinoma, that typically occurs in young patients.[21] Similar to biliary-enteric drainage, the pathophysiology of this increased risk is thought to stem from anomalous junction of the pancreatic and biliary ducts, allowing for reflux of pancreatic enzymes into the biliary tree, resulting in chronic inflammation and cystic degeneration.[22]

CLINICAL PRESENTATION AND DIAGNOSIS

Common symptoms of distal cholangiocarcinoma at presentation are listed in **Box 1**.

Radiographic Evaluation

Ultrasonography has limited utility in the diagnosis of distal cholangiocarcinoma, however, can be useful in ruling out choledocholithiasis as the cause of cholestatic symptoms and can also demonstrate dilated bile ducts in periductal infiltrating and intraductal tumors.[6,8] Contrast-enhanced computed tomography is commonly used to characterize liver masses, although, like ultrasonography, has restricted utility in imaging distal cholangiocarcinoma, because evaluation of tumor spread along and within bile ducts is limited. However, biliary dilation, lymphadenopathy, vascular invasion, and the presence of metastases may be well characterized using this imaging modality.[23]

MRI is the modality of choice for diagnosis and staging of cholangiocarcinoma. MRI provides high-quality soft tissue evaluation for the identification of infiltrating tumors, and magnetic resonance cholangiopancreatography is the most accurate noninvasive evaluation of intraductal tumoral spread.[6] Periductal-infiltrating tumors appear as irregular circumferential wall thickening, which can sometimes be seen as enhancing rings, with dilation of proximal bile ducts that enhance slowly, peaking on delayed phases. Intraductal cholangiocarcinoma appears as a polypoid or sessile mass within the biliary system with proximal ductal dilation and heterogeneous enhancement, beginning early and peaking on delayed phase images.[6,24,25]

Endoscopic Evaluation

Endoscopic retrograde cholangiopancreatography (ERCP) allows for tissue sampling via brush cytology or biopsy. Unfortunately, however, sensitivity of these modalities in detecting cholangiocarcinoma remains limited and varies widely, ranging from 20% to 80%, although most studies quote sensitivity between 20% and 50%. Specificity of these tests is close to 100% across studies.[26–30] Fluorescence in situ hybridization and flow cytometry have been shown to augment the sensitivity of brush cytology to 35% to 60%; however, these techniques are not universally available, and the improvement in sensitivity remains modest.[31,32] Given this limited sensitivity, negative results of brush cytology or biopsy often result in additional procedures to obtain a tissue diagnosis for patients in whom there is a high suspicion for malignancy. ERCP also importantly allows for the therapeutic benefit of biliary stenting in patients with obstructive cholestasis and the collection of bile for microbiological fluid or proteomic analysis.[33,34]

Box 1
Common symptoms at presentation

- Painless jaundice
- Abdominal pain
- Weight loss
- Cholestatic symptoms, including
  - Pruritis
  - Clay-colored stools
  - Dark urine
  - Malabsorption
  - Cholangitis

Endoscopic ultrasound provides visualization of the extrahepatic biliary tree, gall-bladder, regional lymph nodes, and vascular structures. Particularly useful for distal lesions, as they are the most accessible, fine needle aspiration (FNA) may allow for tissue diagnosis in patients with negative brush cytology, with sensitivity reported to be 59% in patients with negative brush cytology, and 80% in patients with mass lesions.[32,35] There is some controversy over the risk of tumor seeding with FNA biopsy however, although the precise risk or likelihood of this occurring remains unclear.[36-38]

Transpapillary cholangioscopy allows for complete visualization of the biliary mucosa via passage of a 10-F scope through and endoscope channel.[8,32] Targeted biopsies have a high accuracy in diagnosing cholangiocarcinoma. However, cholangioscopy is technically challenging, especially if tight distal strictures and obstruction are present, and is associated with a higher rate of cholangitis compared with ERCP alone.[39,40]

Intraductal ultrasound, the insertion of a high-frequency probe into the bile ducts, can be used to assess depth of invasion, longitudinal extension of tumor through the bile duct, and vascular invasion; however, the differentiation of inflammation and malignant tissue is challenging, leading to limited use of this modality.[8,32]

Serum Tumor Markers

Conventional serum markers for cholangiocarcinoma include carcinoembryonic antigen (CEA) and carbohydrate antigen 19-9 (CA19-9); however, these markers have limited utility in both screening and diagnosis of cholangiocarcinoma. Individually, CA19-9 has a sensitivity of 53% to 92% and specificity of 45% to 80%, whereas CEA has a sensitivity of 38% to 53% and specificity of 86% to 100%.[41-45] The utility of these markers is increased when considered together, however, and even further when considered with brush cytology and DNA analysis.[46]

Serum p53 antibodies are present in approximately 20% of patients with extrahepatic cholangiocarcinoma and may be a useful marker in early detection of these tumors.[47,48] Seropositivity is correlated with increasing rates of p53 expression and independent of CEA and CA19-9 expression, possibly allowing for earlier detection of tumors in patients who are negative for conventional tumor markers. Serum p53 antibodies have not been shown to be associated with recurrence or survival, and the use of this marker as a prognostic indicator is limited.[47]

Preoperative Differentiation Between Distal Cholangiocarcinoma and Pancreatic Ductal Adenocarcinoma

Distal cholangiocarcinoma and pancreatic ductal adenocarcinoma (PDAC) are difficult to distinguish preoperatively and are often grouped together and treated as 1 entity, as "periampullary tumors."[49] Final definitive diagnosis is generally made postoperatively on pathologic evaluation. However, this leaves a gap in ability to discern best treatment of patients with unresectable disease, give cholangiocarcinoma-specific neoadjuvant therapy, and titrate surgical planning, because the lymph node spread may differ between distal cholangiocarcinoma and PDAC. Yokoyama and colleagues[50] investigated perioperative characteristics of both tumor types in patients who underwent resection at a single high-volume institution. Preoperatively, they found the coronal diameter of the pancreatic neck to be significantly greater in patients with distal cholangiocarcinoma, 23 mm versus 20 mm, and the main pancreatic duct diameter to be significantly smaller in patients with distal cholangiocarcinoma, 2.1 mm versus 5 mm. They also found CEA and CA19-9 levels to be significantly higher in patients with PDAC (CEA: 2.9 vs 2.3; CA19-9: 137 vs 41). There were no differences in rate of positive biliary cytology or positive bile duct biopsy between distal cholangiocarcinoma and PDAC patients.[50] This study was performed in a single institution and only in patients with resectable disease; further investigation into preoperative differentiation of these 2 distinct disease processes is needed.

STAGING

A novel T-stage classification system has also been proposed taking into account tumor size and lymphovascular invasion, rather than tumor invasion as per American Joint Committee on Cancer (AJCC) guidelines. Postlewait and colleagues[51] analyzed retrospective data from a multi-institutional collaborative and found that the seventh edition AJCC T-staging system inadequately distinguished patients by survival. They proposed a new T-stage classification system, presented in **Table 1**, that did stratify patients with resected distal cholangiocarcinoma by survival. Patients with T1 tumors had a median overall survival of 38 months compared with 22 months for patients with T2 tumors and 8 months for T3 tumors ($P = .005$).[51] Tumor size and lymphovascular invasion have not yet been included in AJCC staging guidelines, but appear to be important prognostic markers.

TREATMENT/OUTCOMES
Surgical Management

Surgical management, generally with pancreatoduodenectomy, and rarely in more proximal tumors with bile duct resection and hepaticojejunostomy, is the mainstay of treatment of resectable disease, and the only potential for cure. Criteria for resectability generally follow those for other periampullary tumors. Patients must otherwise be able to tolerate a major operation, without distant metastatic disease, and without significant vascular involvement (>180° involvement of the hepatic or superior mesenteric artery and/or >2 cm involvement of the portal or superior mesenteric vein).[52] Although portal vein resection during pancreatoduodenectomy is often performed for PDAC, portal vein invasion in distal cholangiocarcinoma has been shown to be associated with locally advanced disease and negative prognostic factors, including high T stage, lymphatic invasion, perineural invasion, pancreatic invasion, and lymph node metastases as well as poor overall survival after curative resection (5-year overall survival 15%).[53]

Survival following curative intent resection is superior to that for PDAC; large retrospective analysis has shown median disease-specific survival after resection to be 39.8 months with 5-year disease-specific survival of 42%.[49] Both resection margin and the presence of lymph node metastases greatly impact survival. Patients with an R0 resection have a median overall survival of 48 months, compared with a median overall survival of 9 months in patients with an R1 resection.[54] Patients with lymph node metastases have a median disease-specific survival of 29.7 months compared

Table 1		
Proposed new T-stage classification system for distal cholangiocarcinoma		
T Stage	**Description**	
T1	Tumor size <3 cm and LVI negative	
T2	Tumor size <3 cm and LVI positive OR tumor size ≥3 cm and LVI negative	
T3	Tumor size ≥3 cm and LVI positive	

Abbreviation: LVI, Lymphovascular invasion.
From Postlewait LM, Ethun CG, Le N, et al. Proposal for a new T-stage classification system for distal cholangiocarcinoma: a 10-institution study from the U.S. Extrahepatic Biliary Malignancy Consortium. HPB (Oxford). 2016;18(10):793-799; with permission.

with 60.5 months in lymph node–negative patients.[49] Given the impact of these factors on survival, specifically that of margin status, patient selection before proceeding with an operation and emphasis on an R0 resection are paramount.

Adjuvant Treatment: Chemotherapy

There is no clear consensus regarding optimal neoadjuvant or adjuvant treatment of distal cholangiocarcinoma. Guidelines from the National Comprehensive Cancer Network (NCCN) offer a range of options for adjuvant therapy for extrahepatic cholangiocarcinoma, including fluoropyrimidine chemoradiation or fluoropyrimidine or gemcitabine-based chemotherapy or a combination of these 2 modalities while encouraging clinical trial participation and acknowledging limited clinical trial data available defining a standard regimen.[55]

A systematic review and metaanalysis conducted by Horgan and colleagues[56] analyzed 20 studies involving 6712 patients, of whom 1797 received adjuvant therapy, to attempt to elucidate the impact of adjuvant therapy on survival. Overall, receipt of adjuvant therapy was not associated with improved overall survival compared with surgery alone; however, on treatment-specific analysis, patients who received chemotherapy or chemoradiotherapy had improved overall survival compared with patients who received radiotherapy alone. In addition, certain subgroups of patients appeared to derive greater benefit from adjuvant therapy. Patients with R1 resections had improved overall survival after receipt of adjuvant radiation; however, patients with R0 resections did not. Similarly, patients with lymph node–positive disease appeared to derive benefit from adjuvant chemotherapy compared with patients with lymph node–negative disease. It is important to note that this metaanalysis included patients with cholangiocarcinoma of all sites as well as gallbladder cancer.[56]

Takada and colleagues[57] performed the first phase 3 randomized clinical trial investigating the use of adjuvant chemotherapy in pancreatobiliary cancers stratified by disease site. Patients were randomized to receive Mitomycin C and 5-fluorouracil (5-FU) or surgery alone. There was no significant difference between groups for patients with cholangiocarcinoma in 5-year overall or disease-free survival.[57] Without clear guidelines and benefit regarding a particular chemotherapy regimen for cholangiocarcinoma, gemcitabine was increasingly used because of its benefit in pancreatic cancer.[58] Gemcitabine and cisplatin were studied in phase 2 and 3 trials in locally advanced and metastatic cholangiocarcinoma, and the combination was found to have a benefit in progression-free (6-month progression-free survival 57.1% vs 47.7%) and overall survival (median overall survival 11.7 months vs 8.1 months) compared with gemcitabine alone.[58,59] These findings in locally advanced and metastatic cholangiocarcinoma guided subsequent studies in the adjuvant setting.

The European Study Group for Pancreatic Cancer-3 trial investigated the effect of adjuvant 5-FU and leucovorin or gemcitabine in patients with resected periampullary cancers.[60] There was no overall survival difference between patients who received adjuvant therapy and patients who were observed, nor was there an overall survival difference between patients who received 5-FU and leucovorin and those who received gemcitabine. However, on multivariable analysis accounting for tumor site and prognostic markers, receipt of chemotherapy was associated with improved overall survival (hazard ratio [HR] 0.75; 95% confidence interval [CI] 0.57–0.98; $P = .03$) compared with observation, and gemcitabine was associated with improved overall survival compared with 5-FU and leucovorin and observation (gemcitabine: HR 0.70; 95% CI 0.51–0.97; $P = .03$; 5-FU: HR 0.79; 95% CI 0.58–18; $P = .13$).[60]

The recently published BILCAP trial investigated adjuvant capecitabine compared with observation in patients with resected cholangiocarcinoma.[61] Although overall survival was not significantly improved in patients in intent-to-treat analysis, in per-protocol analysis patients who received capecitabine had a median overall survival of 53 months compared with 36 months in the observation group with an HR of 0.71 (95% CI 0.55–0.92; P = .010), suggesting that capecitabine could be considered standard of care for adjuvant treatment of cholangiocarcinoma.[61] This trial has largely formed the basis for the American Society of Clinical Oncology clinical practice guidelines for adjuvant therapy after resection of biliary tract malignancies.[62]

Adjuvant Treatment: Radiation

Regarding adjuvant radiotherapy alone, no clinical trials have demonstrated clear benefit; retrospective analyses have contributed mixed results; and have largely been conducted in intrahepatic and perihilar tumors, or without differentiating tumor site.[63,64] Heron and colleagues[65] performed a retrospective analysis in patients with extrahepatic cholangiocarcinoma. They found an association with improved overall survival in patients with perihilar tumors who received adjuvant radiation compared with those who received surgery alone; however, no difference in overall survival in patients with distal cholangiocarcinoma was observed between those who did and those who did not receive adjuvant radiation. However, median follow-up was 58 months for patients who received surgery alone compared with 82 months for patients who received adjuvant radiation. This analysis was limited by sample size; only 3 patients received adjuvant radiation alone. Given lack of convincing data, adjuvant radiotherapy alone does not play a standard role in adjuvant treatment of distal cholangiocarcinoma.[5]

Adjuvant Treatment: Chemoradiation

There are no randomized clinical trials demonstrating benefit of adjuvant chemoradiation; however, retrospective studies indicate potential benefit. Similar to the systematic review and metaanalysis performed by Horgan and colleagues[56] that demonstrated improved overall survival in patients who received adjuvant chemotherapy or chemoradiotherapy as opposed to adjuvant radiotherapy, a retrospective multicenter analysis performed in Korea likewise demonstrated an association between improved overall survival and receipt of chemotherapy (HR 0.21; 95% CI 0.08–0.53; P = .001) and chemoradiation (HR 0.25; 95% CI 0.08–0.83; P = .024) compared with surgery alone in patients with distal cholangiocarcinoma who underwent an R0 resection. As seen previously, adjuvant radiotherapy was associated with worse overall survival compared with surgery alone (HR 2.38; 95% CI 1.04–5.43; P = .040) in these patients.[66] Of note, this analysis was limited by sample size, because only 9 patients received adjuvant radiotherapy alone. A single-arm phase 2 cooperative group study demonstrated the feasibility of concurrent chemoradiation after resection of extrahepatic biliary malignancy and gallbladder cancer.[67] In this study, the survival and toxicity were reasonable, and patients with a margin positive resection had similar outcomes as those with negative margins, suggesting a benefit of radiation. Patients with distal cholangiocarcinoma comprised a minority in this study, and thus, further investigations in all adjuvant treatment modalities are needed to determine best practices for patients with distal cholangiocarcinoma. Ongoing or recently completed clinical trials investigating adjuvant therapy for distal cholangiocarcinoma are listed in **Table 2**.

Neoadjuvant Treatment

There is no consensus or randomized controlled trial regarding neoadjuvant therapy for distal cholangiocarcinoma, and neoadjuvant treatment is not mentioned in the NCCN

Table 2
Current active, recruiting, recently completed, or unknown status clinical trials for adjuvant treatment of resectable extrahepatic cholangiocarcinoma

Study	N	Arms	Status
Phase III Multicenter Randomized Study Comparing the Effect of Adjuvant Chemotherapy for Six Months with Gemcitabine-Oxaliplatin 85 mg/m^2 (GEMOX85) to Observation in Patients Who Underwent Surgery for Cancer of the Bile Ducts France (*PRODIGE 12*) [NCT01313377]	190	Observation vs GEMOX85	No benefit
Capecitabine compared with observation in resected biliary tract cancer (BILCAP): a randomized, controlled, multicenter, phase 3 study UK (*BILCAP*) [NCT00363584]	360	Observation vs Capecitabine	Benefit
Adjuvant Chemotherapy with Gemcitabine and Cisplatin Compared to Standard of Care After Curative Intent Resection of Biliary Tract Cancer Europe (*ACTICCA-1*) [NCT02170090]	781	Observation vs Cisplatin + Gemcitabine	Design revised to Capecitabine vs Cisplatin + Gemcitabine
A Randomized Phase III Trial of Adjuvant S-1 Therapy vs Observation Alone in Resected Biliary Tract Cancer Japan (*JCOG1202*) [UMIN000011688]	350	Observation vs S-1	Completed accrual
Clinical Trial of Adjuvant Chemotherapy Followed by Concurrent Chemoradiotherapy Compared with Adjuvant Chemotherapy Alone in Patients with Gallbladder Carcinoma and Extrahepatic Cholangiocarcinoma China [NCT02798510]	140	Gemcitabine + Capecitabine + Capecitabine/ Radiotherapy vs Gemcitabine + Capecitabine	Unknown, anticipated completion April 2019
Adjuvant Capecitabine vs Gemcitabine Plus Cisplatin in Resected Extrahepatic Cholangiocarcinoma Korea [NCT03079427]	100	Capecitabine vs Gemcitabine + Cisplatin	Recruiting

guidelines.[68] Furthermore, the difficulty in differentiating distal cholangiocarcinoma from PDAC in the head of the pancreas preoperatively complicates neoadjuvant treatment decisions. However, retrospective single-institution analyses have demonstrated potential benefit to neoadjuvant therapy. McMasters and colleagues[69] reported their institution's experience with neoadjuvant chemoradiation for extrahepatic cholangiocarcinoma from 1983 to 1996. Nine patients (5 perihilar, 4 distal) received neoadjuvant chemoradiation. Three had a pathologic complete response, and the R0 resection rate was 100% in patients who received neoadjuvant therapy compared with 54% for patients who did not (*P*<.01). In contrast, Kato and colleagues[70] conducted a retrospective review to determine the association of neoadjuvant chemotherapy alone with resectability of locally advanced cholangiocarcinoma. Of 8 patients with extrahepatic cholangiocarcinoma, only one had tumor downsizing by RECIST criteria, and no patients underwent surgical resection. Prospective clinical trials are needed to determine the impact of neoadjuvant treatment on survival and resectability of distal cholangiocarcinoma, although improvement in preoperative discrimination between distal cholangiocarcinoma and PDAC will ultimately be necessary to inform clinical trial design and provide the best possible care to each distinct group of patients.

SUMMARY

Distal cholangiocarcinoma is a rare malignancy with a dismal prognosis. Because of its location and aggressive nature, patients often present with locally advanced or metastatic disease, and effective treatment options are limited. For patients with resectable disease, surgery is the only chance for cure, but achieving an R0 resection is paramount. Optimal adjuvant therapy in resectable disease remains under investigation; however, retrospective analyses have seen improved outcomes with the use of adjuvant chemoradiation, and the recently published BILCAP trial provided the first randomized controlled evidence that chemotherapy with capecitabine has overall survival benefit in the adjuvant setting.[61] Randomized controlled trials investigating neoadjuvant therapy and its impact on resectability and long-term outcomes are needed to continue to improve the outcomes of patients with distal cholangiocarcinoma.

REFERENCES

1. Hoyos S, Navas MC, Restrepo JC, et al. Current controversies in cholangiocarcinoma. Biochim Biophys Acta Mol Basis Dis 2018;1864(4 Pt B):1461–7.
2. International Agency for Research on Cancer (IARC). GLOBOCAN 2012: estimated cancer incidence, mortality, and prevalence worldwide in 2012 2012. Available at: http://globocan.iarc.fr/Default.aspx. Accessed April 15, 2019.
3. American Cancer Society. Cancer Facts & Figures 2018 2018. Available at: https://www.cancer.org/cancer/bile-duct-cancer/about/key-statistics.html. Accessed April 15, 2019.
4. DeOliveira ML, Cunningham SC, Cameron JL, et al. Cholangiocarcinoma: thirty-one-year experience with 564 patients at a single institution. Ann Surg 2007; 245(5):755–62.
5. Razumilava N, Gores GJ. Cholangiocarcinoma. Lancet 2014;383(9935):2168–79.
6. Jhaveri KS, Hosseini-Nik H. MRI of cholangiocarcinoma. J Magn Reson Imaging 2015;42(5):1165–79.
7. Lim JH. Cholangiocarcinoma: morphologic classification according to growth pattern and imaging findings. AJR Am J Roentgenol 2003;181(3):819–27.
8. Lad N, Kooby DA. Distal cholangiocarcinoma. Surg Oncol Clin N Am 2014;23(2): 265–87.
9. Bergquist A, Ekbom A, Olsson R, et al. Hepatic and extrahepatic malignancies in primary sclerosing cholangitis. J Hepatol 2002;36(3):321–7.
10. Chapman MH, Webster GJ, Bannoo S, et al. Cholangiocarcinoma and dominant strictures in patients with primary sclerosing cholangitis: a 25-year single-centre experience. Eur J Gastroenterol Hepatol 2012;24(9):1051–8.
11. Claessen MM, Vleggaar FP, Tytgat KM, et al. High lifetime risk of cancer in primary sclerosing cholangitis. J Hepatol 2009;50(1):158–64.
12. Donato F, Gelatti U, Tagger A, et al. Intrahepatic cholangiocarcinoma and hepatitis C and B virus infection, alcohol intake, and hepatolithiasis: a case-control study in Italy. Cancer Causes Control 2001;12(10):959–64.
13. El-Serag HB, Engels EA, Landgren O, et al. Risk of hepatobiliary and pancreatic cancers after hepatitis C virus infection: a population-based study of U.S. veterans. Hepatology 2009;49(1):116–23.

14. Lee TY, Lee SS, Jung SW, et al. Hepatitis B virus infection and intrahepatic cholangiocarcinoma in Korea: a case-control study. Am J Gastroenterol 2008;103(7): 1716–20.
15. Shaib YH, El-Serag HB, Davila JA, et al. Risk factors of intrahepatic cholangiocarcinoma in the United States: a case-control study. Gastroenterology 2005;128(3): 620–6.
16. Welzel TM, Mellemkjaer L, Gloria G, et al. Risk factors for intrahepatic cholangiocarcinoma in a low-risk population: a nationwide case-control study. Int J Cancer 2007;120(3):638–41.
17. Zhou YM, Yin ZF, Yang JM, et al. Risk factors for intrahepatic cholangiocarcinoma: a case-control study in China. World J Gastroenterol 2008;14(4):632–5.
18. Hakamada K, Sasaki M, Endoh M, et al. Late development of bile duct cancer after sphincteroplasty: a ten- to twenty-two-year follow-up study. Surgery 1997; 121(5):488–92.
19. Strong RW. Late bile duct cancer complicating biliary-enteric anastomosis for benign disease. Am J Surg 1999;177(6):472–4.
20. Tocchi A, Mazzoni G, Liotta G, et al. Late development of bile duct cancer in patients who had biliary-enteric drainage for benign disease: a follow-up study of more than 1,000 patients. Ann Surg 2001;234(2):210–4.
21. Soreide K, Korner H, Havnen J, et al. Bile duct cysts in adults. Br J Surg 2004; 91(12):1538–48.
22. Dickson PV, Behrman SW. Distal cholangiocarcinoma. Surg Clin North Am 2014; 94(2):325–42.
23. Tillich M, Mischinger HJ, Preisegger KH, et al. Multiphasic helical CT in diagnosis and staging of hilar cholangiocarcinoma. AJR Am J Roentgenol 1998;171(3): 651–8.
24. Sainani NI, Catalano OA, Holalkere NS, et al. Cholangiocarcinoma: current and novel imaging techniques. Radiographics 2008;28(5):1263–87.
25. Vanderveen KA, Hussain HK. Magnetic resonance imaging of cholangiocarcinoma. Cancer Imaging 2004;4(2):104–15.
26. Farrell RJ, Jain AK, Brandwein SL, et al. The combination of stricture dilation, endoscopic needle aspiration, and biliary brushings significantly improves diagnostic yield from malignant bile duct strictures. Gastrointest Endosc 2001;54(5): 587–94.
27. Fogel EL, deBellis M, McHenry L, et al. Effectiveness of a new long cytology brush in the evaluation of malignant biliary obstruction: a prospective study. Gastrointest Endosc 2006;63(1):71–7.
28. Jailwala J, Fogel EL, Sherman S, et al. Triple-tissue sampling at ERCP in malignant biliary obstruction. Gastrointest Endosc 2000;51(4 Pt 1):383–90.
29. Kitajima Y, Ohara H, Nakazawa T, et al. Usefulness of transpapillary bile duct brushing cytology and forceps biopsy for improved diagnosis in patients with biliary strictures. J Gastroenterol Hepatol 2007;22(10):1615–20.
30. Smoczynski M, Jablonska A, Matyskiel A, et al. Routine brush cytology and fluorescence in situ hybridization for assessment of pancreatobiliary strictures. Gastrointest Endosc 2012;75(1):65–73.
31. Lindberg B, Enochsson L, Tribukait B, et al. Diagnostic and prognostic implications of DNA ploidy and S-phase evaluation in the assessment of malignancy in biliary strictures. Endoscopy 2006;38(6):561–5.
32. Voigtlander T, Lankisch TO. Endoscopic diagnosis of cholangiocarcinoma: from endoscopic retrograde cholangiography to bile proteomics. Best Pract Res Clin Gastroenterol 2015;29(2):267–75.

33. Lankisch TO, Metzger J, Negm AA, et al. Bile proteomic profiles differentiate cholangiocarcinoma from primary sclerosing cholangitis and choledocholithiasis. Hepatology 2011;53(3):875–84.

34. Negm AA, Schott A, Vonberg RP, et al. Routine bile collection for microbiological analysis during cholangiography and its impact on the management of cholangitis. Gastrointest Endosc 2010;72(2):284–91.

35. Navaneethan U, Njei B, Venkatesh PG, et al. Endoscopic ultrasound in the diagnosis of cholangiocarcinoma as the etiology of biliary strictures: a systematic review and meta-analysis. Gastroenterol Rep (Oxf) 2015;3(3):209–15.

36. El Chafic AH, Dewitt J, Leblanc JK, et al. Impact of preoperative endoscopic ultrasound-guided fine needle aspiration on postoperative recurrence and survival in cholangiocarcinoma patients. Endoscopy 2013;45(11):883–9.

37. Heimbach JK, Sanchez W, Rosen CB, et al. Trans-peritoneal fine needle aspiration biopsy of hilar cholangiocarcinoma is associated with disease dissemination. HPB (Oxford) 2011;13(5):356–60.

38. Khan SA, Davidson BR, Goldin RD, et al. Guidelines for the diagnosis and treatment of cholangiocarcinoma: an update. Gut 2012;61(12):1657–69.

39. Kalaitzakis E, Sturgess R, Kaltsidis H, et al. Diagnostic utility of single-user peroral cholangioscopy in sclerosing cholangitis. Scand J Gastroenterol 2014; 49(10):1237–44.

40. Sethi A, Chen YK, Austin GL, et al. ERCP with cholangiopancreatoscopy may be associated with higher rates of complications than ERCP alone: a single-center experience. Gastrointest Endosc 2011;73(2):251–6.

41. Buffet C, Fourre C, Altman C, et al. Bile levels of carcino-embryonic antigen in patients with hepatopancreatobiliary disease. Eur J Gastroenterol Hepatol 1996; 8(2):131–4.

42. Gores GJ. Early detection and treatment of cholangiocarcinoma. Liver Transpl 2000;6(6 Suppl 2):S30–4.

43. Nichols JC, Gores GJ, LaRusso NF, et al. Diagnostic role of serum CA 19-9 for cholangiocarcinoma in patients with primary sclerosing cholangitis. Mayo Clin Proc 1993;68(9):874–9.

44. Patel AH, Harnois DM, Klee GG, et al. The utility of CA 19-9 in the diagnoses of cholangiocarcinoma in patients without primary sclerosing cholangitis. Am J Gastroenterol 2000;95(1):204–7.

45. Ramage JK, Donaghy A, Farrant JM, et al. Serum tumor markers for the diagnosis of cholangiocarcinoma in primary sclerosing cholangitis. Gastroenterology 1995; 108(3):865–9.

46. Lindberg B, Arnelo U, Bergquist A, et al. Diagnosis of biliary strictures in conjunction with endoscopic retrograde cholangiopancreaticography, with special reference to patients with primary sclerosing cholangitis. Endoscopy 2002;34(11): 909–16.

47. Okada R, Shimada H, Otsuka Y, et al. Serum p53 antibody as a potential tumor marker in extrahepatic cholangiocarcinoma. Surg Today 2017;47(12):1492–9.

48. Shimada H, Ochiai T, Nomura F, Japan p53 Antibody Research Group. Titration of serum p53 antibodies in 1,085 patients with various types of malignant tumors: a multiinstitutional analysis by the Japan p53 Antibody Research Group. Cancer 2003;97(3):682–9.

49. Ethun CG, Lopez-Aguiar AG, Pawlik TM, et al. Distal cholangiocarcinoma and pancreas adenocarcinoma: are they really the same disease? A 13-institution study from the US extrahepatic biliary malignancy consortium and the central pancreas consortium. J Am Coll Surg 2017;224(4):406–13.

50. Yokoyama Y, Ebata T, Igami T, et al. Different clinical characteristics between distal cholangiocarcinoma and pancreatic head carcinoma with biliary obstruction. Pancreas 2017;46(10):1322–6.

51. Postlewait LM, Ethun CG, Le N, et al. Proposal for a new T-stage classification system for distal cholangiocarcinoma: a 10-institution study from the U.S. Extrahepatic Biliary Malignancy Consortium. HPB (Oxford) 2016;18(10):793–9.

52. Schulick RD. Criteria of unresectability and the decision-making process. HPB (Oxford) 2008;10(2):122–5.

53. Maeta T, Ebata T, Hayashi E, et al. Pancreatoduodenectomy with portal vein resection for distal cholangiocarcinoma. Br J Surg 2017;104(11):1549–57.

54. Chua TC, Mittal A, Arena J, et al. Resection margin influences survival after pancreatoduodenectomy for distal cholangiocarcinoma. Am J Surg 2017;213(6):1072–6.

55. NCCN clinical practice guidelines in oncology: hepatobiliary cancers, Version 2. Available at: https://www.nccn.org/professionals/physician_gls/pdf/hepatobiliary.pdf. Accessed April 15, 2019.

56. Horgan AM, Amir E, Walter T, et al. Adjuvant therapy in the treatment of biliary tract cancer: a systematic review and meta-analysis. J Clin Oncol 2012;30(16):1934–40.

57. Takada T, Amano H, Yasuda H, et al. Is postoperative adjuvant chemotherapy useful for gallbladder carcinoma? A phase III multicenter prospective randomized controlled trial in patients with resected pancreaticobiliary carcinoma. Cancer 2002;95(8):1685–95.

58. Valle J, Wasan H, Palmer DH, et al. Cisplatin plus gemcitabine versus gemcitabine for biliary tract cancer. N Engl J Med 2010;362(14):1273–81.

59. Valle JW, Wasan H, Johnson P, et al. Gemcitabine alone or in combination with cisplatin in patients with advanced or metastatic cholangiocarcinomas or other biliary tract tumours: a multicentre randomised phase II study–the UK ABC-01 study. Br J Cancer 2009;101(4):621–7.

60. Neoptolemos JP, Moore MJ, Cox TF, et al. Effect of adjuvant chemotherapy with fluorouracil plus folinic acid or gemcitabine vs observation on survival in patients with resected periampullary adenocarcinoma: the ESPAC-3 periampullary cancer randomized trial. JAMA 2012;308(2):147–56.

61. Primrose JN, Fox RP, Palmer DH, et al. Capecitabine compared with observation in resected biliary tract cancer (BILCAP): a randomised, controlled, multicentre, phase 3 study. Lancet Oncol 2019;20(5):663–73.

62. Shroff RT, Kennedy EB, Bachini M, et al. Adjuvant therapy for resected biliary tract cancer: ASCO clinical practice guideline. J Clin Oncol 2019;37(12):1015–27.

63. Pitt HA, Nakeeb A, Abrams RA, et al. Perihilar cholangiocarcinoma. Postoperative radiotherapy does not improve survival. Ann Surg 1995;221(6):788–97 [discussion 797–8].

64. Shinohara ET, Mitra N, Guo M, et al. Radiation therapy is associated with improved survival in the adjuvant and definitive treatment of intrahepatic cholangiocarcinoma. Int J Radiat Oncol Biol Phys 2008;72(5):1495–501.

65. Heron DE, Stein DE, Eschelman DJ, et al. Cholangiocarcinoma: the impact of tumor location and treatment strategy on outcome. Am J Clin Oncol 2003;26(4):422–8.

66. Kim YS, Hwang IG, Park SE, et al. Role of adjuvant therapy after R0 resection for patients with distal cholangiocarcinoma. Cancer Chemother Pharmacol 2016;77(5):979–85.

67. Ben-Josef E, Guthrie KA, El-Khoueiry AB, et al. SWOG S0809: a phase II intergroup trial of adjuvant capecitabine and gemcitabine followed by radiotherapy and concurrent capecitabine in extrahepatic cholangiocarcinoma and gallbladder carcinoma. J Clin Oncol 2015;33(24):2617–22.
68. National Comprehensive Cancer Network clinical practice guidelines in oncology: breast cancer version 1.2019. 2019. Available at: https://www.nccn.org/professionals/physician_gls/pdf/breast.pdf. Accessed April 15, 2019.
69. McMasters KM, Tuttle TM, Leach SD, et al. Neoadjuvant chemoradiation for extrahepatic cholangiocarcinoma. Am J Surg 1997;174(6):605–8 [discussion 608–9].
70. Kato A, Shimizu H, Ohtsuka M, et al. Surgical resection after downsizing chemotherapy for initially unresectable locally advanced biliary tract cancer: a retrospective single-center study. Ann Surg Oncol 2013;20(1):318–24.

Evolving Surgical Options for Hepatocellular Carcinoma

Gregory C. Wilson, MD, David A. Geller, MD*

KEYWORDS

- Hepatocellular carcinoma • Barcelona Clinic Liver Cancer
- Laparoscopic liver resection • Radiofrequency ablation • Liver transplant

KEY POINTS

- Liver resection remains the cornerstone of treatment of hepatocellular carcinoma in patients without cirrhosis or early cirrhosis without portal hypertension.
- The role of laparoscopic liver resection for hepatocellular carcinoma continues to expand, with equivalent oncologic outcomes and improvements in perioperative care.
- Liver transplant remains the best treatment option for patients with hepatocellular carcinoma within Milan criteria and cirrhosis.

INTRODUCTION

Hepatocellular carcinoma (HCC) is the most common primary malignancy of the liver.[1] It has a high incidence, especially in Asia, and is considered the sixth most common type of cancer worldwide, and the fourth leading cause of cancer-related death.[1,2] Treatment options with curative intent include liver transplant, resection, and ablation. Liver transplant is the gold standard treatment of cirrhotic patients associated with the lowest recurrence rates and also addresses the background liver disease, which is present in more than 80% of patients with HCC.[2] However, with the increasing incidence of HCC and limited number of available organs, liver transplant is not a practical treatment option for many patients.[2,3]

Diagnosis and staging of HCC are complex topics not covered in this article. HCC is unique to other malignancies in that treatment allocation must account for not only tumor stage but also the patient's liver function and performance status. The Barcelona Clinic Liver Cancer (BCLC) classification system accounts for each of these aspects and provides treatment recommendations based on each component, and it remains

Disclosure: The authors have no financial disclosures to report.
Department of Surgery, Liver Cancer Center, University of Pittsburgh Medical Center, 3471 Fifth Avenue, Suite 300, Pittsburgh, PA, USA
* Corresponding author.
E-mail address: gellerda@upmc.edu

Surg Oncol Clin N Am 28 (2019) 645–661
https://doi.org/10.1016/j.soc.2019.06.006
1055-3207/19/© 2019 Elsevier Inc. All rights reserved.

surgonc.theclinics.com

the most widely used staging system for HCC.[4] Surgical resection is recommended for patients with solitary tumors and preserved liver function without portal hypertension or hyperbilirubinemia. Patients with advanced cirrhosis, increased portal pressures, or multiple tumors should be evaluated for liver transplant.[3–5] Advanced tumors, including multifocal disease not within Milan criteria, tumors with major vascular invasion, extrahepatic extension, or distant metastases, are not candidates for surgical therapy and treatment options are addressed in other articles. The focus of this article is on the evolving surgical options for management of HCC, with a particular focus on laparoscopic versus open resection. In addition, it examines the role of radiofrequency ablation (RFA) versus resection for small HCCs and liver transplant, including a discussion on the pros/cons of resection versus transplant for patients that would be candidates for both.

SURGICAL RESECTION OF HEPATOCELLULAR CARCINOMA

Liver resection is an excellent treatment option for selected patients with HCC.[6] Both the European Association for the Study of the Liver (EASL) and American Association for the Study of Liver Diseases (AASLD) guidelines recommend surgical resection for HCC in patients with noncirrhotic livers and should be considered for patients with early, compensated cirrhosis.[3,5] However, in cirrhotic patients, resection can lead to significant morbidity, including worsening ascites and liver failure and even death.[7] Extreme caution should be exercised when considering resection for cirrhotic patients, and patients with signs of advanced cirrhosis are potentially better served with liver transplant. When feasible, anatomic resections (ARs) should be performed, as opposed to nonanatomic, parenchymal-sparing resections (NARs). Meta-analysis of 18 studies including more than 9000 patients with HCC showed improved 5-year survival (54.4% in NAR group vs 62% in AR group, relative risk of 1.14, $P = .001$) and improved 5-year disease-free survival (27.5% in NAR group vs 38.1% in AR group, relative risk of 1.38, $P<.001$) with AR.[8]

Surgical dogma has always viewed traditional open surgery as being more suitable for liver resections. Early fears with incorporating laparoscopy into liver surgery included the risk of gas embolization during parenchymal transection. However, this complication was shown to occur with rare frequency.[9,10] In addition, the concern of uncontrolled hemorrhage during laparoscopic liver resection (LLR), caused by the inability to apply manual compression on bleeding vessels, was also invalidated. Most reports show that LLR is associated with less blood loss and lower transfusion needs. Similar to other technological advances in surgery, proponents of LLR first had to prove this approach was not inferior to standard open liver resections (OLRs) before the advantages of LLR could be established.[11,12]

The first report in the literature on LLR for HCC was by Hashizume and colleagues[13] in 1995. Not long after, multiple reports and case series with increasing cases of LLR emerged. With continued technological advancements, improvements in the understanding of liver anatomy, and better preoperative liver imaging, there has been a paradigm shift, with tremendous growth in the number of LLRs performed worldwide.

Two international LLR consensus conferences have been convened, the first in Louisville, Kentucky, in 2008,[14] and the second in Morioka, Japan, in 2014.[15] Recommendations from this first meeting established baseline terminology and efficacy of LLR.[14] The first conference concluded that minor LLRs are safe and should be considered for minor hepatic resections in carefully selected patients. In addition, patient safety and procedure efficacy should be monitored with a centralized registry. Six years later, the Second International Consensus Conference convened in Morioka and recommendations were given by a 9-member independent jury and an expert panel of surgeons. Major LLR was considered an innovative procedure, still in the exploration or learning phase with incompletely defined risks. Minor resections, consisting of resection of 2 or fewer Couinaud segments, were standard clinical practice.[15] The recommendations of these consensus conferences were based on a large number of reports, including series with propensity score matching as well as meta-analyses, almost all of which showed not only noninferiority of LLR compared with OLR but also superiority of LLR in several parameters, as discussed in detail later.

The role of LLR has continued to expand and now includes all types of liver diseases and conditions, including laparoscopic live donor hepatectomies. In 2009, Nguyen and colleagues[16] published a world literature review that included 127 articles on LLR, accounting for 2804 patients. Fifty percent of LLRs reviewed were for malignancy, and 75% were totally laparoscopic, with wedge resections and/or segmentectomy being most frequently performed (45%). Mortality was 0.3% (9 of 2804 patients), and morbidity was 10.5%, with no intraoperative deaths reported. Regarding oncologic outcomes, negative margins (R0 resection) were achieved in 82% to 100% of the reported series. Five-year overall and disease-free survival rates after LLR for HCC ranged from 50% to 75% and 31% to 38.2%, respectively. This review was the first to summarize outcomes from a large number of LLRs and showed the safety and feasibility of LLR.

As this article continues to focus on LLR for HCC, reported short-term and long-term outcomes directly comparing LLR and OLR will be discussed in further detail. **Table 1** outlines long-term outcomes including overall survival from 16 studies and 3 meta-analysis comparing 5-year overall survival in LLR versus OLR in matched patients. Five-year overall survival ranged from 50% to 90% in LLR, and no study showed worse 5-year overall survival for LLR compared with OLR. **Table 2** summarizes the short-term and perioperative outcomes comparing LLR with OLR. In general, patients undergoing LLR had less blood loss, fewer transfusions, less postoperative morbidity, and shorter length of stay compared with OLR cases.[17]

Surgical Margins

Negative resection (R0) margins are the cornerstone of oncologic surgery. They have been correlated with long-term outcomes and disease recurrence in cancer types. Chang and colleagues[18] reported that an R0 resection was achieved in 97% of patients with LLR, similar to OLR. Several reports have shown that LLR was able to achieve wider resection margins compared with OLR.[17,19] Most case-match series have shown equivalent resection margins to OLR, and no study has shown compromised R0 resection rates for LLR compared with OLR. These equivalent R0 resection rates also explain the similar local recurrence rates between LLR and OLR in some studies.[17,18]

Intraoperative Blood Loss and Transfusion Requirements

One persistent finding in most published series is that LLR is associated with less intraoperative blood loss and less transfusion requirement even in matched cohorts.[17–30] Naysayers hold onto a claim of selection bias, but these findings leave little doubt that LLR is not inferior, if not superior, to OLR regarding intraoperative blood loss. The importance of these data is that they eliminate early concerns about loss of control and excessive hemorrhage during laparoscopic parenchymal transection. In addition, a later report from Chen and colleagues[20] took this notion one step further and showed that this is true not only for minor laparoscopic resections but also for major LLR, compared with major OLR.

Table 1
Five-year survival comparison between laparoscopic liver resection and open liver resection

Study (Lead Author)	Number of Patients with LLR/OLR	Year of Publication	Country	5-y Overall Survival LLR/OLR		Statistical Significance
Sotiropoulos et al,[17] 2017[a]	2112/3019	2017	Greece	HR, 0.97 (95% CI 0.82–1.14)		NS
Cheung et al,[21] 2016	110/330	2016	China	52%	48%	NS
Chang et al,[18] 2016	30/30	2016	Singapore	59%	65%	NS
Takahara et al,[27] 2015	387/387	2105	Japan	77%	71%	NS
Kim et al,[89] 2014	29/29	2014	Korea	92%	88%	NS
Yin et al,[29] 2013[a]	485/753	2013	China	HR, 0.99 (95% CI 0.74–1.33)		NS
Cheung et al,[90] 2013	32/64	2013	China	77%	57%	NS
Ker et al,[91] 2011	116/208	2011	Taiwan	62%	72%	NS
Truant et al,[92] 2011	35/53	2011	France	70%	46%	NS
Zhou et al,[30] 2011[a]	213/281	2011	China	HR, 1.64 (95% CI 0.92–2.93)		NS
Fancellu et al,[22] 2011[a]	227/363	2011	Italy	63%	56%	NS
Lee et al,[93] 2011	33/50	2011	China	76%	76%	NS
Hu et al,[94] 2011	30/30	2011	China	50%	53%	NS
Tranchart et al,[57] 2010	42/42	2010	France	60%	47%	NS
Sarpel et al,[95] 2009	20/56	2009	USA	95%	75%	NS
Endo et al,[96] 2009	10/11	2009	Japan	57%	48%	NS
Cai et al,[97] 2008	31-31	2008	China	50%	51%	NS
Kaneko et al,[98] 2005	30/28	2005	Japan	61%	62%	NS
Shimada et al,[99] 2001	17/38	2001	Japan	50%	38%	NS

Abbreviations: CI, confidence interval; HR, hazard ratio; NS, no statistical significance.
[a] Denotes study is a meta-analysis.

Table 2
Comparison of intraoperative and postoperative outcomes between LLR and OLR

Study (Lead Author)	Number of Patients LLR/OLR	Operative Blood Loss	Transfusion Requirements	Operative Time	Overall Morbidity	LOS	R0 Resection Rate
Chang et al,[18] 2016	30/30	Favors LLR	Not reported	Not reported	Not reported	Favors LLR	Equivalent
Takahara et al,[27] 2015	387/387	Favors LLR	Favors LLR	Favors OLR	Favors LLR	Favors LLR	Not reported
Chen et al,[19] 2015	281/547	Favors LLR	Favors LLR	Equivalent	Not reported	Favors LLR	Favors LLR
Cheung et al,[21] 2016	110/330	Favors LLR	Equivalent	Favors LLR	Equivalent	Favors LLR	Not reported
Komatsu et al,[60] 2016	38/38	Equivalent	Equivalent	Favors OLR	Favors LLR	Equivalent	Equivalent
Xu et al,[59] 2018	32/32	Favors LLR	Equivalent	Favors OLR	Equivalent	Equivalent	Not reported
Sotiropoulos et al,[17] 2017[a]	2112/3019	Favors LLR	Favors LLR	Equivalent	Favors LLR	Favors LLR	Favors LLR
Chen et al,[20] 2017	225/291	Favors LLR	Favors LLR	Minor resections: favor LLR Major resections: favor OLR	Equivalent	Favors LLR	Not reported
Xiong et al,[28] 2012[a]	234/316	Favors LLR	Favors LLR	Equivalent	Favors LLR	Favors LLR	Equivalent
Li et al,[24] 2012[a]	244/383	Favors LLR	Favors LLR	Equivalent	Favors LLR	Favors LLR	Equivalent
Mizuguchi et al,[100] 2011[a]	232/253	Favors LLR	Not reported	Equivalent	Favors LLR	Favors LLR	Not reported
Yin et al,[29] 2013[a]	485/753	Favors LLR	Favors LLR	Equivalent	Favors LLR	Favors LLR	Equivalent
Zhou et al,[30] 2011[a]	213/281	Favors LLR	Favors LLR	Equivalent	Favors LLR	Favors LLR	Equivalent
Fancellu et al,[22] 2011[a]	227/363	Favors LLR	Favors LLR	Equivalent	Favors LLR	Favors LLR	Favors LLR

Abbreviations: LOS, length of stay; OR, operating room.
[a] Denotes study is a meta-analysis.

One obvious aspect present during LLR and likely in part responsible for these findings is the presence of pneumoperitoneum during LLR. Standard pneumoperitoneum pressure is set to 12 to 15 mm Hg, which is considerably higher than the average central venous pressure (intentionally maintained at 5 mm Hg or less before liver transection) during parenchymal transection. This positive pressure gradient occludes tiny venous branches at the cut surface of the liver that would otherwise be a constant source of blood loss during OLR.[31–34] One other additional explanation for the decreased intraoperative blood loss with LLR is the magnification and visualization provided by the laparoscope, allowing for better identification and ligation of small vessels. Furthermore, modern laparoscopic instruments have shown excellent hemostatic capabilities.[35] Additional technologic advances with the electronically powered staplers allows smoother and less jerky stapling of the intrahepatic structures, providing better stapled lines and improved hemostasis.[36,37] Achieving better hemostasis becomes even more paramount for oncologic resections. Several studies have shown the negative effects that excessive blood loss and transfusion requirements have on short-term and long-term outcomes, including survival and disease recurrence.[38,39]

Operative Time

In contrast with blood loss, for which there is wide agreement in the literature about the superiority of LLR compared with OLR, when it comes to operative duration, the reports differ considerably. There is wide variability in reported operative times for LLR compared with OLR and is likely multifactorial based on institution experience, surgeon experience, and patient-specific factors. Cheung and colleagues[21] reported a shorter operation time with LLR. Chen and colleagues[20] reached a similar conclusion, but only in patients undergoing minor LLR. However, operative times with the laparoscopic approach were significantly longer for major liver resections. These findings are consistent with the clinical practice of experienced laparoscopic surgeons. Minor LLRs are more established and surgeons have more experience with the technique. Minor LLRs also do not involve complete liver mobilization, nor do they require gaining vascular control, steps that require advanced laparoscopic skills and more operative time. With minor LLR, the resections are usually straightforward and can be accomplished with energy devices alone, such as ultrasonic shears. Significant time is also saved with closure compared with OLR. In contrast, major LLRs are still in the innovative phase. Experience is significantly more limited and they require full mobilization and retraction of the liver, which are technically challenging when performed laparoscopically. Several other reports have shown no significant difference in operative time between LLR and OLR,[17] whereas still others showed significantly longer operative time with LLR compared with OLR.[27] There is no question that operative time is directly influenced by multiple factors, including surgical skill/experience, background training of the surgeon, institutional volume, and location on the learning curve for these procedures.

Postoperative Course, Including Length of Stay and Complications

Consistent with other complex surgical procedures, the laparoscopic approach is almost always associated with significantly shorter hospital length of stay compared with the traditional open approach. In a multi-institutional Japanese study with propensity score matching, Takahara and colleagues[27] reported shorter hospital stay for patients undergoing LLR for HCC by as many as 4 days compared with patients undergoing OLR. Similar findings have also been shown by several other studies.[17–21,23] This finding has been established for both minor and major LLRs.[20]

It is well established that the smaller incisions and lesser associated abdominal wall trauma during laparoscopic abdominal surgery lead to less postoperative pain, quicker patient mobility, fewer pulmonary complications, fewer wound infections, and decreased incidence of wound dehiscence.[40,41] All of these factors contribute to improved recovery and decreased hospital length of stay. Each of these contribute to the improved outcomes associated with LLR. The standard incision for OLR is usually a large subcostal or hockey-stick incision that transects the abdominal wall musculature, resulting in increased postoperative pain and painful pulmonary toileting. Also, the laparoscopic approach minimizes the extensive retraction of the lower ribs that is standard practice with OLR. It is likely a combination of all these factors that contribute to decreased postoperative pain and enhanced recovery after LLR that leads to decreased hospital length of stay.

Similar results have been shown with major LLRs that require larger incisions for specimen extraction. During these procedures in which a larger incision is necessary for specimen retrieval, these extraction sites are typically created in the lower abdomen, minimizing postoperative pain and pulmonary complications associated with a right upper quadrant incision. One of the most common extraction sites used in laparoscopic resections is the Pfannenstiel incision, which provides good cosmetic results and low morbidity, with incisional hernia rates reported between 0% and 2%.[42,43] Although most reports reviewed showed lower overall complication rates in LLR than in OLR,[19,23,27] other reports showed equivalent overall complication rates between the two groups.[20,21]

Long-Term Outcomes

Despite the benefits documented with regard to short-term outcomes, it was critical that long-term outcomes were not compromised for LLR to be considered a viable option in the treatment of HCC. Most reports in the literature show equivalent overall and disease-free survival rates between LLR and OLR.[17,18,23,27] These findings of equivalent oncologic outcomes provided further support for the role of LLR in the management of HCC. Some reports have shown superior results with LLR. Chen and colleagues[19] reported a better 5-year survival rate with LLR compared with OLR (Relative Risk = 1.28, 95% confidence interval [CI] 1.01–1.62, $P = .04$). Cheung and colleagues[21] reported statistically significant 1-year, 3-year, and 5-year overall survival improvements with LLR compared with OLR, with reported survival rates of 98.9%, 89.8%, and 83.7% in the LLR group, and 94%, 79.3%, and 67.4% in the OLR group ($P = .033$). The 1-year, 3-year, and 5-year disease-free survival rates were also better for the LLR group, at 87.7%, 65.8%, and 52.2%, and 75.2%, 56.3%, and 47.9% in the OLR group ($P = .141$). The two groups had similar cancer staging on final pathology. On subgroup analysis by HCC stage, the survival differences were significant with stage-II HCC, but not in patients with stage-I HCC, with a 5-year disease-free survival of 54.2% in the LLR group with stage-II HCC, versus 40.1% in the OLR group with the same stage ($P = .045$). The investigators attributed these results to 2 factors: (1) less blood loss in the LLR group, because blood loss is known to be a risk factor for HCC recurrence[44]; and (2) unlike the conventional open approach used, which includes significant mobilization and tissue manipulation before parenchymal transection, the laparoscopic resections used the anterior approach, with parenchymal transection taking place before any significant mobilization and providing a no-touch technique to the resection, which could theoretically lead to better oncological outcomes, and reduced hematogenous dissemination of tumor cells during surgical resection/manipulation.[45,46]

Perhaps not surprising, overall recurrence-free survival after LLR for HCC has been shown to be shorter in patients with advanced cirrhosis compared with patients with early cirrhosis (43 vs 55 months respectively, $P = .034$).[47] However, when examined carefully, the rate of recurrence at the resection margin or in the same segment was not different between the two groups. Hence, the higher recurrence rate in advanced cirrhotic livers probably reflects the carcinogenic effect of advanced cirrhosis, being more prominent than in less cirrhotic livers, which is well established in the literature.[48,49]

Laparoscopic Liver Resection in Cirrhotic Patients

Nearly 80% of HCCs arise in the setting of cirrhotic livers.[6] Hepatectomy in patients with cirrhosis is associated with higher complication rates, including infection, pleural effusion, ascites decompensation, and liver failure,[50–52] thus deterring many surgeons from performing liver resections in patients with signs of advanced cirrhosis. Additional factors adding increased complexity to liver resections in cirrhotic patients include a firm and friable liver parenchyma, portal hypertension and variceal formation, thrombocytopenia, and decreased synthetic function, all of which make hemostasis and resection more challenging. As a result of all these complicating factors, liver resection in cirrhotic patients has been linked to high rates of postoperative mortality, ranging from 1% to 4%, even at high-volume centers.[53–55] Therefore, LLR in the setting of advanced cirrhosis is higher risk, especially given the lack of manual control frequently required for hemostasis in difficult livers. In most centers, Child-Pugh B patients are not considered for LLR.

Despite this, select centers are challenging this dogma and "pushing the envelope" with selection criteria for LLR including patients with signs of advanced cirrhosis. Cipriani and colleagues[47] compared LLR in early well-compensated Child-Pugh A cirrhotic patients with LLR in patients with signs of advanced, decompensated, Child-Pugh B cirrhosis. There was no significant difference between the two groups in blood loss, blood transfusions, operative time, Pringle maneuver duration, overall morbidity, and postoperative mortality. Even liver-specific complications, such as ascites decompensation and postoperative liver failure, were similar between the two groups. Disease-free intervals were significantly shorter in the Child-Pugh B cirrhotic patients compared with the Child A cohort, but overall survival was not significantly different between these two groups. Obviously, these patients should be individually selected for LLR and general recommendations cannot be made based solely on the available data.

Overall it seems that LLR is associated with lower rates of postoperative liver failure and ascites, even in Child B cirrhotics when carefully selected.[52,56,57] Whether this is purely a patient selection phenomenon or a protective effect of the laparoscopic approach remains unknown. Theoretically, the laparoscopic approach could minimize disruption of the collateral circulation by avoiding the large abdominal incision and extensive liver mobilization standard in the open approach.

The safety and efficacy of LLR in cirrhotic patients have been shown in numerous reports.[19,21] Compared with OLR, LLR is associated with a lower incidence of postoperative ascites, decompensation, and liver failure.[52,58] There is some evidence that this may also pertain to major hepatectomies. Xu and colleagues[59] compared patients undergoing major liver resections with either a laparoscopic or open approach. The LLR group had a significantly longer operative time (255 vs 200 min, $P<.001$) but had similar intraoperative blood loss, transfusion requirements, and rates of postoperative complications. One interesting finding was that the incidence of postoperative ascites was significantly less in the LLR group versus the OLR group (9.4 vs 31.3%, $P = .030$). Oncologic outcomes were comparable between the two groups, with similar overall and disease-free survival. Similar findings were seen in a study by

Komatsu and colleagues[60] between patients undergoing open or laparoscopic major hepatectomies. There were no differences in blood loss, transfusion requirements, overall survival, and disease-free survival between the two groups. The biggest difference was seen in overall complication rates, which were significantly higher in the OLR group, with the most common complications being surgical site infection, ascites, decompensation, and liver failure.[60]

Another report, by Beard and colleagues[61] compared LLR for HCC in 80 patients with early (Child A) cirrhosis with 26 patients with advanced cirrhosis (20 Child B and 6 Child C). There were no significant differences between the two patient groups in terms of blood loss, conversion, negative margin rates, length of stay, perioperative complications, 30-day mortality, and 90-day mortality. There was a trend toward longer survival in the early cirrhosis cohort but this did not reach statistical significance (50 vs 21 months, $P = .077$). This finding again shows that LLR can be safely performed in the setting of advanced cirrhosis when patients are carefully selected.

Laparoscopic Resection of Hepatocellular Carcinoma Located in Difficult Segments

As experience with LLR continues to expand, the limits of LLR are continually being pushed. In addition to performing major hepatectomies laparoscopically, which is now standard in select centers, lesions in those difficult, inaccessible segments of the liver are being resected via a laparoscopic approach. Guro and colleagues[62] compared LLR with OLR for HCC located in segments 7 and 8. LLR was associated with less blood loss and shorter hospital stay. There were no statistically significant differences between the two groups in operative time, postoperative complications, rate of negative resection margins, and 3-year overall and disease-free survival rates.

Robotic Approach for Minimally Invasive Liver Resection

With technical feasibility and oncologic safety of LLR for HCC established, robotic liver resections are now increasing. The flexibility and versatility given by the robotic platform make larger and difficultly located tumors amenable to a straightforward minimally invasive resection. In one report, Lai and Tang[63] compared the long-term oncological outcomes of robotic and laparoscopic hepatectomy for HCC. The success rate of major liver resections and resection of posterosuperior segments was significantly higher in the robotic group compared with the laparoscopic group (27% vs 2.9%, and 29% vs 0%, respectively). There were no differences in blood loss, morbidity, mortality, R0 resection rates, or overall and disease-free survival between the two groups. Another series published in 2014 compared robotic (n = 57) and laparoscopic (n = 114) approaches for liver resection in matched cohorts.[64] There were no significant differences between the two groups regarding blood loss, R0 resection rates, postoperative peak bilirubin levels, intensive care unit admission rate, hospital length of stay, and 90-day mortality. The 1 disadvantage noted in the robotic cohort was significantly longer operative time compared with laparoscopic resections (253 vs 199 minutes). However, in the robotic group, significantly more major resections were performed in a purely minimally invasive approach, compared with the laparoscopic resections, which were associated with higher rates of hand-port or hybrid assistance. These emerging data show the safety and efficacy of the robotic approach for liver resection and the authors believe this platform will continue to have an expanding role in the future of liver surgery.

Additional Benefits of Laparoscopic Liver Resection

The risk of recurrence of HCC after liver resection is always a concern and is common with the diseased liver remaining in situ. Therefore, patients may require repeat resections. It is well established that LLR makes future resections easier, because of decreased adhesion formation compared with OLR.[65,66] Some reports have also shown that redo LLRs are associated with better short-term outcomes.[56,67-69] In addition, in general, laparoscopic resections are associated with improved cosmetic results, lower rates of incisional hernias, and quicker return to the patient's life.

Randomized Data

A recent randomized trial directly compared laparoscopic versus open liver resection for HCC.[70] All patients reviewed at a single institution were considered for inclusion if they met the following criteria: solitary HCC less than 5 cm, Child A cirrhosis, tumor located in the peripheral segments (segments 2–6), substantial distance from line of transection, hepatic hilum and vena cava, and able to be treated with limited resections.[70] Ultimately 50 patients were randomized. The study was designed to assess short-term outcomes including margin but also attempted to evaluate recurrence rates. LLR had decreased length of hospital stay. R0 resection rates and complication rates were similar between the two groups. Although not powered to specifically address long-term oncologic outcomes, there were similar recurrence rates and disease-free survival between the two groups. Although small in study size, this study adds additional level 1 evidence for equivalent oncologic outcomes with LLR.

Resection Versus Radiofrequency Ablation for Small Hepatocellular Carcinoma

Local ablation remains a viable treatment option for smaller HCCs for which technical resection is not feasible. For patients with early-stage HCC and early cirrhosis (Child-Pugh class A) the AASLD guidelines recommend resection rather than ablation.[5] The EASL treatment guidelines recommend ablation or resection for patients with solitary HCC less than 2 cm and with preserved liver function and good performance status, whereas tumors between 2 and 5 cm should undergo resection in those patients with preserved liver function and good performance status.[3] The concern with RFA has also been local recurrence and incomplete ablation. This question was addressed in a meta-analysis that evaluated the results of 95 independent series including more than 5000 treated tumors.[71] The local recurrence rate was 3.6% for HCC less than or equal to 3 cm, 21.7% for tumors between 3 and 5 cm, and 50% for tumors greater than 5 cm in diameter.[71] There were 2 particularly interesting findings from this meta-analysis: (1) local recurrence rates are much higher for percutaneous ablation compared with open/laparoscopic at all sizes, and (2) local recurrence rates are prohibitively high for tumors larger than 3 cm in diameter.

To date there have been 4 randomized controlled trials (RCTs) directly comparing surgical resection with ablation.[72-75] In each of these studies overall survival and recurrence-free survival were examined. Two of these studies found no differences in 3-year overall survival (74.8%, 77.5% for resection and 67.2%, 82.5% for ablation) or 3-year recurrence-free survival (61.1%, 41.3% for resection and 49.6%, 55.4% for ablation). Both of these studies included patients with Child A or B cirrhosis and early HCC (1 or 2 tumors, none greater than 4 cm[74]; 3 or fewer tumors, none greater than 3 cm[73]). One additional study found similar results in Child A cirrhotic patients with solitary HCC less than 5 cm with no differences in 4-year overall survival (64% for resection and 65.9% for ablation) or 4-year recurrence-free survival (51.6% for resection and 48.2% for ablation).[72] The largest RCT to date includes 230 patients with HCC within Milan criteria and Child A or B cirrhosis.[75] This study found significantly better 5-year overall survival (75.65% for resection and 54.87% for ablation) and 5-year recurrence-free survival (51.3% for resection and 28.69% for ablation).[75] In a subgroup analysis, overall survival and recurrence-free survival were better with resection for all sizes of HCC (<3 cm, 3–5 cm, multifocal HCC <3 cm).[75] One important point regarding all these RCT data is that the patients included are predominantly Asian with a high prevalence of hepatitis B virus infection. It is unclear how applicable these findings are to the remainder of patients throughout the world.

There are no randomized data available comparing ablation and resection of HCC from Western centers. Recent studies from both the United States and Europe have attempted to address this question but more importantly provide a glimpse of current practice patterns in western institutions. An analysis from the National Cancer Database examined all available patients with solitary HCC less than or equal to 3 cm treated with curative intent.[76] Almost 70% of the approximately 3000 patients underwent local ablation rather than resection. Patients with underlying cirrhosis and increased alpha-fetoprotein levels were more likely to be treated with ablation. In a propensity score–matched cohort there was a significant survival benefit with surgical resection (5-year survival of 54% for resection vs 36% for ablation; hazard ratio = 0.63, 95% CI 0.48–0.81, $P<.001$).[76] A similar study was reported on from 15 different Italian centers examining long-term outcomes of resection versus ablation for solitary HCC less than or equal to 3 cm in patients with Child A cirrhosis. The ablation cohort had a higher incidence of portal hypertension, increased alpha-fetoprotein and total bilirubin levels, and overall lower platelet counts.[77] There were no statistical differences in overall survival or recurrence-free survival between the two groups despite propensity score–matched cohorts. However, local tumor progression was found in 20% of the ablation cohort compared with less than 1% of the resection cohort.

LIVER TRANSPLANT FOR HEPATOCELLULAR CARCINOMA

Liver transplant has the unique advantage of treating both the malignancy as well as the underlying diseased liver, which is ripe for decompensation and HCC recurrence. Selection criteria to optimize the use of available allografts has been an ongoing debate and continues to evolve. Most consensus statements agree that liver transplant should be considered for cirrhotic patients with tumors within Milan criteria (solitary tumor <5 cm or up to 3 tumors not exceeding 3 cm in diameter) that are not candidates for surgical resection.[78] These Milan criteria are currently used as the benchmark for recommendations made in the selection criteria for liver transplant in patients with HCC.[3,5,79,80] Five-year survival after liver transplant for HCC is approximately 70%.[79] Despite complete removal of the native liver, HCC recurrence still occurs in 8% to 20% of recipients.[81]

Liver Transplant Versus Surgical Resection

The decision to pursue liver transplant for treatment of HCC is easy when the underlying liver disease precludes safe surgical resection. Controversy exists over the role of liver transplant in patients that are also candidates for liver resection. There have been 3 large meta-analyses that have examined the available literature comparing outcomes of liver transplant versus liver resection for HCC.[82–84] Five-year overall survival for liver transplant ranged from 61% to 65%, compared with 49% to 56% for liver resection. However, a large portion of the available literature has not been done on an intention-to-treat analysis and therefore important factors such as waitlist mortality and disease progression are not always accounted for. When evaluating the literature performed with an intention-to-treat analysis, there was no difference in 5-year overall survival between liver transplant and resection (56% vs 59%; odds ratio (OR) = 1.19 [0.78–1.8], $P = .42$)[84] and (57.3% vs 58.3%; OR = 0.84 [0.48–1.48], $P = .55$).[83] However, there does seem to be an advantage of liver transplant compared with resection in 5-year disease-free survival (54% vs 49%; OR = 0.75 [0.57–1.0], P = .05).[84]

Dropout rates while awaiting transplant are as high as 25% at 6 months and 38% at 12 months.[85,86] Current treatment strategies attempt to address the increased dropout rates of potential transplant candidates while on the waitlist. The most recent revision of the Organ Procurement and Transplantation Network outlines the exception scores for patients with HCC listed for liver transplant in the United States. Exception points are given for patients with at least 2-cm HCC in the setting of cirrhosis. After 6 months of listing, patients within these criteria are granted exception points and are listed with a Model for End-stage Liver Disease (MELD) score of 28. These patients continue to receive exception points to their MELD score every 6 months but are capped at a MELD score of 34. In addition, locoregional therapy with ablation, transarterial chemoembolization, or yttrium-90 can be used as bridging therapy to avoid disease progression while awaiting transplant.[3,5,79,87] The use of live donor liver transplant has continued to increase over recent years and early reports show excellent outcomes as well lower waitlist dropout rates and decreased wait times.[88]

REFERENCES

1. Bray F, Ferlay J, Soerjomataram I, et al. Global cancer statistics 2018: GLOBOCAN estimates of incidence and mortality worldwide for 36 cancers in 185 countries. CA Cancer J Clin 2018;68(6):394–424.
2. Forner A, Reig M, Bruix J. Hepatocellular carcinoma. Lancet 2018;391(10127): 1301–14.
3. European Association for the Study of the Liver. EASL clinical practice guidelines: management of hepatocellular carcinoma. J Hepatol 2018;69(1):182–236.
4. Llovet JM, Bru C, Bruix J. Prognosis of hepatocellular carcinoma: the BCLC staging classification. Semin Liver Dis 1999;19(3):329–38.
5. Heimbach JK, Kulik LM, Finn RS, et al. AASLD guidelines for the treatment of hepatocellular carcinoma. Hepatology 2018;67(1):358–80.
6. Forner A, Reig ME, de Lope CR, et al. Current strategy for staging and treatment: the BCLC update and future prospects. Semin Liver Dis 2010;30(1): 61–74.
7. Ishizawa T, Hasegawa K, Kokudo N, et al. Risk factors and management of ascites after liver resection to treat hepatocellular carcinoma. Arch Surg 2009; 144(1):46–51.
8. Cucchetti A, Cescon M, Ercolani G, et al. A comprehensive meta-regression analysis on outcome of anatomic resection versus nonanatomic resection for hepatocellular carcinoma. Ann Surg Oncol 2012;19(12):3697–705.
9. Tang CN, Tsui KK, Ha JP, et al. A single-centre experience of 40 laparoscopic liver resections. Hong Kong Med J 2006;12(6):419–25.
10. Bazin JE, Gillart T, Rasson P, et al. Haemodynamic conditions enhancing gas embolism after venous injury during laparoscopy: a study in pigs. Br J Anaesth 1997;78(5):570–5.
11. Wakabayashi G, Cherqui D, Geller DA, et al. Laparoscopic hepatectomy is theoretically better than open hepatectomy: preparing for the 2nd International Consensus Conference on laparoscopic liver resection. J Hepatobiliary Pancreat Sci 2014;21(10):723–31.
12. Nguyen KT, Marsh JW, Tsung A, et al. Comparative benefits of laparoscopic vs open hepatic resection: a critical appraisal. Arch Surg 2011;146(3):348–56.

13. Hashizume M, Takenaka K, Yanaga K, et al. Laparoscopic hepatic resection for hepatocellular carcinoma. Surg Endosc 1995;9(12):1289–91.
14. Buell JF, Cherqui D, Geller DA, et al. The international position on laparoscopic liver surgery: the Louisville Statement, 2008. Ann Surg 2009;250(5):825–30.
15. Wakabayashi G, Cherqui D, Geller DA, et al. Recommendations for laparoscopic liver resection: a report from the second international consensus conference held in Morioka. Ann Surg 2015;261(4):619–29.
16. Nguyen KT, Gamblin TC, Geller DA. World review of laparoscopic liver resection-2,804 patients. Ann Surg 2009;250(5):831–41.
17. Sotiropoulos GC, Prodromidou A, Kostakis ID, et al. Meta-analysis of laparoscopic vs open liver resection for hepatocellular carcinoma. Updates Surg 2017;69(3):291–311.
18. Chang SK, Tay CW, Shen L, et al. Long-term oncological safety of minimally invasive hepatectomy in patients with hepatocellular carcinoma: a case-control study. Ann Acad Med Singapore 2016;45(3):91–7.
19. Chen J, Bai T, Zhang Y, et al. The safety and efficacy of laparoscopic and open hepatectomy in hepatocellular carcinoma patients with liver cirrhosis: a systematic review. Int J Clin Exp Med 2015;8(11):20679–89.
20. Chen J, Li H, Liu F, et al. Surgical outcomes of laparoscopic versus open liver resection for hepatocellular carcinoma for various resection extent. Medicine 2017;96(12):e6460.
21. Cheung TT, Dai WC, Tsang SH, et al. Pure laparoscopic hepatectomy versus open hepatectomy for hepatocellular carcinoma in 110 patients with liver cirrhosis: a propensity analysis at a single center. Ann Surg 2016;264(4):612–20.
22. Fancellu A, Rosman AS, Sanna V, et al. Meta-analysis of trials comparing minimally-invasive and open liver resections for hepatocellular carcinoma. J Surg Res 2011;171(1):e33–45.
23. Han DH, Choi SH, Park EJ, et al. Surgical outcomes after laparoscopic or robotic liver resection in hepatocellular carcinoma: a propensity-score matched analysis with conventional open liver resection. Int J Med Robot 2016;12(4):735–42.
24. Li N, Wu YR, Wu B, et al. Surgical and oncologic outcomes following laparoscopic versus open liver resection for hepatocellular carcinoma: A meta-analysis. Hepatol Res 2012;42(1):51–9.
25. Mirnezami R, Mirnezami AH, Chandrakumaran K, et al. Short- and long-term outcomes after laparoscopic and open hepatic resection: systematic review and meta-analysis. HPB (Oxford) 2011;13(5):295–308.
26. Parks KR, Kuo YH, Davis JM, et al. Laparoscopic versus open liver resection: a meta-analysis of long-term outcome. HPB (Oxford) 2014;16(2):109–18.
27. Takahara T, Wakabayashi G, Beppu T, et al. Long-term and perioperative outcomes of laparoscopic versus open liver resection for hepatocellular carcinoma with propensity score matching: a multi-institutional Japanese study. J Hepatobiliary Pancreat Sci 2015;22(10):721–7.
28. Xiong JJ, Altaf K, Javed MA, et al. Meta-analysis of laparoscopic vs open liver resection for hepatocellular carcinoma. World J Gastroenterol 2012;18(45):6657–68.
29. Yin Z, Fan X, Ye H, et al. Short- and long-term outcomes after laparoscopic and open hepatectomy for hepatocellular carcinoma: a global systematic review and meta-analysis. Ann Surg Oncol 2013;20(4):1203–15.
30. Zhou YM, Shao WY, Zhao YF, et al. Meta-analysis of laparoscopic versus open resection for hepatocellular carcinoma. Dig Dis Sci 2011;56(7):1937–43.

31. Belli G, Fantini C, D'Agostino A, et al. Laparoscopic liver resection without a Pringle maneuver for HCC in cirrhotic patients. Chir Ital 2005;57(1):15–25 [in Italian].

32. Cherqui D, Husson E, Hammoud R, et al. Laparoscopic liver resections: a feasibility study in 30 patients. Ann Surg 2000;232(6):753.

33. Jayaraman S, Khakhar A, Yang H, et al. The association between central venous pressure, pneumoperitoneum, and venous carbon dioxide embolism in laparoscopic hepatectomy. Surg Endosc 2009;23(10):2369–73.

34. Otsuka Y, Katagiri T, Ishii J, et al. Gas embolism in laparoscopic hepatectomy: what is the optimal pneumoperitoneal pressure for laparoscopic major hepatectomy? J Hepatobiliary Pancreat Sci 2013;20(2):137–40.

35. Chiappa A, Bertani E, Biffi R, et al. Effectiveness of LigaSure diathermy coagulation in liver surgery. Surg Technol Int 2008;17:33–8.

36. Gayet B, Cavaliere D, Vibert E, et al. Totally laparoscopic right hepatectomy. Am J Surg 2007;194(5):685–9.

37. Gumbs AA, Gayet B. Totally laparoscopic left hepatectomy. Surg Endosc 2007; 21(7):1221.

38. Jarnagin WR, Gonen M, Fong Y, et al. Improvement in perioperative outcome after hepatic resection: analysis of 1,803 consecutive cases over the past decade. Ann Surg 2002;236(4):397–406 [discussion: 406–97].

39. Kooby DA, Stockman J, Ben-Porat L, et al. Influence of transfusions on perioperative and long-term outcome in patients following hepatic resection for colorectal metastases. Ann Surg 2003;237(6):860.

40. Milsom JW, Böhm B, Hammerhofer KA, et al. A prospective, randomized trial comparing laparoscopic versus conventional techniques in colorectal cancer surgery: a preliminary report. J Am Coll Surg 1998;187(1):46–54.

41. Oshikiri T, Yasuda T, Kawasaki K, et al. Hand-assisted laparoscopic surgery (HALS) is associated with less-restrictive ventilatory impairment and less risk for pulmonary complication than open laparotomy in thoracoscopic esophagectomy. Surgery 2016;159(2):459–66.

42. Domajnko B, Park J, Marecik S, et al. Incisional hernia, midline versus low transverse incision: what is the ideal incision for specimen extraction and hand-assisted laparoscopy? Surg Endosc 2011;25(4):1031–6.

43. Kisielinski K, Conze J, Murken A, et al. The Pfannenstiel or so called "bikini cut": still effective more than 100 years after first description. Hernia 2004;8(3): 177–81.

44. Katz SC, Shia J, Liau KH, et al. Operative blood loss independently predicts recurrence and survival after resection of hepatocellular carcinoma. Ann Surg 2009;249(4):617–23.

45. Hayashi N, Egami H, Kai M, et al. No-touch isolation technique reduces intraoperative shedding of tumor cells into the portal vein during resection of colorectal cancer. Surgery 1999;125(4):369–74.

46. Liu C-L, Fan S-T, Lo C-M, et al. Anterior approach for major right hepatic resection for large hepatocellular carcinoma. Ann Surg 2000;232(1):25.

47. Cipriani F, Fantini C, Ratti F, et al. Laparoscopic liver resections for hepatocellular carcinoma. Can we extend the surgical indication in cirrhotic patients? Surg Endosc 2018;32(2):617–26.

48. Poon RTP, Fan ST, Ng IOL, et al. Different risk factors and prognosis for early and late intrahepatic recurrence after resection of hepatocellular carcinoma. Cancer 2000;89(3):500–7.

49. Taura K, Ikai I, Hatano E, et al. Influence of coexisting cirrhosis on outcomes after partial hepatic resection for hepatocellular carcinoma fulfilling the Milan criteria: an analysis of 293 patients. Surgery 2007;142(5):685–94.
50. Chirica M, Scatton O, Massault P-P, et al. Treatment of stage IVA hepatocellular carcinoma: should we reappraise the role of surgery? Arch Surg 2008;143(6): 538–43.
51. Farges O, Malassagne B, Flejou JF, et al. Risk of major liver resection in patients with underlying chronic liver disease: a reappraisal. Ann Surg 1999;229(2):210.
52. Kanazawa A, Tsukamoto T, Shimizu S, et al. Impact of laparoscopic liver resection for hepatocellular carcinoma with F4-liver cirrhosis. Surg Endosc 2013; 27(7):2592–7.
53. Belghiti J, Hiramatsu K, Benoist S, et al. Seven hundred forty-seven hepatectomies in the 1990s: an update to evaluate the actual risk of liver resection1. J Am Coll Surg 2000;191(1):38–46.
54. Fan S. Problems of hepatectomy in cirrhosis. Hepatogastroenterology 1998; 45(3):1288–90.
55. Vauthey J-N, Dixon E, Abdalla EK, et al. Pretreatment assessment of hepatocellular carcinoma: expert consensus statement. HPB (Oxford) 2010;12(5):289–99.
56. Belli G, Fantini C, D'agostino A, et al. Laparoscopic versus open liver resection for hepatocellular carcinoma in patients with histologically proven cirrhosis: short-and middle-term results. Surg Endosc 2007;21(11):2004–11.
57. Tranchart H, Di Giuro G, Lainas P, et al. Laparoscopic resection for hepatocellular carcinoma: a matched-pair comparative study. Surg Endosc 2010;24(5): 1170–6.
58. Morise Z, Ciria R, Cherqui D, et al. Can we expand the indications for laparoscopic liver resection? A systematic review and meta-analysis of laparoscopic liver resection for patients with hepatocellular carcinoma and chronic liver disease. J Hepatobiliary Pancreat Sci 2015;22(5):342–52.
59. Xu H-W, Liu F, Li H-Y, et al. Outcomes following laparoscopic versus open major hepatectomy for hepatocellular carcinoma in patients with cirrhosis: a propensity score-matched analysis. Surg Endosc 2018;32(2):712–9.
60. Komatsu S, Brustia R, Goumard C, et al. Laparoscopic versus open major hepatectomy for hepatocellular carcinoma: a matched pair analysis. Surg Endosc 2016;30(5):1965–74.
61. Beard RE, Wang Y, Khan S, et al. Laparoscopic liver resection for hepatocellular carcinoma in early and advanced cirrhosis. HPB (Oxford) 2018;20(6):521–9.
62. Guro H, Cho JY, Han H-S, et al. Laparoscopic liver resection of hepatocellular carcinoma located in segments 7 or 8. Surg Endosc 2018;32(2):872–8.
63. Lai EC, Tang CN. Long-term survival analysis of robotic versus conventional laparoscopic hepatectomy for hepatocellular carcinoma: a comparative study. Surg Laparosc Endosc Percutan Tech 2016;26(2):162–6.
64. Tsung A, Geller DA, Sukato DC, et al. Robotic versus laparoscopic hepatectomy: a matched comparison. Ann Surg 2014;259(3):549–55.
65. Laurent A, Tayar C, Andréoletti M, et al. Laparoscopic liver resection facilitates salvage liver transplantation for hepatocellular carcinoma. J Hepatobiliary Pancreat Surg 2009;16(3):310–4.
66. Soubrane O, Goumard C, Laurent A, et al. Laparoscopic resection of hepatocellular carcinoma: a French survey in 351 patients. HPB (Oxford) 2014;16(4): 357–65.
67. Hu M, Zhao G, Xu D, et al. Laparoscopic repeat resection of recurrent hepatocellular carcinoma. World J Surg 2011;35(3):648–55.

68. Kazaryan AM, Marangos IP, Rosseland AR, et al. Laparoscopic liver resection for malignant and benign lesions: ten-year Norwegian single-center experience. Arch Surg 2010;145(1):34–40.

69. Shelat V, Serin K, Samim M, et al. Outcomes of repeat laparoscopic liver resection compared to the primary resection. World J Surg 2014;38(12):3175–80.

70. El-Gendi A, El-Shafei M, El-Gendi S, et al. Laparoscopic versus open hepatic resection for solitary hepatocellular carcinoma less than 5 cm in cirrhotic patients: a randomized controlled study. J Laparoendosc Adv Surg Tech A 2018;28(3):302–10.

71. Mulier S, Ni Y, Jamart J, et al. Local recurrence after hepatic radiofrequency coagulation: multivariate meta-analysis and review of contributing factors. Ann Surg 2005;242(2):158–71.

72. Chen MS, Li JQ, Zheng Y, et al. A prospective randomized trial comparing percutaneous local ablative therapy and partial hepatectomy for small hepatocellular carcinoma. Ann Surg 2006;243(3):321–8.

73. Fang Y, Chen W, Liang X, et al. Comparison of long-term effectiveness and complications of radiofrequency ablation with hepatectomy for small hepatocellular carcinoma. J Gastroenterol Hepatol 2014;29(1):193–200.

74. Feng K, Yan J, Li X, et al. A randomized controlled trial of radiofrequency ablation and surgical resection in the treatment of small hepatocellular carcinoma. J Hepatol 2012;57(4):794–802.

75. Huang J, Yan L, Cheng Z, et al. A randomized trial comparing radiofrequency ablation and surgical resection for HCC conforming to the Milan criteria. Ann Surg 2010;252(6):903–12.

76. Miura JT, Johnston FM, Tsai S, et al. Surgical resection versus ablation for hepatocellular carcinoma ≤ 3 cm: a population-based analysis. HPB (Oxford) 2015; 17(10):896–901.

77. Pompili M, Saviano A, de Matthaeis N, et al. Long-term effectiveness of resection and radiofrequency ablation for single hepatocellular carcinoma ≤3 cm. Results of a multicenter Italian survey. J Hepatol 2013;59(1):89–97.

78. Mazzaferro V, Regalia E, Doci R, et al. Liver transplantation for the treatment of small hepatocellular carcinomas in patients with cirrhosis. N Engl J Med 1996; 334(11):693–9.

79. Clavien PA, Lesurtel M, Bossuyt PM, et al. Recommendations for liver transplantation for hepatocellular carcinoma: an international consensus conference report. Lancet Oncol 2012;13(1):e11–22.

80. Jarnagin W, Chapman WC, Curley S, et al. Surgical treatment of hepatocellular carcinoma: expert consensus statement. HPB (Oxford) 2010;12(5):302–10.

81. Zimmerman MA, Ghobrial RM, Tong MJ, et al. Recurrence of hepatocellular carcinoma following liver transplantation: a review of preoperative and postoperative prognostic indicators. Arch Surg 2008;143(2):182–8 [discussion: 188].

82. Dhir M, Lyden ER, Smith LM, et al. Comparison of outcomes of transplantation and resection in patients with early hepatocellular carcinoma: a meta-analysis. HPB (Oxford) 2012;14(9):635–45.

83. Proneth A, Zeman F, Schlitt HJ, et al. Is resection or transplantation the ideal treatment in patients with hepatocellular carcinoma in cirrhosis if both are possible? A systematic review and metaanalysis. Ann Surg Oncol 2014;21(9): 3096–107.

84. Rahman A, Assifi MM, Pedroso FE, et al. Is resection equivalent to transplantation for early cirrhotic patients with hepatocellular carcinoma? A meta-analysis. J Gastrointest Surg 2012;16(10):1897–909.

85. Park SJ, Freise CE, Hirose R, et al. Risk factors for liver transplant waitlist dropout in patients with hepatocellular carcinoma. Clin Transplant 2012;26(4): E359–64.
86. Yao FY, Bass NM, Nikolai B, et al. A follow-up analysis of the pattern and predictors of dropout from the waiting list for liver transplantation in patients with hepatocellular carcinoma: implications for the current organ allocation policy. Liver Transpl 2003;9(7):684–92.
87. Heckman JT, Devera MB, Marsh JW, et al. Bridging locoregional therapy for hepatocellular carcinoma prior to liver transplantation. Ann Surg Oncol 2008; 15(11):3169–77.
88. Goldaracena N, Gorgen A, Doyle A, et al. Live donor liver transplantation for patients with hepatocellular carcinoma offers increased survival vs. deceased donation. J Hepatol 2019;70(4):666–73.
89. Kim H, Suh K-S, Lee K-W, et al. Long-term outcome of laparoscopic versus open liver resection for hepatocellular carcinoma: a case-controlled study with propensity score matching. Surg Endosc 2014;28(3):950–60.
90. Cheung TT, Poon RT, Yuen WK, et al. Long-term survival analysis of pure laparoscopic versus open hepatectomy for hepatocellular carcinoma in patients with cirrhosis: a single-center experience. Ann Surg 2013;257(3):506–11.
91. Ker C, Chen J, Kuo K, et al. Liver surgery for hepatocellular carcinoma: laparoscopic versus open approach. Int J Hepatol 2011;2011:596792.
92. Truant S, Bouras A, Hebbar M, et al. Laparoscopic resection vs. open liver resection for peripheral hepatocellular carcinoma in patients with chronic liver disease: a case-matched study. Surg Endosc 2011;25(11):3668–77.
93. Lee KF, Chong CN, Wong J, et al. Long-term results of laparoscopic hepatectomy versus open hepatectomy for hepatocellular carcinoma: a case-matched analysis. World J Surg 2011;35(10):2268.
94. Hu B-S, Chen K, Tan H-M, et al. Comparison of laparoscopic vs open liver lobectomy (segmentectomy) for hepatocellular carcinoma. World J Gastroenterol 2011;17(42):4725.
95. Sarpel U, Hefti M, Wisnievsky J, et al. Outcome for patients treated with laparoscopic versus open resection of hepatocellular carcinoma: case-matched analysis. Ann Surg Oncol 2009;16(6):1572–7.
96. Endo Y, Ohta M, Sasaki A, et al. A comparative study of the long-term outcomes after laparoscopy-assisted and open left lateral hepatectomy for hepatocellular carcinoma. Surg Laparosc Endosc Percutan Tech 2009;19(5):e171–4.
97. Cai XJ, Yang J, Yu H, et al. Clinical study of laparoscopic versus open hepatectomy for malignant liver tumors. Surg Endosc 2008;22(11):2350–6.
98. Kaneko H, Takagi S, Otsuka Y, et al. Laparoscopic liver resection of hepatocellular carcinoma. Am J Surg 2005;189(2):190–4.
99. Shimada M, Hashizume M, Maehara S, et al. Laparoscopic hepatectomy for hepatocellular carcinoma. Surg Endosc 2001;15(6):541–4.
100. Mizuguchi T, Kawamoto M, Meguro M, et al. Laparoscopic hepatectomy: a systematic review, meta-analysis, and power analysis. Surg Today 2011;41(1): 39–47.

Staging of Biliary and Primary Liver Tumors
Current Recommendations and Workup

Geoffrey W. Krampitz, MD, PhD[a],
Thomas A. Aloia, MD, MHCM, FACS[b],*

KEYWORDS

- Hepatobiliary • Cholangiocarcinoma • Hepatocellular • Gallbladder • Liver • Cancer
- Carcinoma • Staging

KEY POINTS

- Patients with hepatobiliary malignancies may present with vague abdominal symptoms that require a high index of suspicion to make a timely diagnosis.
- Serum tumor markers carbohydrate antigen (CA) 19 to 9, carcinoembryonic antigen (CEA), and alpha-fetoprotein (AFP) should be obtained as part of the initial workup and surveillance but are not diagnostic.
- Contrast-enhanced multiphasic computed tomography (CT), MRI, MRI with cholangio-pancreatocholangiography (MRI/MRCP), and in some instances, fluorodeoxyglucose positron emission tomography (FDG-PET-CT) are useful imaging modalities in preoperative staging evaluation.
- Definitive tissue pathologic diagnosis is not always necessary in patients for whom surgery is planned but is often required before chemotherapy or radiation therapy.
- Surgical staging may identify occult metastatic disease that precludes radical resection, and adequate lymphadenectomy may better inform prognosis and treatment.

INTRODUCTION

Hepatobiliary cancers are a diverse group of malignant neoplasms involving the liver, gallbladder, and bile ducts. Biliary tract cancers arise from the biliary ductal and gallbladder epithelium and include intrahepatic cholangiocarcinomas, extrahepatic (perihilar or distal) cholangiocarcinomas, and gallbladder carcinomas.[1,2] Hepatocellular carcinoma is the most common primary liver malignancy and arises from hepatocytes.

Disclosures: None.
[a] Department of Surgery, Thomas Jefferson University, 1015 Walnut Street, Curtis Building, Suite 620, Philadelphia, PA 19107, USA; [b] Department of Surgical Oncology, University of Texas, MD Anderson Cancer Center, 1440 Pressler Street, Unit 1484, Houston, TX 77030, USA
* Corresponding author.
E-mail address: TAAloia@mdanderson.org

Surg Oncol Clin N Am 28 (2019) 663–683
https://doi.org/10.1016/j.soc.2019.06.007
1055-3207/19/Published by Elsevier Inc.

surgonc.theclinics.com

Hepatobiliary cancers are the second leading cause of cancer-related deaths worldwide.[3] The causes of these cancers are multifactorial and include germline mutations, genotoxic substances, inherited diseases, steatohepatic disease, and infectious agents. The incidence of these cancers is increasing in large part as a result of improved recognition of risk factors and enhanced methods for disease detection. Nevertheless, the overall prognosis of these tumors remains poor because many patients present with advanced disease at diagnosis. A critical step in the management of patients with hepatobiliary cancers is performing a proper workup and obtaining accurate staging to guide appropriate treatment.

HEPATOCELLULAR CARCINOMA
Incidence and Outcomes

Hepatocellular carcinoma is the fifth most common cancer and has the third highest mortality of any cancer worldwide.[4] Although the burden of hepatocellular carcinoma is highest in developing countries, the incidence is rising in the United States and is expected to continue to rise for the next 2 decades.[5–7] Approximately one-third of patients with cirrhosis due to hepatitis C will eventually develop hepatocellular carcinoma.[8] Obesity also appears to be an emerging significant risk factor for the development of hepatocellular carcinoma and interacts synergistically with both alcohol and tobacco use to further increase the risk.[9,10] For patients affected by this often-devastating disease, surgical therapy represents the only hope for cure.

Patient Presentation and Initial Workup

Patients with hepatocellular carcinoma may present with sequelae of cirrhosis, including fatigue, coagulopathies, anorexia, ascites, peripheral edema, weight loss, pruritis, and jaundice. Preexisting cirrhosis is found in more than 80% of patients diagnosed with hepatocellular carcinoma.[11] Consequently, patients with cirrhosis are at highest risk for developing hepatocellular carcinoma and should undergo surveillance consisting of liver ultrasound with or without alpha-fetoprotein (AFP) every 6 months.[12] If a screening liver ultrasound identifies a lesion measuring ≥10 mm, further investigation is warranted. A 10-mm threshold is used because lesions smaller than 10 mm are rarely malignant, whereas lesions ≥10 mm have a substantial likelihood of being malignant.[13] AFP levels more than 20 ng/mL should also prompt further investigation, whereas those less than 20 ng/mL are considered negative.[14] A threshold of 20 ng/mL provides a sensitivity of approximately 60% and a specificity of approximately 90%.[14]

Staging Imaging

The diagnosis of hepatocellular carcinoma can be established, and treatment rendered, based on characteristic findings on cross-sectional imaging studies and without biopsy confirmation. In at-risk patients with abnormal surveillance test results or a clinical suspicion of hepatocellular carcinoma, multiphase computed tomography (CT) or MRI is recommended for initial diagnostic testing. The American College of Radiology CT/MRI Liver Imaging Reporting And Data System (CT/MRI LI-RADS) provides guidelines for how multiphase CT and MR examinations should be performed, interpreted, and reported (**Fig. 1**).[15] Lesions >10 mm visible on multiphase studies are assigned category codes reflecting their relative probability of being benign, hepatocellular carcinoma, or other hepatic malignant neoplasm. LI-RADS 1 indicates definitely benign lesions, such as cysts and typical hemangiomas. LI-RADS 2 indicates probably benign lesions, such as atypical hemangiomas and focal parenchymal

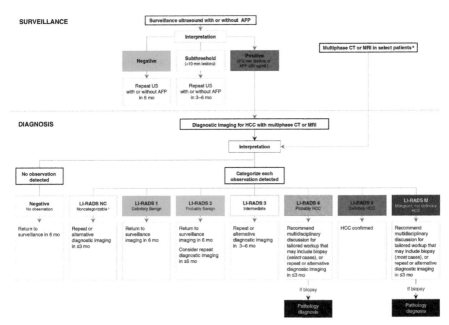

Fig. 1. American Association for the Study of Liver Diseases (AASLD) surveillance and diagnostic algorithm. HCC, hepatocellular carcinoma; US, ultrasound. [a] Multiphase CT or MRI in select patients: Some high-risk patients may undergo multiphase CT or MRI for HCC surveillance (depending on patient body habitus, visibility of liver at ultrasound, being on the transplant waiting list, and other factors). [b] Noncategorizable: These are due to technical problem such as image omission or severe degradation. (*From* J. Marrero, L. Kulik, C. Sirlin, et all. Diagnosis, Staging, and Management of Hepatocellular Carcinoma: 2018 Practice Guidance by the American Association for the Study of Liver Diseases. 2019; with permission.)

abnormalities likely attributable to underlying cirrhosis. LI-RADS 3 corresponds to a low probability of hepatocellular carcinoma, including benign and malignant entities. LI-RADS 4 indicates probable hepatocellular carcinoma. Imaging features diagnostic of hepatocellular carcinoma (LI-RADS 5) include size $\geq$20 mm with arterial phase hyperenhancement and either nonperipheral "washout," enhancing capsule, or an increase in size by $\geq$50% in $\leq$6 months. In addition, smaller lesions (10–19 mm) with all of the previously mentioned features are also highly suspicious. LI-RADS M corresponds to lesions with features highly suggestive or even diagnostic of malignancy, but not specific for hepatocellular carcinoma. The average probabilities of hepatocellular carcinoma for LI-RADS 1, 2, 3, 4, 5, and M are 0%, 11%, 33%, 80%, 96%, and 42%, respectively.[16–21] Furthermore, cross-sectional imaging is important in identifying possible extrahepatic disease.

Pathologic Diagnosis

Liver biopsy should be considered in patients with a liver mass whose appearance is not typical for hepatocellular carcinoma on multiphasic contrast-enhanced imaging (LI-RADS 4 or M). The histologic evaluation of hepatocellular carcinoma is challenging, as often it arises in equivocal nodular lesions, such as dysplastic nodules in the cirrhotic liver and are highly differentiated in the early stages. The classic histomorphologic features of hepatocellular carcinoma are well vascularized tumors with wide trabeculae (>3 cells), prominent acinar pattern, small cell changes, cytologic atypia, mitotic activity, vascular invasion, absence of Kupffer cells, and the loss of the reticulin network.[22] Immunostaining for several biomarkers, including glypican-3 (GPC3), heat shock protein 70 (HSP70), and glutamine synthetase may be helpful to distinguish hepatocellular carcinoma from high-grade dysplastic nodules.[23,24]

Staging Classification

The Barcelona-Clinic Liver Cancer (BCLC) staging system incorporates tumor-related variables (number, size, presence of vascular invasion, involvement of lymph nodes, and presence of metastases), liver function (Child-Pugh score), and patient functional status (Eastern Cooperative Oncology Group [ECOG]) to classify patients into 5 stages (0, A, B, C, and D) and recommend appropriate treatment strategies for specific prognostic classifications (**Fig. 2**).[25–27] Consequently, it is the preferred clinical staging system for the management of hepatocellular carcinoma. Patients classified as stage 0 are Child-Pugh A with an ECOG of 0 and have a single tumor <2 cm in size. Such patients are appropriate candidates for liver resection. Stage A patients are Child-Pugh A or B with a performance status of 0 and have 1 to 3 tumors, all ≤3 cm. These patients are candidates for resection, liver transplantation, or ablative therapies.

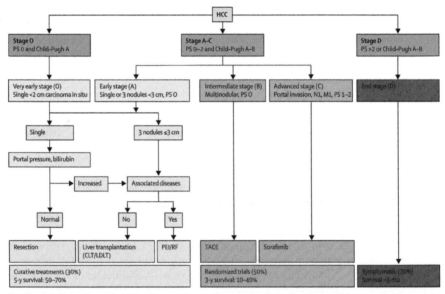

Fig. 2. BCLC staging classification and treatment schedule. Patients with very early hepatocellular carcinoma (HCC) (stage 0) are optimal candidates for resection. Patients with early hepatocellular carcinoma (stage A) are candidates for radical therapy (resection, liver transplantation [LT], or local ablation via percutaneous ethanol injection [PEI] or radiofrequency [RF] ablation). Patients with intermediate hepatocellular carcinoma (stage B) benefit from transarterial chemoembolization (TACE). Patients with advanced hepatocellular carcinoma, defined as presence of macroscopic vascular invasion, extrahepatic spread, or cancer-related symptoms (ECOG performance status 1 or 2) (stage C), benefit from sorafenib. Patients with end-stage disease (stage D) will receive symptomatic treatment. Treatment strategy will transition from one stage to another on treatment failure or contraindications for the procedures. CLT, cadaveric liver transplantation; LDLT, living donor liver transplantation; PS, performance status. (*Reprinted with permission from* Elsevier (The Lancet, Bruix J, Llovet JM. Major achievements in hepatocellular carcinoma. Lancet. 2009;373(9664):614–616.))

Together these 2 groups of patients have an expected median overall survival of 60 months or longer.[27] Stage B patients are also Child-Pugh A-B with a performance status of 0, but have multinodular tumors and so are not candidates for curative therapy and have an expected median overall survival of approximately 20 months. Patients in this class are most frequently treated with chemoembolization. Patients who are stage C are also Child-Pugh A-B, but have a lower performance status of 1 to 2 and have portal vein invasion, positive lymph nodes, or metastatic disease and, thus, have an expected median overall survival of only 11 months. Such patients would be considered for treatment with sorafenib.[27] Stage D patients are terminal patients with a performance status greater than 2 and Child-Pugh C, have a limited survival of less than 3 months, and should be treated with best supportive care.[27]

Determining Resectability

Most patients with hepatocellular carcinoma have some degree of compromised liver function that may represent a contraindication to an otherwise anatomically feasible resection. Consequently, a careful preoperative assessment is critical for these patients and must include an evaluation of medical comorbidities, tumor location, baseline liver function, and tumor biology.

In general, liver tumors are technically resectable if they can be removed with negative margins while preserving a sufficient liver remnant with adequate hepatic arterial and portal venous inflow, venous outflow, biliary drainage, and sufficient parenchyma to support critical liver functions.[28] However, determination of what constitutes "sufficient remnant parenchyma" necessitates an understanding of the baseline liver function of patients with hepatocellular carcinoma. Patients with fibrosis or cirrhosis, encompassing most patients with hepatocellular carcinoma, have increased risk of death following major hepatectomy compared with patients with normal background liver parenchyma.[29] Previous studies evaluating the percent functional liver remnant relative to the standardized liver volume required for preventing postoperative liver-related mortality advocate persevering a minimum 20% for patients with normal livers and 40% for patients with cirrhosis.[30–33] Although these thresholds are useful guidelines, they are not a direct reflection of liver function. Some investigators advocate using indocyanine green retention testing as a direct measure of liver function. In the absence of this test, patients with marginal functional liver remnant are recommended to have preoperative portal vein embolization performed, as this allows the surgeon to test the regenerative capacity of the liver before operative intervention.

The presence of portal hypertension in cirrhotic patients being considered for possible liver resection should be carefully evaluated, as it is one of the strongest predictors of poor outcome.[25,34] A thorough history in patients with advanced cirrhosis and portal hypertension may reveal encephalopathy, gastrointestinal bleeding, easy bruisability, and ascites. Prothrombin time and serum albumin should be obtained to determine a Childs-Turcotte-Pugh score.[35] Portal hypertension is also characterized by a hepatic venous pressure gradient ≥ 10 mm Hg, the presence of esophageal varices or splenomegaly, and thrombocytopenia (platelet count $<100,000/mm^3$). Preoperative imaging should be carefully evaluated for the presence of varices and/or splenomegaly and in patients at high risk of portal hypertension, direct measurement of the hepatic venous pressure gradient should be considered.[36]

The Model for End-Stage Liver Disease score incorporating serum creatinine, bilirubin, and international normalized ratio is predictive of survival in patients with cirrhosis and has been adopted as a means of prioritizing patients for liver transplantation.[37] Although it does not account for tumor characteristics, its powerful stratification of severity of liver disease makes it useful for most patients with hepatocellular carcinoma.[38,39]

The presence of extrahepatic disease precluding surgical intervention should be evaluated using MRI and/or CT.[34] Furthermore, preoperative MRI should be examined to determine the number and location of tumors, as well as the relationship of the lesions to major vascular structures within the liver.[34] In addition, intraoperative ultrasound should be used to confirm the number and location of the tumor(s) as well as the anatomy of the major vascular structures within the liver immediately before resection.

INTRAHEPATIC CHOLANGIOCARCINOMA
Incidence and Outcomes

Cholangiocarcinoma is an aggressive epithelial malignancy of the bile ducts and is the second most common primary liver tumor.[40] Cholangiocarcinoma can arise from anywhere in the biliary tract and is subclassified anatomically, with intrahepatic cholangiocarcinoma arising from within the liver and extrahepatic cholangiocarcinoma arising from the extrahepatic bile ducts. Intrahepatic cholangiocarcinoma makes up 8% to 10% of cholangiocarcinoma and 10% to 20% of all primary liver tumors. A recent 40-year analysis of trends in cholangiocarcinoma determined that the incidence of intrahepatic cholangiocarcinoma is increasing, whereas the incidence of extrahepatic cholangiocarcinoma has remained relatively stable.[41] Currently, the incidence of intrahepatic cholangiocarcinoma is 1.18 cases per 100,000 population in the United States. There are a number of risk factors associated with intrahepatic cholangiocarcinoma, including chemical exposure, liver flukes, biliary tract disease, viral hepatitis, metabolic syndrome, lifestyle factors, and cirrhosis. Nevertheless, a substantial number of patients do not have any identifiable risk factors. Overall, patients with intrahepatic cholangiocarcinoma have a poor prognosis, in large part because most patients present with advanced disease that is not amenable to surgical resection. Unresectable intrahepatic cholangiocarcinoma has a median survival of only 6 to 9 months.[42–44] Although complete resection is the only hope of long-term cure, the 5-year overall survival of patients after resection ranged from 20% to 39% in a number of series.[45–49]

Patient Presentation and Initial Workup

Patients with early-stage disease are usually asymptomatic. Patients may present with nonspecific symptoms such as abdominal discomfort and malaise. With advanced disease, patients may develop weight loss, hepatomegaly, or palpable abdominal mass. Because patients with intrahepatic cholangiocarcinoma typically do not develop biliary tract obstruction, preliminary laboratory studies may not show any abnormality. Plasma serum tumor markers carbohydrate antigen (CA) 19-9 and carcinoembryonic antigen (CEA) have a high specificity but low sensitivity for intrahepatic cholangiocarcinoma. Although they should be included in the initial workup for intrahepatic cholangiocarcinoma, normal results are not sufficiently sensitive to definitively diagnose or rule out intrahepatic cholangiocarcinoma.[50,51] A typical patient presentation will prompt an abdominal ultrasound that usually will show a hypoechoic mass and may be associated with peripheral ductal dilatation. Hyperenhancement on contrast-enhanced ultrasound can identify tumors but lack specificity for intrahepatic cholangiocarcinoma.[52]

Staging Imaging

Multiphasic CT is often the first cross-sectional imaging modality used to evaluate patients presenting with intrahepatic cholangiocarcinoma. Tumors typically appear as a hypodense hepatic mass with irregular margins in the unenhanced phase, peripheral rim enhancement in the arterial phase, and progressive hyperattenuation on venous and delayed phases.[53] The progressive contrast uptake from the arterial to the venous phase with increased update in the delayed phase is characteristic of intrahepatic cholangiocarcinoma and may reflect fibrosis that is slow to enhance but retains the intravenous contrast agent. On MRI, intrahepatic cholangiocarcinoma appears as hypointense on T1-weighted imaging and hyperintense, often with a central hypointensity corresponding to areas of fibrosis, on T2-weighted imaging.[54] MRI with cholangiopancreatography (MRI/MRCP) may be helpful in delineating the ductal system and vascular structures and thus determining the anatomic extent of the tumor. Because intrahepatic cholangiocarcinoma is almost always (up to 90%) FDG-avid, PET-CT has a high sensitivity for detecting mass-forming intrahepatic cholangiocarcinoma; however, PET-CT is less useful in detecting infiltrating intrahepatic cholangiocarcinoma tumors. Some studies have suggested the use of PET-CT may identify occult metastatic disease in up to 20% to 30% of patients and may help to rule out an occult primary tumor.[55–57] However, the routine use of PET-CT in the absence of questionable or concerning features on CT or MRI remains controversial.

Pathologic Diagnosis

Although definitive diagnosis requires pathologic evidence of intrahepatic cholangiocarcinoma, obtaining a tissue biopsy is not routinely recommended or necessary in all patients for whom surgery is planned. Often, clinical suspicion, laboratory analysis, and radiologic evaluation is all that is required to proceed with surgical removal. This is in contrast to patients with unresectable tumors undergoing systemic chemotherapy or radiation therapy, in which a tissue diagnosis is required. A "negative" biopsy does not necessarily exclude intrahepatic cholangiocarcinoma given the potential for sampling error. Typically, pathologic analysis of biopsy specimens reveals adenocarcinoma, and the challenge is differentiating primary intrahepatic cholangiocarcinoma from metastasis from other gastrointestinal or pancreatic primary tumors, often requiring additional immunohistochemical evaluation.

When pathologic evaluation with extended immunohistochemical analysis corresponds with imaging characteristic to support a diagnosis of intrahepatic cholangiocarcinoma, proceeding expeditiously to definitive treatment is recommended. However, when the results of pathology and imaging are incongruous and cannot distinguish between primary intrahepatic cholangiocarcinoma and metastatic disease, additional workup is necessary to rule out metastatic disease from an occult primary tumor. Cross-sectional imaging of the chest, abdomen, and pelvis; colonoscopy; and upper endoscopy are recommended to rule out a primary gastrointestinal tumor. Careful evaluation of the pancreas and portal and celiac lymph nodes on cross-sectional imaging is warranted, and any abnormality should be followed with an endoscopic ultrasound (EUS) with fine-needle aspiration (FNA). In women, a mammogram should be performed to evaluate for breast cancer as well as a transvaginal ultrasound for gynecologic malignancy.

Staging Classification

Historically, intrahepatic cholangiocarcinoma was staged according to the criteria derived for patients with hepatocellular carcinoma. Recognition of the biological and epidemiologic differences between hepatocellular carcinoma and intrahepatic cholangiocarcinoma led to the development of a distinct tumor, node, metastasis (TNM) staging system for intrahepatic cholangiocarcinoma that has been updated in the Eighth Edition of the American Joint Commission on Cancer (AJCC) Cancer

Staging Manual.[58] T1a tumors are solitary, ≤5 cm, and without vascular invasion. T1b tumors are solitary, larger than 5 cm, and without vascular invasion. T2 tumors are solitary tumors with intrahepatic vascular invasion or multiple tumors with or without vascular invasion. T3 tumors perforate the visceral peritoneum. T4 tumors involve local extrahepatic structures by direct invasion. N0 indicates no regional lymph node metastasis, whereas N1 corresponds to the presence of regional lymph node metastasis. M0 corresponds to the absence of distant metastasis, whereas M1 indicates distant metastasis including involvement of N2 nodal basins. Stage IA corresponds to T1a N0 M0. Stage IB corresponds to T1b N0 M0. Stage II corresponds to T2 N0 M0. Stage IIIA corresponds to T3 N0 M0. Stage IIIB corresponds to T4 N0 M0 or Any T N1 M0. Stage IV corresponds to Any T Any N M1.[59] The prognostic significance of the most recent staging system has been independently validated.[60–62]

Surgical Staging

Staging laparoscopy identified occult metastatic disease precluding surgical resection in 25% to 36% of patients with intrahepatic cholangiocarcinoma.[63,64] Consequently, a substantial number of patients with unresectable disease would benefit from staging laparoscopy. Thus, staging laparoscopy with or without the use of laparoscopic ultrasound should be routinely used in patients with high-risk features for occult metastatic disease. These features include multicentric disease, high CA 19-9 levels, questionable vascular invasion, or suspicion of peritoneal disease that may be optimally evaluated with laparoscopy or laparoscopic ultrasound.

Lymph node metastases may be present in up to 25% to 50% of patients undergoing resection for intrahepatic cholangiocarcinoma and is one of the strongest predictors of early disease recurrence and poor outcomes.[65–67] The regional lymph node stations most likely to be involved depend on the laterality of the tumor within the liver.[68] Intrahepatic cholangiocarcinoma of the left liver primarily drains to the inferior phrenic, hilar (common bile duct, hepatic artery, portal vein, and cystic duct), and gastrohepatic lymph nodes. In contrast, intrahepatic cholangiocarcinomas of the right liver preferentially drain to the hilar, periduodenal, and peripancreatic lymph node basins.[69] For all intrahepatic cholangiocarcinomas, spread to the celiac, periaortic, and/or pericaval lymph nodes is considered distant metastatic disease (M1). Because of the prognostic importance of nodal disease status, routine lymphadenectomy at the time of hepatic resection for intrahepatic cholangiocarcinoma is strongly recommended.[70–73]

Determining Resectability

Tumors that may be completely removed with negative histologic margins while preserving a sufficient liver remnant (minimum of 2 contiguous segments with adequate vascular inflow/outflow and biliary drainage) and without any evidence of extrahepatic disease are potentially resectable.[74–76] Involvement of lymph nodes beyond the regional lymph node basins and into the celiac, periaortic, and/or pericaval lymph nodes is considered metastatic disease and a contraindication to resection. In addition, patients with bilateral multifocal or multicentric disease are considered unresectable.[77,78] Given these criteria, negative-margin (R0) resection rates can approach 85% with an aggressive surgical approach that often involves a major or extended hepatectomy (in up to 70% of cases) or a concomitant bile duct (in up to 20% of cases) or vascular resection (in up to 5% of cases).[74] With proper patient selection, rates of 5-year survival following resection range from 30% to 40%.[45,74,78–80]

PERIHILAR CHOLANGIOCARCINOMA
Incidence and Outcomes

Cholangiocarcinoma may arise anywhere within the biliary tree, but tumors involving the biliary confluence (perihilar cholangiocarcinoma) are the most common, accounting for 60% of cholangiocarcinoma, with approximately 3000 cases annually in the United States. Most cases of cholangiocarcinoma are sporadic, although a number of conditions confer an increased risk. Among the risk factors for cholangiocarcinoma are primary biliary sclerosis, an autoimmune periductal inflammation resulting in multifocal strictures of the intrahepatic and extrahepatic bile ducts, congenital biliary cystic disease, hepatolithiasis, and biliary parasites (*Clonorchis sinensis*, *Opisthorchis viverrini*). Complete surgical resection offers the only chance at cure; however, patients with cholangiocarcinoma typically present with unresectable, advanced disease resulting in a poor prognosis. Even after surgical resection, the 5-year survival for perihilar cholangiocarcinoma ranges from 10% to 40%, with recurrence rates as high as 50% to 70% even after R0 resection.[81]

Patient Presentation and Initial Workup

Patients typically present with cachexia, fatigue, and jaundice, often reflecting locally advanced or metastatic disease. The vast majority of patients present with painless jaundice, and up to 10% will have concomitant cholangitis. The objectives of the preoperative evaluation are to rule out benign causes of hilar obstruction, distinguish surgical candidates who would benefit from resection from patients with unresectable disease, and provide appropriate biliary drainage in a neoadjuvant or palliative setting. Cholangiocarcinoma has 3 pathologic subtypes, including sclerosing (>70%), nodular (20%), and papillary (5%–10%), with papillary having the most favorable prognosis due to an endobiliary growth pattern.

The workup for patients suspected of having perihilar cholangiocarcinoma begins with laboratory studies including the tumor marker CA 19-9. Levels of CA 19-9 may be falsely elevated in the setting of biliary obstruction, cholangitis, and hyperbilirubinemia. However, obtaining baseline levels of the tumor marker are useful to monitor response to treatment and disease recurrence and progression. Abdominal ultrasonography may demonstrate intrahepatic biliary dilatation with a decompressed distal bile duct and gallbladder, localizing the obstruction to the common hepatic duct and/ or hilum.

Staging Imaging

Cross-sectional imaging before biliary ductal instrumentation is the single most important step to establishing an accurate diagnosis and staging. Multiphasic high-resolution CT with at least arterial and portovenous phases may accurately predict resectability in most perihilar cholangiocarcinoma.[82] Radiological evaluation should focus on the location and extent of biliary involvement (Bismuth-Corlette classification), involvement of the hepatic arteries, portal veins, peritoneum and adjacent structures, and intrahepatic metastases. MRI/MRCP better evaluates nonmalignant etiologies of hilar obstruction and provides a clearer delineation of the intrahepatic extension of the tumor within the bile ducts compared with CT. However, MRI/ MRCP lacks resolution for determining vascular invasion and therefore resectability. Because perihilar cholangiocarcinoma is usually not FDG-avid, PET-CT has a low sensitivity for the diagnosis of perihilar cholangiocarcinoma and is generally not recommended.

Endobiliary Procedures and Pathologic Diagnosis

Because patients with perihilar cholangiocarcinoma often present with hyperbilirubi-nemia in the setting of jaundice, cholangitis, malnutrition, hepatic or renal insuffi-ciency, or will require portal venous embolization, many patients undergo biliary drainage during the preoperative phase, which may provide the opportunity for brush biopsy to confirm the diagnosis of perihilar cholangiocarcinoma; however, brushings alone yield a definitively result in only 40% of patients with perihilar cholangiocarci-noma.[83] However, fluorescent in situ hybridization analysis for chromosomal aberra-tions associated with perihilar cholangiocarcinoma can significantly enhance the sensitivity of brush biopsy, up to 90%.[84] In patients with suspected perihilar cholan-giocarcinoma, preoperative pathologic confirmation is not required before surgical resection or transplantation, although confirmation is mandatory before chemo-therapy or radiation. Patients with suspicious regional lymphadenopathy should be considered for EUS or laparoscopic FNA of any suspicious nodes to rule out unresect-able disease. However, in patients who may be candidates for liver transplantation, percutaneous or laparoscopic biopsy of the primary tumor is not recommended because of the high risk of disease dissemination.[85]

Staging Classification

Bismuth and Corlette[86] categorized perihilar cholangiocarcinoma based on the extent to which the common hepatic duct, duct confluence, and left and right hepatic ducts were involved by tumor (**Fig. 3**). The Bismuth-Corlette classification is widely used because it correlates with the operations required for complete removal of the tumor and reestablishing biliary continuity. Jarnagin and colleagues[87] subsequently

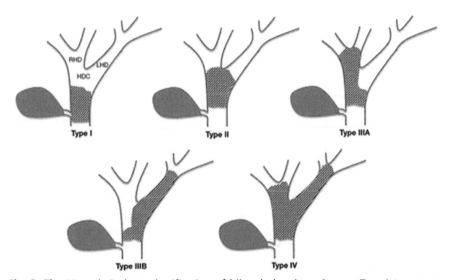

Fig. 3. The Bismuth-Corlette classification of hilar cholangiocarcinoma. Type I tumors are distal to the hepatic duct confluence (HDC), whereas type II neoplasms extend to and involve the HDC. Type III tumors involve the HDC and either the proximal right hepatic duct (type IIIA) or proximal left hepatic duct (type IIIB). Type IV tumors extend into the bilat-eral proximal hepatic ducts up to the segmental bile ducts. LHD, left hepatic duct; RHD, right hepatic duct. (*From* Soares KC, Kamel I, Cosgrove DP, Herman JM, Pawlik TM. Hilar cholan-giocarcinoma: diagnosis, treatment options, and management. *Hepatobiliary Surg Nutr.* 2014;3(1):18-34; with permission.)

developed a classification system that incorporates vascular involvement by the tumor, resulting in lobar atrophy, and extension to secondary biliary radicles, which is useful for defining the resectability of hilar lesions. The Mayo Clinic classification system includes the size and multifocality of the primary tumor, the nodal and extraregional metastatic burden, and clinical features such as jaundice and performance status. The AJCC Cancer Staging Manual Eighth Edition adopts a TNM staging system for perihilar cholangiocarcinoma.[88] T1 tumors are confined to the bile duct, with extension up to the muscle layer or fibrous tissue. T2a tumors invade beyond the wall of the bile duct to surrounding adipose tissue. T2b tumors invade adjacent hepatic parenchyma. T3 tumors invade unilateral branches of the portal vein or hepatic artery. T4 tumors invade the main portal vein or its branches bilaterally, or the common hepatic artery, or unilateral second-order biliary radicals with contralateral portal vein or hepatic artery involvement. N0 indicates no regional lymph node metastasis. N1 corresponds to 1 to 3 positive lymph nodes typically involving the hilar, cystic duct, common bile duct, hepatic artery, posterior pancreaticoduodenal, and portal vein lymph nodes. N2 designates involvement of 4 or more positive lymph nodes. M0 indicates no distant metastasis, whereas M1 corresponds to distant metastasis, including lymph node metastasis distant to the hepatoduodenal ligament. Stage I corresponds to T1 N0 M0, stage II corresponds to T2a-b N0 M0, stage IIIa corresponds to T3 N0 M0, stage IIIb corresponds to T4 N0 M0, stage IIIc corresponds to Any T N1 M0, stage IVa corresponds to Any T N2 M0, and stage IVb corresponds to Any T Any N M1.

Surgical Staging

Staging laparoscopy is recommended in all patients with perihilar cholangiocarcinoma undergoing resection to exclude metastatic disease, especially in patients with advanced disease or suspicious radiographic findings. The most significant prognostic factors for patients undergoing resection for perihilar cholangiocarcinoma are the status of the resection margin and involvement of lymph node metastases, which occur in 23% to 33% of patients.[89–92] Regional lymphadenectomy of the porta hepatis, from the level of the common hepatic artery on the left and the retroduodenal area on the right and extending upward to the base of the liver, with examination of 7 to 9 lymph nodes is required for appropriate staging.[66,89,93,94] However, extended lymphadenectomy beyond the regional basin does not improve staging accuracy or survival.[94]

Determining Resectability

In general, surgical resectability is possible if the involved intrahepatic and extrahepatic bile ducts and associated hepatic and caudate lobes can be removed, with suitable reconstruction options for sufficient vascular inflow/outflow and biliary drainage, and a plan permitting an adequate future liver remnant. Because of the stringent criteria for resectability, late presentation of disease, and anatomic proximity of critical structures in the hepatic hilum, many patients present with unresectable disease and have dismal outcomes. Even following resection, 5-year survival rates generally range from 25% to 50%, with regional metastasis limiting long-term survival.[87,95–97] Survival following resection is highly correlated with resection margin status, with the median survival and 5-year survival among patients with a negative-margin (R0) resection range from 27 months to 58 months and from 27% to 45%, respectively. Among patients with a positive microscopic (R1) or gross margin (R2), median survival and 5-year survival are markedly worse, ranging from 12 months to 21 months and from 0% to 23%, respectively.[87,98–101]

GALLBLADDER CARCINOMA
Incidence and Outcomes

More than 12,000 new cases of biliary cancers are diagnosed annually in the United States, of which 40% are gallbladder cancers. Incidence rates of gallbladder cancer are 66% higher in women than in men. Most gallbladder cancers are found incidentally in patients undergoing exploration for cholelithiasis. More than 600,000 cholecystectomies are performed in the United States annually, most of which are for benign gallbladder disease. However, invasive cancer is found in 1% to 2% of gallbladder pathology specimens. Survival for gallbladder cancer is dependent on the stage of disease. Nevertheless, due to the anatomic location of the gallbladder and the nonspecificity of symptoms, patients with gallbladder cancer present with advanced disease and consequently have poor prognoses. Only 10% to 25% of patients will undergo potentially curative surgery, and overall just 16% will survive for more than 5 years. The 5-year survival rates for people with gallbladder cancer are 80%, 50%, 28%, 7% to 8%, and 2% to 4% for stages 0, I, II, III, and IV, respectively. As a result, an important feature of the clinical workup is accurate pathologic and imaging staging to direct appropriate treatment strategies.

Patient Presentation and Initial Workup

Patients typically present with vague symptoms associated most commonly with benign gallbladder disease (nausea, vomiting, abdominal pain); however, in some advanced cases, patients present with weight loss and jaundice. The initial workup begins with laboratory studies (including liver function tests) and a preoperative transcutaneous ultrasound examination with Doppler flow studies that is useful in characterizing potential masses or polyps and determining their vascularity.

Although most polypoid masses of the gallbladder are small cholesterol or fibromyoglandular lesions that are benign,[102] true intra-cholecystic papillary tubular neoplasms harbor malignant potential thought to be proportional to their overall size and degree of vascularity. Although gallbladder polyps smaller than 1.0 cm in diameter are seldom malignant, most polyps larger than 2.0 cm contain invasive cancer. Consequently, polyps larger than 1.0 cm in diameter or with a vascular pedicle, as determined by preoperative transcutaneous ultrasound examination with Doppler flow studies, are generally referred for cholecystectomy.[103,104]

Staging Imaging

If suspicious masses are identified preoperatively, contrast-enhanced abdominal CT is necessary to interrogate portal nodes, peritoneal implants, and vascular invasion, making it the most accurate modality with which to determine resectability.[105] The diagnostic and staging accuracy of CT may be augmented by gadolinium-enhanced MRI, which can provide more detailed evaluation of the common hepatic duct, common bile duct, and liver parenchyma, especially in patients with concomitant liver steatosis or cirrhosis. The presence of lymph node metastases in gallbladder cancer is often difficult to determine preoperatively; abdominal CT and MRI are reported to facilitate a detection rate of 24%.[106] Although PET-CT is useful in identifying occult peritoneal, omental, and/or lymph node metastases with a sensitivity of 56% in patients with known or suspected gallbladder cancer,[107] it should be selectively used when there are questionable or concerning features apparent on CT or MRI.

Staging Classification

The AJCC Cancer Staging Manual Eighth Edition adopts a TNM staging system for gallbladder cancer.[58] T1a tumors invade the lamina propria, whereas T1b tumors invade the muscularis. T2a tumors invade the perimuscular connective tissue on the peritoneal side without involvement of the visceral peritoneum. T2b tumors invade the perimuscular connective tissue on the hepatic side without extension into the liver. T3 tumors perforate the serosa (visceral peritoneum) or invade the liver or one other adjacent organ or structure. T4 tumors invade the main portal vein or hepatic artery or invades 2 or more extrahepatic organs or structures. N0 describes the absence of regional lymph node metastasis. N1 refers to metastasis in 1 to 3 regional lymph nodes, including the common bile duct, hepatic artery, portal vein, and cystic duct lymph nodes. N2 corresponds to metastasis in 4 or more regional lymph nodes. M1 indicates no distant metastasis, whereas M1 corresponds to the presence of distant metastasis. Stage I corresponds to T1 N0 M0, stage IIA corresponds to T2a N0 M0, stage IIB corresponds to T2b N0 M0, stage IIIA corresponds to T3 N0 M0, stage IIIB corresponds to T1-3, N1 M0, stage IVA corresponds to T4 N0-1 M0, and stage IVB corresponds to Any T N2 M0 or Any T Any N M1. The prognostic significance of the most recent staging system has been independently validated.[108]

Surgical Staging

If imaging identifies suspicious intrahepatic masses, regional lymphadenopathy, and/ or peritoneal implants, then endoscopic, percutaneous, or laparoscopic biopsy should be performed before resection for accurate staging to rule out unresectable disease. In some patients with suspected gallbladder cancer, definitive preoperative pathologic diagnosis may be elusive. Staging laparoscopy (with or without laparoscopic ultrasound) with extensive intraoperative core needle biopsy with immediate frozen-section analysis is recommended for all instances of suspected or proven gallbladder cancer before committing to radical resection.[63,109,110]

Due to the lymphatic drainage of the biliary tract, gallbladder cancer has a propensity to spread from the gallbladder to the periportal lymph nodes to the aortocaval station, and may cross to the celiac nodal station before advancing to more distant axial sites. Complete surgical resection may result in long-term survival for patients found to have involvement of the pancreaticoduodenal and hepatic artery lymph nodes (N1). However, up to 26% of patients with gallbladder cancer have involved para-aortic, celiac, or superior mesenteric artery nodes (N2), for whom radical surgical resection provides no survival benefit.[111,112] Consequently, aortocaval lymph node sampling should be performed routinely at the initiation of the operation.

Pathologic Evaluation of Gallbladder Specimens

Because cholecystectomy for benign gallbladder disease is so common, stepwise pathology sampling protocol has been proposed to identify malignancy in 1% to 2% of pathology specimens for patients in whom there is no clinical or imaging suspicion of gallbladder cancer.[113,114] In gallbladders that appear normal on gross examination, a minimum of 3 random areas and the cystic duct margin should be submitted for microscopic assessment. Furthermore, a finding of dysplasia or neoplasia on initial random sampling prompts a complete sampling of the gallbladder due to the increased possibility of harboring invasive cancer. Increased sampling of the gallbladder also is indicated in patients with high-risk features associated with gallbladder cancer, such as choledochal cysts, anomalous unions of the pancreatobiliary ducts, primary sclerosing cholangitis, and hyalinizing cholecystitis. Suspicious mass lesions in gallbladder specimens require complete analysis, with particular attention to distinguishing early (muscle-confined) from advanced (through the tunica muscularis) cancer due to the prognostic significance.[113] In addition, laterality of involvement is an important prognostic factor, as involvement of the hepatic versus the free peritoneal surface of the gallbladder appears to have worse outcomes.[115] Moreover, determining whether the cystic duct margin is involved with cancer is potentially important in planning subsequent surgical interventions.

Re-resection for Incidental Gallbladder Cancer

Gallbladder cancer is frequently diagnosed as an incidental finding following cholecystectomy. The imaging and surgical staging workup is the same as previously discussed. The rationale for re-resection following cholecystectomy is based on the incidence of residual disease, accurate staging, and improving survival. The incidence of finding residual disease at any site varies by T-stage of the primary tumor, and may be as high as 37.5%, 56.7%, and 77.3% for T1, T2, and T3 tumors, respectively.[116] The 5-year survival rate for patients who underwent re-resection was 41% compared with only 15% in those who did not.[117] When assessed by T-stage classification, re-resection was associated with improved survival in T1b, T2, and T3, but not T1a, tumors.[117–119] Thus, re-resection is indicated for T1b, T2, and T3 incidentally discovered gallbladder cancer.

The goal of liver resection is to obtain negative margins. More extensive resections have not been associated with increased morbidity without any survival advantage.[117,120–122] Thus, a lesser resection is recommended, as long as negative margins are achieved. The incidence of lymph node involvement varies by T-stage, and may be as high as 12%, 31%, and 45% in patients with T1b, T2, and T3 tumors, respectively.[116] Radical resection with lymphadenectomy of at least 5 to 6 lymph nodes results in improved survival and more accurate staging compared with lesser lymphadenectomy or resection alone.[122–124] Although biopsy of N2-level nodes may provide prognostic benefit, extending lymph node excision to the N2 level is not associated with improved outcomes because involvement of these distant nodes represents distant metastatic disease.[122] Consequently, formal lymph adenectomy should be limited to the hepatoduodenal ligament (N1) lymph nodes. Although resection of the laparoscopic port sites has been advocated by some investigators, the practice has been associated with significant complications without any survival advantage, and thus is not indicated.[117,125]

SUMMARY

Here, we discuss the incidence, outcomes, patient presentation, initial workup, pathologic diagnoses, staging classification, imaging and surgical staging, and determinants of resectability for hepatocellular carcinoma, intrahepatic cholangiocarcinoma, perihilar cholangiocarcinoma, and gallbladder adenocarcinoma. The overall prognosis for patients with hepatobiliary malignancies is generally poor, and complete surgical extirpation is the only chance at a long-term cure, underlining the importance of expeditious and accurate workup and staging to guide appropriate treatment.

REFERENCES

1. Razumilava N, Gores GJ. Cholangiocarcinoma. Lancet 2014;383(9935): 2168–79.
2. Aloia TA, Jarufe N, Javle M, et al. Gallbladder cancer: expert consensus statement. HPB (Oxford) 2015;17(8):681–90.

3. Ferlay J, Soerjomataram I, Dikshit R, et al. Cancer incidence and mortality world-wide: sources, methods and major patterns in GLOBOCAN 2012. Int J Cancer 2015;136(5):E359–86.

4. Ferlay J, Shin HR, Bray F, et al. Estimates of worldwide burden of cancer in 2008: GLOBOCAN 2008. Int J Cancer 2010;127(12):2893–917.

5. Razavi H, El Khoury A, Elbasha E, et al. Chronic hepatitis C virus (HCV) disease burden and cost in the United States. Hepatology 2013;57(6):2164–70.

6. Bosch FX, Ribes J, Diaz M, et al. Primary liver cancer: worldwide incidence and trends. Gastroenterology 2004;127(5 Suppl 1):S5–16.

7. Deuffic-Burban S, Poynard T, Sulkowski MS, et al. Estimating the future health burden of chronic hepatitis C and human immunodeficiency virus infections in the United States. J Viral Hepat 2007;14(2):107–15.

8. Sangiovanni A, Prati GM, Fasani P, et al. The natural history of compensated cirrhosis due to hepatitis C virus: a 17-year cohort study of 214 patients. Hepatology 2006;43(6):1303–10.

9. Calle EE, Rodriguez C, Walker-Thurmond K, et al. Overweight, obesity, and mortality from cancer in a prospectively studied cohort of U.S. adults. N Engl J Med 2003;348(17):1625–38.

10. Marrero JA, Fontana RJ, Fu S, et al. Alcohol, tobacco and obesity are synergistic risk factors for hepatocellular carcinoma. J Hepatol 2005;42(2):218–24.

11. Bruix J, Sherman M, American Association for the Study of Liver Diseases. Management of hepatocellular carcinoma: an update. Hepatology 2011;53(3): 1020–2.

12. Simmons O, Fetzer DT, Yokoo T, et al. Predictors of adequate ultrasound quality for hepatocellular carcinoma surveillance in patients with cirrhosis. Aliment Pharmacol Ther 2017;45(1):169–77.

13. Willatt JM, Hussain HK, Adusumilli S, et al. MR imaging of hepatocellular carcinoma in the cirrhotic liver: challenges and controversies. Radiology 2008; 247(2):311–30.

14. Gupta S, Bent S, Kohlwes J. Test characteristics of alpha-fetoprotein for detecting hepatocellular carcinoma in patients with hepatitis C. A systematic review and critical analysis. Ann Intern Med 2003;139(1):46–50.

15. Tang A, Bashir MR, Corwin MT, et al. Evidence supporting LI-RADS major features for CT- and MR imaging-based diagnosis of hepatocellular carcinoma: a systematic review. Radiology 2018;286(1):29–48.

16. Abd Alkhalik Basha M, Abd El Aziz El Sammak D, El Sammak AA. Diagnostic efficacy of the Liver Imaging-Reporting and Data System (LI-RADS) with CT imaging in categorising small nodules (10-20 mm) detected in the cirrhotic liver at screening ultrasound. Clin Radiol 2017;72(10):901.e1–11.

17. Minamoto N, Oki K, Tomita M, et al. Isolation and characterization of rotavirus from feral pigeon in mammalian cell cultures. Epidemiol Infect 1988;100(3): 481–92.

18. Choi SH, Byun JH, Kim SY, et al. Liver imaging reporting and data system v2014 with gadoxetate disodium-enhanced magnetic resonance imaging: validation of LI-RADS category 4 and 5 criteria. Invest Radiol 2016;51(8):483–90.

19. Lee SE, An C, Hwang SH, et al. Extracellular contrast agent-enhanced MRI: 15-min delayed phase may improve the diagnostic performance for hepatocellular carcinoma in patients with chronic liver disease. Eur Radiol 2018;28(4):1551–9.

20. Liu W, Qin J, Guo R, et al. Accuracy of the diagnostic evaluation of hepatocellular carcinoma with LI-RADS. Acta Radiol 2018;59(2):140–6.

21. Kim YY, An C, Kim S, et al. Diagnostic accuracy of prospective application of the liver imaging reporting and data system (LI-RADS) in gadoxetate-enhanced MRI. Eur Radiol 2018;28(5):2038–46.

22. Shafizadeh N, Kakar S. Diagnosis of well-differentiated hepatocellular lesions: role of immunohistochemistry and other ancillary techniques. Adv Anat Pathol 2011;18(6):438–45.

23. Chen IP, Ariizumi S, Nakano M, et al. Positive glypican-3 expression in early hepatocellular carcinoma predicts recurrence after hepatectomy. J Gastroenterol 2014;49(1):117–25.

24. Tremosini S, Forner A, Boix L, et al. Prospective validation of an immunohistochemical panel (glypican 3, heat shock protein 70 and glutamine synthetase) in liver biopsies for diagnosis of very early hepatocellular carcinoma. Gut 2012;61(10):1481–7.

25. European Association for the Study of the Liver, European Organisation for Research and Treatment of Cancer. EASL-EORTC clinical practice guidelines: management of hepatocellular carcinoma. J Hepatol 2012;56(4):908–43.

26. Llovet JM, Bru C, Bruix J. Prognosis of hepatocellular carcinoma: the BCLC staging classification. Semin Liver Dis 1999;19(3):329–38.

27. Llovet JM, Di Bisceglie AM, Bruix J, et al. Design and endpoints of clinical trials in hepatocellular carcinoma. J Natl Cancer Inst 2008;100(10):698–711.

28. Adams RB, Aloia TA, Loyer E, et al. Selection for hepatic resection of colorectal liver metastases: expert consensus statement. HPB (Oxford) 2013;15(2):91–103.

29. Farges O, Malassagne B, Flejou JF, et al. Risk of major liver resection in patients with underlying chronic liver disease: a reappraisal. Ann Surg 1999;229(2):210–5.

30. Abdalla EK, Barnett CC, Doherty D, et al. Extended hepatectomy in patients with hepatobiliary malignancies with and without preoperative portal vein embolization. Arch Surg 2002;137(6):675–80 [discussion: 680–1].

31. Kishi Y, Abdalla EK, Chun YS, et al. Three hundred and one consecutive extended right hepatectomies: evaluation of outcome based on systematic liver volumetry. Ann Surg 2009;250(4):540–8.

32. Belghiti J, Ogata S. Assessment of hepatic reserve for the indication of hepatic resection. J Hepatobiliary Pancreat Surg 2005;12(1):1–3.

33. Abdalla EK, Hicks ME, Vauthey JN. Portal vein embolization: rationale, technique and future prospects. Br J Surg 2001;88(2):165–75.

34. Vauthey JN, Dixon E, Abdalla EK, et al. Pretreatment assessment of hepatocellular carcinoma: expert consensus statement. HPB (Oxford) 2010;12(5):289–99.

35. Van Deusen MA, Abdalla EK, Vauthey JN, et al. Staging classifications for hepatocellular carcinoma. Expert Rev Mol Diagn 2005;5(3):377–83.

36. Marrero JA, Fontana RJ, Barrat A, et al. Prognosis of hepatocellular carcinoma: comparison of 7 staging systems in an American cohort. Hepatology 2005;41(4):707–16.

37. Malinchoc M, Kamath PS, Gordon FD, et al. A model to predict poor survival in patients undergoing transjugular intrahepatic portosystemic shunts. Hepatology 2000;31(4):864–71.

38. Teh SH, Christein J, Donohue J, et al. Hepatic resection of hepatocellular carcinoma in patients with cirrhosis: model of end-stage liver disease (MELD) score predicts perioperative mortality. J Gastrointest Surg 2005;9(9):1207–15 [discussion: 1215].

39. Delis SG, Bakoyiannis A, Biliatis I, et al. Model for end-stage liver disease (MELD) score, as a prognostic factor for post-operative morbidity and mortality in cirrhotic patients, undergoing hepatectomy for hepatocellular carcinoma. HPB (Oxford) 2009;11(4):351–7.

40. Ramia JM. Hilar cholangiocarcinoma. World J Gastrointest Oncol 2013;5(7): 113–4.

41. Saha SK, Zhu AX, Fuchs CS, et al. Forty-year trends in cholangiocarcinoma incidence in the U.S.: intrahepatic disease on the rise. Oncologist 2016;21(5): 594–9.

42. Weimann A, Varnholt H, Schlitt HJ, et al. Retrospective analysis of prognostic factors after liver resection and transplantation for cholangiocellular carcinoma. Br J Surg 2000;87(9):1182–7.

43. Chu KM, Lai EC, Al-Hadeedi S, et al. Intrahepatic cholangiocarcinoma. World J Surg 1997;21(3):301–5 [discussion: 305–6].

44. Berdah SV, Delpero JR, Garcia S, et al. A western surgical experience of peripheral cholangiocarcinoma. Br J Surg 1996;83(11):1517–21.

45. de Jong MC, Nathan H, Sotiropoulos GC, et al. Intrahepatic cholangiocarcinoma: an international multi-institutional analysis of prognostic factors and lymph node assessment. J Clin Oncol 2011;29(23):3140–5.

46. Paik KY, Jung JC, Heo JS, et al. What prognostic factors are important for resected intrahepatic cholangiocarcinoma? J Gastroenterol Hepatol 2008;23(5): 766–70.

47. Choi SB, Kim KS, Choi JY, et al. The prognosis and survival outcome of intrahepatic cholangiocarcinoma following surgical resection: association of lymph node metastasis and lymph node dissection with survival. Ann Surg Oncol 2009;16(11):3048–56.

48. Lang H, Sotiropoulos GC, Fruhauf NR, et al. Extended hepatectomy for intrahepatic cholangiocellular carcinoma (ICC): when is it worthwhile? Single center experience with 27 resections in 50 patients over a 5-year period. Ann Surg 2005;241(1):134–43.

49. Shimada K, Sano T, Nara S, et al. Therapeutic value of lymph node dissection during hepatectomy in patients with intrahepatic cholangiocellular carcinoma with negative lymph node involvement. Surgery 2009;145(4):411–6.

50. Dodson RM, Weiss MJ, Cosgrove D, et al. Intrahepatic cholangiocarcinoma: management options and emerging therapies. J Am Coll Surg 2013;217(4): 736–50.e4.

51. Maithel SK, Gamblin TC, Kamel I, et al. Multidisciplinary approaches to intrahepatic cholangiocarcinoma. Cancer 2013;119(22):3929–42.

52. Xu HX, Chen LD, Liu LN, et al. Contrast-enhanced ultrasound of intrahepatic cholangiocarcinoma: correlation with pathological examination. Br J Radiol 2012;85(1016):1029–37.

53. Valls C, Guma A, Puig I, et al. Intrahepatic peripheral cholangiocarcinoma: CT evaluation. Abdom Imaging 2000;25(5):490–6.

54. Hamrick-Turner J, Abbitt PL, Ros PR. Intrahepatic cholangiocarcinoma: MR appearance. AJR Am J Roentgenol 1992;158(1):77–9.

55. Kim YJ, Yun M, Lee WJ, et al. Usefulness of 18F-FDG PET in intrahepatic cholangiocarcinoma. Eur J Nucl Med Mol Imaging 2003;30(11):1467–72.

56. Chong YS, Kim YK, Lee MW, et al. Differentiating mass-forming intrahepatic cholangiocarcinoma from atypical hepatocellular carcinoma using gadoxetic acid-enhanced MRI. Clin Radiol 2012;67(8):766–73.

57. Corvera CU, Blumgart LH, Akhurst T, et al. 18F-fluorodeoxyglucose positron emission tomography influences management decisions in patients with biliary cancer. J Am Coll Surg 2008;206(1):57–65.

58. Amin MB, American Joint Committee on Cancer, American Cancer Society. AJCC cancer staging manual. editor-in-chief, Amin MB; editors, Edge SB and 16 others; Gress DM, Technical editor; Meyer LR, Managing editor. In: American Joint Committee on Cancer. 8th edition. Chicago: Springer; 2017.

59. Lee AJ, Chun YS. Intrahepatic cholangiocarcinoma: the AJCC/UICC 8th edition updates. Chin Clin Oncol 2018;7(5):52.

60. Kim Y, Moris DP, Zhang XF, et al. Evaluation of the 8th edition American Joint Commission on Cancer (AJCC) staging system for patients with intrahepatic cholangiocarcinoma: a surveillance, epidemiology, and end results (SEER) analysis. J Surg Oncol 2017;116(6):643–50.

61. Spolverato G, Bagante F, Weiss M, et al. Comparative performances of the 7th and the 8th editions of the American Joint Committee on Cancer staging systems for intrahepatic cholangiocarcinoma. J Surg Oncol 2017;115(6):696–703.

62. Kang SH, Hwang S, Lee YJ, et al. Prognostic comparison of the 7th and 8th editions of the American Joint Committee on Cancer staging system for intrahepatic cholangiocarcinoma. J Hepatobiliary Pancreat Sci 2018;25(4):240–8.

63. Goere D, Wagholikar GD, Pessaux P, et al. Utility of staging laparoscopy in subsets of biliary cancers: laparoscopy is a powerful diagnostic tool in patients with intrahepatic and gallbladder carcinoma. Surg Endosc 2006;20(5):721–5.

64. D'Angelica M, Fong Y, Weber S, et al. The role of staging laparoscopy in hepatobiliary malignancy: prospective analysis of 401 cases. Ann Surg Oncol 2003; 10(2):183–9.

65. Amini N, Ejaz A, Spolverato G, et al. Management of lymph nodes during resection of hepatocellular carcinoma and intrahepatic cholangiocarcinoma: a systematic review. J Gastrointest Surg 2014;18(12):2136–48.

66. Guglielmi A, Ruzzenente A, Campagnaro T, et al. Patterns and prognostic significance of lymph node dissection for surgical treatment of perihilar and intrahepatic cholangiocarcinoma. J Gastrointest Surg 2013;17(11):1917–28.

67. Zhang XF, Beal EW, Bagante F, et al. Early versus late recurrence of intrahepatic cholangiocarcinoma after resection with curative intent. Br J Surg 2018;105(7): 848–56.

68. Rouvière H. Anatomie des lymphatiques de l'homme, vol. 1. Paris: Mason; 1932.

69. Shimada M, Yamashita Y, Aishima S, et al. Value of lymph node dissection during resection of intrahepatic cholangiocarcinoma. Br J Surg 2001;88(11): 1463–6.

70. Bartella I, Dufour JF. Clinical diagnosis and staging of intrahepatic cholangiocarcinoma. J Gastrointestin Liver Dis 2015;24(4):481–9.

71. Uenishi T, Yamamoto T, Takemura S, et al. Surgical treatment for intrahepatic cholangiocarcinoma. Clin J Gastroenterol 2014;7(2):87–93.

72. Uenishi T, Yamazaki O, Yamamoto T, et al. Serosal invasion in TNM staging of mass-forming intrahepatic cholangiocarcinoma. J Hepatobiliary Pancreat Surg 2005;12(6):479–83.

73. Zhang XF, Chen Q, Kimbrough CW, et al. Lymphadenectomy for intrahepatic cholangiocarcinoma: has nodal evaluation been increasingly adopted by surgeons over time? A national database analysis. J Gastrointest Surg 2018; 22(4):668–75.

74. Ribero D, Pinna AD, Guglielmi A, et al. Surgical approach for long-term survival of patients with intrahepatic cholangiocarcinoma: a multi-institutional analysis of 434 patients. Arch Surg 2012;147(12):1107–13.

75. Endo I, Gonen M, Yopp AC, et al. Intrahepatic cholangiocarcinoma: rising frequency, improved survival, and determinants of outcome after resection. Ann Surg 2008;248(1):84–96.

76. Hyder O, Hatzaras I, Sotiropoulos GC, et al. Recurrence after operative management of intrahepatic cholangiocarcinoma. Surgery 2013;153(6):811–8.

77. Sulpice L, Rayar M, Boucher E, et al. Treatment of recurrent intrahepatic cholangiocarcinoma. Br J Surg 2012;99(12):1711–7.

78. Farges O, Fuks D, Boleslawski E, et al. Influence of surgical margins on outcome in patients with intrahepatic cholangiocarcinoma: a multicenter study by the AFC-IHCC-2009 study group. Ann Surg 2011;254(5):824–9 [discussion: 830].

79. Lang H, Sotiropoulos GC, Sgourakis G, et al. Operations for intrahepatic cholangiocarcinoma: single-institution experience of 158 patients. J Am Coll Surg 2009;208(2):218–28.

80. Jonas S, Thelen A, Benckert C, et al. Extended liver resection for intrahepatic cholangiocarcinoma: a comparison of the prognostic accuracy of the fifth and sixth editions of the TNM classification. Ann Surg 2009;249(2):303–9.

81. Soares KC, Kamel I, Cosgrove DP, et al. Hilar cholangiocarcinoma: diagnosis, treatment options, and management. Hepatobiliary Surg Nutr 2014;3(1):18–34.

82. Aloia TA, Charnsangavej C, Faria S, et al. High-resolution computed tomography accurately predicts resectability in hilar cholangiocarcinoma. Am J Surg 2007;193(6):702–6.

83. De Bellis M, Sherman S, Fogel EL, et al. Tissue sampling at ERCP in suspected malignant biliary strictures (Part 1). Gastrointest Endosc 2002;56(4):552–61.

84. Halling KC, Kipp BR. Fluorescence in situ hybridization in diagnostic cytology. Hum Pathol 2007;38(8):1137–44.

85. Heimbach JK, Sanchez W, Rosen CB, et al. Trans-peritoneal fine needle aspiration biopsy of hilar cholangiocarcinoma is associated with disease dissemination. HPB (Oxford) 2011;13(5):356–60.

86. Bismuth H, Corlette MB. Intrahepatic cholangioenteric anastomosis in carcinoma of the hilus of the liver. Surg Gynecol Obstet 1975;140(2):170–8.

87. Jarnagin WR, Fong Y, DeMatteo RP, et al. Staging, resectability, and outcome in 225 patients with hilar cholangiocarcinoma. Ann Surg 2001;234(4):507–17 [discussion: 517–9].

88. Gaspersz MP, Buettner S, van Vugt JLA, et al. Evaluation of the new American Joint Committee on Cancer Staging Manual 8th Edition for perihilar cholangiocarcinoma. J Gastrointest Surg 2019. [Epub ahead of print].

89. Rocha FG, Matsuo K, Blumgart LH, et al. Hilar cholangiocarcinoma: the Memorial Sloan-Kettering Cancer Center experience. J Hepatobiliary Pancreat Sci 2010;17(4):490–6.

90. Nagino M, Ebata T, Yokoyama Y, et al. Evolution of surgical treatment for perihilar cholangiocarcinoma: a single-center 34-year review of 574 consecutive resections. Ann Surg 2013;258(1):129–40.

91. Bhuiya MR, Nimura Y, Kamiya J, et al. Clinicopathologic factors influencing survival of patients with bile duct carcinoma: multivariate statistical analysis. World J Surg 1993;17(5):653–7.

92. DeOliveira ML, Cunningham SC, Cameron JL, et al. Cholangiocarcinoma: thirty-one-year experience with 564 patients at a single institution. Ann Surg 2007;245(5):755–62.

93. Ito K, Ito H, Allen PJ, et al. Adequate lymph node assessment for extrahepatic bile duct adenocarcinoma. Ann Surg 2010;251(4):675–81.

94. Kambakamba P, Linecker M, Slankamenac K, et al. Lymph node dissection in resectable perihilar cholangiocarcinoma: a systematic review. Am J Surg 2015;210(4):694–701.

95. Kobayashi A, Miwa S, Nakata T, et al. Disease recurrence patterns after R0 resection of hilar cholangiocarcinoma. Br J Surg 2010;97(1):56–64.

96. Lee SG, Song GW, Hwang S, et al. Surgical treatment of hilar cholangiocarcinoma in the new era: the Asan experience. J Hepatobiliary Pancreat Sci 2010;17(4):476–89.

97. Rea DJ, Munoz-Juarez M, Farnell MB, et al. Major hepatic resection for hilar cholangiocarcinoma: analysis of 46 patients. Arch Surg 2004;139(5):514–23 [discussion: 523–5].

98. Hasegawa S, Ikai I, Fujii H, et al. Surgical resection of hilar cholangiocarcinoma: analysis of survival and postoperative complications. World J Surg 2007;31(6): 1256–63.

99. Hemming AW, Reed AI, Fujita S, et al. Surgical management of hilar cholangiocarcinoma. Ann Surg 2005;241(5):693–9 [discussion: 699–702].

100. Hong JC, Jones CM, Duffy JP, et al. Comparative analysis of resection and liver transplantation for intrahepatic and hilar cholangiocarcinoma: a 24-year experience in a single center. Arch Surg 2011;146(6):683–9.

101. Nishio H, Nagino M, Nimura Y. Surgical management of hilar cholangiocarcinoma: the Nagoya experience. HPB (Oxford) 2005;7(4):259–62.

102. Adsay V, Jang KT, Roa JC, et al. Intracholecystic papillary-tubular neoplasms (ICPN) of the gallbladder (neoplastic polyps, adenomas, and papillary neoplasms that are >/=1.0 cm): clinicopathologic and immunohistochemical analysis of 123 cases. Am J Surg Pathol 2012;36(9):1279–301.

103. Eaton JE, Thackeray EW, Lindor KD. Likelihood of malignancy in gallbladder polyps and outcomes following cholecystectomy in primary sclerosing cholangitis. Am J Gastroenterol 2012;107(3):431–9.

104. Ito H, Hann LE, D'Angelica M, et al. Polypoid lesions of the gallbladder: diagnosis and followup. J Am Coll Surg 2009;208(4):570–5.

105. Li B, Xu XX, Du Y, et al. Computed tomography for assessing resectability of gallbladder carcinoma: a systematic review and meta-analysis. Clin Imaging 2013;37(2):327–33.

106. Kokudo N, Makuuchi M, Natori T, et al. Strategies for surgical treatment of gallbladder carcinoma based on information available before resection. Arch Surg 2003;138(7):741–50 [discussion: 750].

107. Rodriguez-Fernandez A, Gomez-Rio M, Medina-Benitez A, et al. Application of modern imaging methods in diagnosis of gallbladder cancer. J Surg Oncol 2006;93(8):650–64.

108. Lee AJ, Chiang YJ, Lee JE, et al. Validation of American Joint Committee on Cancer eighth staging system for gallbladder cancer and its lymphadenectomy guidelines. J Surg Res 2018;230:148–54.

109. Agarwal AK, Kalayarasan R, Javed A, et al. Mass-forming xanthogranulomatous cholecystitis masquerading as gallbladder cancer. J Gastrointest Surg 2013; 17(7):1257–64.

110. Agarwal AK, Kalayarasan R, Javed A, et al. The role of staging laparoscopy in primary gall bladder cancer–an analysis of 409 patients: a prospective study to evaluate the role of staging laparoscopy in the management of gallbladder cancer. Ann Surg 2013;258(2):318–23.

111. Meng H, Wang X, Fong Y, et al. Outcomes of radical surgery for gallbladder cancer patients with lymphatic metastases. Jpn J Clin Oncol 2011;41(8):992–8.
112. Shirai Y, Sakata J, Wakai T, et al. Assessment of lymph node status in gallbladder cancer: location, number, or ratio of positive nodes. World J Surg Oncol 2012;10:87.
113. Adsay NV, Bagci P, Tajiri T, et al. Pathologic staging of pancreatic, ampullary, biliary, and gallbladder cancers: pitfalls and practical limitations of the current AJCC/UICC TNM staging system and opportunities for improvement. Semin Diagn Pathol 2012;29(3):127–41.
114. Adsay V, Saka B, Basturk O, et al. Criteria for pathologic sampling of gallbladder specimens. Am J Clin Pathol 2013;140(2):278–80.
115. de Aretxabala X, Roa I, Hepp J, et al. Early gallbladder cancer: is further treatment necessary? J Surg Oncol 2009;100(7):589–93.
116. Pawlik TM, Gleisner AL, Vigano L, et al. Incidence of finding residual disease for incidental gallbladder carcinoma: implications for re-resection. J Gastrointest Surg 2007;11(11):1478–86 [discussion: 1486–7].
117. Fuks D, Regimbeau JM, Le Treut YP, et al. Incidental gallbladder cancer by the AFC-GBC-2009 Study Group. World J Surg 2011;35(8):1887–97.
118. Abramson MA, Pandharipande P, Ruan D, et al. Radical resection for T1b gallbladder cancer: a decision analysis. HPB (Oxford) 2009;11(8):656–63.
119. Hari DM, Howard JH, Leung AM, et al. A 21-year analysis of stage I gallbladder carcinoma: is cholecystectomy alone adequate? HPB (Oxford) 2013;15(1):40–8.
120. D'Angelica M, Dalal KM, DeMatteo RP, et al. Analysis of the extent of resection for adenocarcinoma of the gallbladder. Ann Surg Oncol 2009;16(4):806–16.
121. Butte JM, Waugh E, Meneses M, et al. Incidental gallbladder cancer: analysis of surgical findings and survival. J Surg Oncol 2010;102(6):620–5.
122. Downing SR, Cadogan KA, Ortega G, et al. Early-stage gallbladder cancer in the Surveillance, Epidemiology, and End Results database: effect of extended surgical resection. Arch Surg 2011;146(6):734–8.
123. Ito H, Ito K, D'Angelica M, et al. Accurate staging for gallbladder cancer: implications for surgical therapy and pathological assessment. Ann Surg 2011;254(2):320–5.
124. Jensen EH, Abraham A, Jarosek S, et al. Lymph node evaluation is associated with improved survival after surgery for early stage gallbladder cancer. Surgery 2009;146(4):706–11 [discussion: 711–3].
125. Maker AV, Butte JM, Oxenberg J, et al. Is port site resection necessary in the surgical management of gallbladder cancer? Ann Surg Oncol 2012;19(2):409–17.

Molecular Characteristics of Biliary Tract and Primary Liver Tumors

Susan Tsai, MD, MHS*, T. Clark Gamblin, MD, MS, MBA, FACS

KEYWORDS

- Intrahepatic cholangiocarcinoma • Hepatocellular carcinoma
- Next-generation sequencing • Gene expression • Molecular subtype

KEY POINTS

- Integrated high-throughput molecular characterization has been performed in hepatocellular carcinoma and cholangiocarcinoma and, less frequently, in gallbladder cancer.
- In hepatocellular carcinoma, there is a high frequency of mutations affecting telomerase function and the WNT signaling pathway.
- In intrahepatic cholangiocarcinoma, unique mutations involving isocitrate dehydrogenase and fibroblast growth factor receptor have been identified.
- Certain molecular signatures reflect etiologic mechanisms of disease (hepatitis B virus, hepatitis C virus, and fluke-related carcinogenesis).

INTRODUCTION

In 2015, the United States launched the Precision Medicine Initiative, which was rooted in the belief that a deeper understanding of the genetic basis of disease would improve the development of better-targeted therapies. The US National Research Council has defined precision medicine as a population-based approach of classifying individuals through genomic, environmental, and social characteristics, with the goal of identifying effective therapies based on a combination of these factors. The development of a molecular taxonomy is particularly germane to cancers of the biliary tract and liver because the pathogenesis of this heterogenous group of diseases are significantly influenced by both environmental factors (alcohol, carcinogenic, viral, or parasitic) and ethnic diversity. In recent years, technological advancements using next-generation sequencing has enabled researchers to gain further insight into the molecular landscape of these tumors. With the ability to perform high-throughput

Disclosures: None.
Division of Surgical Oncology, Department of Surgery, Medical College of Wisconsin, 8701 West Watertown Plank Road, Milwaukee, WI 53226-3596, USA
* Corresponding author.
E-mail address: stsai@mcw.edu

Surg Oncol Clin N Am 28 (2019) 685–693
https://doi.org/10.1016/j.soc.2019.06.004
1055-3207/19/Published by Elsevier Inc.

genomic, epigenetic, and gene expression analyses, there is now the capacity to develop molecular subclassifications of each disease to better understand the drivers of carcinogenesis and identification of novel therapeutic targets. This article provides an overview of the key molecular drivers of biliary tract and primary liver tumors.

Hepatocellular Carcinoma

Like many other solid tumors, hepatocellular carcinomas (HCCs) arise from an accumulation of somatic DNA alterations, including mutations and chromosomal aberrations. Similar to the adenoma–carcinoma transition which has been described for colon cancer, HCCs are believed to arise from a multistep process that progresses from cirrhosis to low-grade and high-grade dysplasia to finally invasive cancer. Integrated next-generation sequencing studies have identified several well-described driver pathways in HCC (see later discussion).

Telomere maintenance

Telomeres are short noncoding DNA repeats localized at the extremity of chromosomes and are coated by sheltering proteins.[1] They protect coding regions from DNA losses and, with each round of cellular replication, telomeres shorten; when they reach a critical point, cell senescence is triggered. The telomerase complex allows the synthesis of telomeres and the most important component of the complex is the catalytic enzyme telomerase reverse transcriptase (TERT). Telomerase reactivation in HCC is a key event and has been reported to occur in up to 90% of cases.[2] There are multiple mutually exclusive mechanisms by which telomerase reactivation can occur. The most common mechanisms involve TERT promoter mutations (50%), followed by hepatitis B virus (HBV) insertion in TERT promoter (10%) and TERT amplification (5%).[3–5] In low-grade dysplasia and high-grade dysplasia, TERT mutations occur at relatively low frequency (6% and 19%, respectively).[3] However, TERT mutations are present in more than 60% of early HCC, suggesting that TERT promoter mutation is among the earliest recurrent somatic genetic alterations. The TERT promoter region has specific target insertion site for both HBV and adeno-associated virus type 2 (AAV2). TERT promoter mutations are frequently associated with mutations in the beta-catenin pathways (ie, catenin, beta-1 [CTNNB1] mutations).[3]

WNT/beta-catenin pathway

The WNT/beta-catenin pathway plays a role in almost every facet of liver biology, including metabolic zonation and regeneration. Aberrant activation is a hallmark of hepatic pathologic abnormality and it is the pathway that is most frequently activated in HCC via either activating mutations in CTNNB1 (30%) or inactivating mutations of AXIN1 (15%) or adenomatous polyposis coli (APC; 2%).[6,7] Both CTNNB1 mutations and deletions of the APC/AXIN1/ glycogen synthase kinase 3-beta (GSK3B) inhibitory complex target a hotspot domain of beta-catenin. Within the context of cirrhosis, WNT/beta-catenin activation is thought to occur following telomerase inactivation. However, in the context of hepatic adenomas, CTNNB1-activating mutations occur early and, in particular, activating mutations in exon 3 have been associated with an increased risk of transformation and are thought to precede changes in TERT promoter mutation.

Tumor protein 53

Tumor protein 53 (TP53) is a master regulator of cellular proliferation and apoptosis and is the most frequently mutated gene in human cancer. Approximately 30% to 50% of patients with HCC have alterations in the p53 cell cycle pathway. Inactivation of tumor suppressors cyclin-dependent kinase inhibitor 2-alpha (CDKN2A; 12%) and retinoblastoma 1 (RB1; 8%) are primarily responsible for dysregulated cell cycle progression.[4,8] TP53 is a large gene and, with the exception of R249S mutations that are specifically related to aflatoxin 1 (AFB1) mycotoxin exposure, there is no identified mutational hotspot. Exposure to AFB1, which is endemic to food products in Asia and Africa, is associated with a specific mutational signature in a hotspot within TP53 (R249S). Additionally, AFB1 exposure in the setting of chronic HBV infection carries an even greater risk of HCC.[9] HBV insertions into the cyclin E1 (CCNE1) and carotenoid cleavage dioxygenase 1 (CCD1) genes occur in 5% of cases; both are key proteins involved in cell cycle progression in HCC.

Epigenetic modifiers

Inactivating mutation of adenine and thymine–rich interaction domain (ARID)-1A (17%) ad ARID2 (18%) are the most frequently altered epigenetic modifiers in HCC. They play a key role in chromatin remodeling complexes, whose primary role is to modify chromatin structure and nucleosome position. Therefore, alterations in histone methylation can affect cellular transcription and carcinogenesis. Epigenetic mutations had unique, disease-specific patterns. For example, mutations in ARID2 were identified in hepatitis C virus (HCV)-related HCC and were correlated with mutations in CTNNB1. These mutations are mutually exclusive with TP53 mutations, which are associated with HBV infection. Mutations in ARID1A have been predominantly associated with HCC arising in the setting of alcoholic cirrhosis.[8]

Genomic subtypes

Multiple genomic profiling studies have been performed, with 2 common subtypes emerging: proliferative and nonproliferative subtypes (**Table 1**). The proliferative subtype is more commonly seen in patients with HBV infection and is associated with an aggressive clinical phenotype, including high serum alpha fetoprotein levels, poorly differentiated tumors, and increased vascular invasion. The molecular characteristics include chromosomal instability, TP53 mutations, and inactivation of oncogenic pathways (including rat sarcoma–mitogen-activated protein kinase [RAS-MAPK] pathway, AKT, and MET). In addition, DNA amplification of chromosome 11q13 has been described (including loci for fibroblast growth factor [FGF]-19, cyclin D1 [CCND1], FGF4). The nonproliferative subtype is associated with alcohol-related and HCV-related HCC and, in general, has a less aggressive clinical phenotype, including

---

Table 1
Hepatocellular carcinoma molecular subtypes

	Proliferative	Nonproliferative
Clinical Characteristics	• HBV infection • High alpha fetoprotein levels • Poorly differentiated tumors • Increased vascular invasion	• Alcohol-related HCC • HCV infection • Lower alpha fetoprotein levels • Well-differentiated tumors
Molecular Characteristics	• TP53 mutations • Chromosomal instability (amplification of chromosome 11q13) • Inactivation of RAS/MEK/ERK, AKT, MET pathways	• TERT promoter mutations • WNT signaling (CTNNB1 mutations) • Overexpression of EGF receptors

Abbreviations: EGF, epidermal growth factor; ERK, extracellular signal-regulated kinase; RAS, rat sarcoma.

more well-differentiated tumors and lower alpha fetoprotein levels. This subtype seems to be driven by the classic WNT signaling pathway (CTNNB1 mutations) and a subset also demonstrates overexpression of epidermal growth factor (EGF) receptors.[10] There are data suggesting that CTNNB1 mutations can induce immune evasion and resistance to anti–programmed death-ligand (PD-L)-1 blockade.[11] Data from CTNNB1-mutated melanomas demonstrate decreased dendritic cell recruitment and decreased CD8 activation. Whether this could be a biomarker for immunotherapeutic agents remains to be seen.

Multiplatform analysis

Recently, The Cancer Genome Atlas Research Network performed a comprehensive and integrative genomic characterization of HCC.[12] In this study, 363 HCCs underwent whole exome sequencing and copy number analysis and 196 HCCs were also characterized by DNA methylation, RNA, microRNA, and proteomic expression. The investigators identified 3 overall subtypes (**Table 2**) and 4 important observations. First, although the most common alterations in HCC included TERT, TP53, AXIN1, RB1, CTNNB1, ARID1A, ARID2, and BAP1, as previously described, 8 novel candidate drivers of HCC were identified: leucine zipper-like transcription regulator 1 (LZTR1), eukaryotic translation elongation factor 1 alpha 1 (EEF1A1), antizyme inhibitor 1 (AZIN1), retinitis pigmentosa-1-like-1(RP1L1), G-patch domain containing 4 (GPATCH4), cyclic AMP-responsive element-binding protein 3-like protein 3 (CREB3L3), AT-hook containing transcription factor 1 (AHCTF1), and histone cluster 1 H1 (HIST1H1). Second, CDKN2A epigenetic silencing was observed in 53% of samples. TERT promoter mutations were associated with a strong cooccurrence with CDKN2A silencing via promoter hypermethylation. Third, a high proportion of HCCs with carbamoyl phosphate synthetase 1 (CPS1) hypermethylation was associated with decreased RNA expression. The CPS1 gene encodes a rate limiting enzyme for the urea cycle, allowing for elimination of ammonia from the body, and suggests a

Table 2
Multiplatform integrative analysis reveals 3 hepatocellular carcinoma subtypes

	Cluster 1	Cluster 2	Cluster 3
Clinical Characteristics	Younger age Asian ethnicity Female gender Normal body weight	Older age Non-Asian Male Gender Normal to overweight	Older age Non-Asian Male Gender Overweight
Histologic Features	Poorly differentiated Microvascular invasion	Moderately differentiated Rare microvascular invasion	Moderately or poorly differentiated Microvascular invasion
Molecular Characteristics	Low CKDN2A mutations Low CTNNB1 mutations Low TERT promoter mutation Overexpression MYBL2, PLK1, MK167	High CDKN2A silencing High TERT promoter mutations High CTNNB1 mutations High HNF1A mutations	High chromosomal instability (17p loss) High TERT promoter mutation High CTNNB1 mutations High TP53 mutations

Abbreviations: HNF1A, hepatic nuclear factor 1 alpha; PLK1, polo-like kinase 1.

Data from Cancer Genome Atlas Research Network. Electronic address wbe, Cancer Genome Atlas Research N. Comprehensive and Integrative Genomic Characterization of Hepatocellular Carcinoma. *Cell.* 2017;169(7):1327-1341 e1323.

mechanism for metabolic reprogramming of the cancer cell to support autonomous growth. Fourth, immunophenotyping of HCC revealed a subset with high levels of immune infiltration and reflects a promising subset of tumors that may respond to immune checkpoint inhibition.

Cholangiocarcinoma

Cholangiocarcinoma (CCA) has historically been classified by gross anatomic location: intrahepatic CCA (iCCA), perihilar CCA (pCCA), and distal CCA (dCCA). Efforts to develop a molecular classification system for CCA have lagged behind that of HCC; however, several studies using next-generation sequencing techniques have been reported in the last decade, particularly for iCCA. This has provided important biologic insight into a heterogenous collection of tumors whose biology is incompletely described based on anatomic classification. Distinct from HCC pathogenesis, CCA have different molecular alterations that vary uniquely based on the etiologic pathogenic exposure (ie, viral *Opisthorchis (0) viverrini*). The most common genetic alterations affect DNA repair (TP53), tyrosine kinase signaling (Kirsten rat sarcoma [KRAS]), FGF receptor 2 (FGFR2), epigenetic (isocitrate dehydrogenase [IDH]-1 and IDH2), and chromatin remodeling factors (ARID1A, activator protein 1 [AP1]).[13] Similar to HCC, integrative genomic and epigenomic characterization has allowed for the classification of CCA molecular subtypes.[14]

Molecular alterations in intrahepatic cholangiocarcinoma
Isocitrate dehydrogenase 1 and isocitrate dehydrogenase 2 Results of next-generation sequencing effort in iCCA are particularly exciting because novel mutations in hot spots of the IDH1 (codon 132) and IDH2 (codon 172) genes in approximately 20% of samples and the presence of IDH mutations were unique to iCCA and not observed in pCCA or dCCA.[15] IDH mutations were almost exclusively found in non–fluke-related iCCA. IDH1 and IDH2 are enzymes that catalyze the oxidative decarboxylation of isocitrate to alpha-ketoglutarate. When an IDH mutation is present, 2-hydroxyglutarte is produced, which is an oncometabolite that contributes to carcinogenesis by inducing widespread epigenetic changes resulting in altered cell differentiation and survival.[16,17] IDH mutations are associated with a clear cell phenotype with poorly differentiated histology.[18] Because IDH mutations are unique to iCCA, the presence of such mutations may assist in the classification of anatomically and histologically indeterminate hepatic tumors. Also, the oncometabolite, 2-hydroxyglutarte, can be detected in serum and could be a valuable biomarker. Studies evaluating IDH1 inhibitors in iCCA are ongoing.

Fibroblast growth factor receptor 2 Another mutation found to be unique to iCCA were FGFR2-fusions, which were identified in 25% of specimens.[15] FGFR2 is a tyrosine kinase protein that acts as a cell-surface receptor for FGFs and plays an essential role in the regulation of cell proliferation, differentiation, migration, and apoptosis.[19,20] FGFR2 fusions were found to be absent in dCCA or pCCA, and HCC. FGFR2 mutant tumors were histologically associated with an intraductal growth pattern and had strong cytokeratin 7 but weak cytokeratin 19 expression.[21] There is also emerging evidence that the presence of FGFR-fusion proteins is a favorable prognostic factor.[22] Importantly, several FGFR selective and nonselective small molecule kinase inhibitors are available, so the presence of FGFR-fusion protein may have important therapeutic implications.

Epigenetic modifiers Similar to HCC, aberrations in chromatin remodeling genes are frequently identified in iCCA. Dysregulated chromatin remodeling was identified in up to 50% of samples and frequently involved ARID1 (36%), BAP1 (9%), and polybromo (PBRM1; 11%).[15,23,24] Loss of ARID1A and PBRM1 were observed to be late events in iCCA carcinogenesis.[25] In general, patients with mutations in any of these genes were observed to have worse overall survival.[24] As with HCC, histone deacetylase inhibitors and DNA methylation transferase inhibitors may be a promising class of therapeutics for iCCA.

Etiologic signatures O viverrini–related tumors had higher rates of somatic mutations (>200) compared with non–fluke-related tumors. This may be attributed in part to the high rate of classic oncogenes and tumor suppressor genes in fluke-related tumors (TP53, 44%; KRAS, 17%; and mothers against decapentaplegic homolog 4 [SMAD4], 17%).[26,27] In particular, non–fluke-related iCCAs have a higher prevalence of IDH1, IDH2, and BAP1 mutations compared with fluke-related iCCAs, which have the highest rates of TP53 and ARID1A mutations. In addition, microsatellite instability was detected in up to 30% of O viverrini–related tumors, whereas in non–fluke-related tumors microsatellite instability was a rare event.[28]

Molecular alterations in perihilar cholangiocarcinoma or distal cholangiocarcinoma
Early flowering 3 Early flowering (ELF)-3 encodes an E26 transformation-specific transcription factor for 2 well-known tumor suppressor genes: transforming growth factor beta receptor 2 (TGFBR2) and EGF1. Inactivating frameshift or nonsense mutations in ELF2 have been identified in approximately 10% of dCCA.[15,29] ELF3 mutations were present at high allele frequencies, suggesting that ELF3 mutations may be a founder mutation and functional studies demonstrated the ELF3 knockdown was associated with increased invasiveness.[30]

Tyrosine kinase pathways Activating mutation in KRAS lead to upregulation of downstream effector pathways, including rapidly accelerated fibrosarcoma (Raf)/ MEK/extracellular signal-regulated kinase (ERK) and PI2K-AKT pathways. KRAS mutations occur in 40% of dCCAs or pCCAs compared with 9% in iCCA.[22] The presence of KRAS mutations has been associated with poor prognosis.[22] Although KRAS is considered an undruggable target, there are many clinical trials that are targeting the downstream MEK/ERK and PI3K-AKT pathways with tyrosine kinase inhibitors.

Cholangiocarcinoma subtypes Recently, comprehensive genomic, epigenomic, and gene expression profiling was performed on 489 CCAs from 10 countries. Importantly, the investigators observed that anatomic site was not correlated with molecular subtype because molecular subtypes were identified within each anatomic site. In addition, tumors at different anatomic sites demonstrated similarities at a molecular level but tumors from a single anatomic site demonstrated a wide variability in molecular profiles. Finally, prognosis was associated with molecular subtype but not anatomic location. Using integrative clustering, 4 distinct subtypes were defined (**Fig. 1**).

Cluster 1 was mostly made up of fluke-related CCA and was characterized by hypermethylation of promoter regions, enrichment of ARID1A, and breast cancer (BRCA)-1 and BRCA 2 mutations. Cluster 2 had both fluke-related and non–fluke-related CCA, with upregulation of CTNNB1, WNT5B, and AKT1 expression and downregulation of eukaryotic initiation factor (EIF) translation initiation factors. Both cluster 1 and 2 were had high TP53 mutations and ERBB2 amplifications. Cluster 3 displayed the highest levels of copy number alterations and upregulation of immune checkpoint genes (PD-L1 PD-L2) and pathways related to antigen presentation

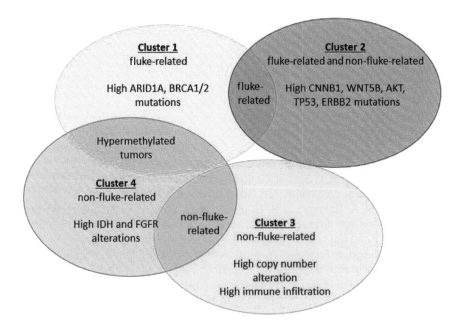

Fig. 1. Integrative cluster analysis of cholangiocarcinoma subtypes. BRCA, breast cancer.

and T-cell activation. Cluster 4 was characterized by BAP1, IDH1 and IDH2 mutations, FGFR alterations, and hypermethylation. Both cluster 3 and 4 consisted of primarily fluke-negative iCCA, whereas clusters 1 and 2 were primarily pCCA and dCCA tumors.

Gallbladder Cancer

Of the cancers of the biliary tract, gallbladder cancer remains the least characterized. The sequence of genetic alterations leading to gallbladder cancer is poorly understood but involves several well-described tumor suppressor and oncogenes. Next-generation sequencing of 17 gallbladder cancers has demonstrated an overall higher rate of somatic mutations compared with iCCA (mean 39 mutations in iCCA vs 91 mutations in gallbladder cancer). TP53was the most frequent somatic mutation, occurring in 63% of cases. Somatic mutations in epigenetic pathways involved PBRM1 and lysine methyltransferase 2C (KMT2C), the latter of which is unique to gallbladder cancer. In addition, phosphatidylinositol 3-kinase (PK3CA) and SMAD4 were also altered; however, no mutations were observed in BAP1, ARID1A, or IDH. Further investigations using high-throughput technologies are needed to confirm these initial observations.

SUMMARY

Integrated analytical approaches have been applied to multiple large data platforms to provide a better understanding of the molecular targets that may lead to improved therapeutic targets for biliary tract and primary liver tumors. These studies have revealed a highly variable and molecularly distinct cancers for which mutagen-specific pathways have been identified. Molecular subclassification of disease based on similarities provides important information regarding biologic and clinical behavior, and may identify novel therapeutic targets.

REFERENCES

1. Calado RT, Young NS. Telomere diseases. N Engl J Med 2009;361(24):2353–65.
2. Rich NE, Hester C, Odewole M, et al. Racial and ethnic differences in presentation and outcomes of hepatocellular carcinoma. Clin Gastroenterol Hepatol 2019; 17(3):551–9.e1.
3. Nault JC, Mallet M, Pilati C, et al. High frequency of telomerase reverse-transcriptase promoter somatic mutations in hepatocellular carcinoma and pre-neoplastic lesions. Nat Commun 2013;4:2218.
4. Totoki Y, Tatsuno K, Covington KR, et al. Trans-ancestry mutational landscape of hepatocellular carcinoma genomes. Nat Genet 2014;46(12):1267–73.
5. Sung WK, Zheng H, Li S, et al. Genome-wide survey of recurrent HBV integration in hepatocellular carcinoma. Nat Genet 2012;44(7):765–9.
6. de La Coste A, Romagnolo B, Billuart P, et al. Somatic mutations of the beta-catenin gene are frequent in mouse and human hepatocellular carcinomas. Proc Natl Acad Sci U S A 1998;95(15):8847–51.
7. Satoh S, Daigo Y, Furukawa Y, et al. AXIN1 mutations in hepatocellular carcinomas, and growth suppression in cancer cells by virus-mediated transfer of AXIN1. Nat Genet 2000;24(3):245–50.
8. Guichard C, Amaddeo G, Imbeaud S, et al. Integrated analysis of somatic mutations and focal copy-number changes identifies key genes and pathways in hepatocellular carcinoma. Nat Genet 2012;44(6):694–8.
9. Bressac B, Kew M, Wands J, et al. Selective G to T mutations of p53 gene in hepatocellular carcinoma from southern Africa. Nature 1991;350(6317):429–31.
10. Boyault S, Rickman DS, de Reynies A, et al. Transcriptome classification of HCC is related to gene alterations and to new therapeutic targets. Hepatology 2007; 45(1):42–52.
11. Spranger S, Bao R, Gajewski TF. Melanoma-intrinsic beta-catenin signalling prevents anti-tumour immunity. Nature 2015;523(7559):231–5.
12. Cancer Genome Atlas Research Network, Electronic address wbe, Cancer Genome Atlas Research Network. Comprehensive and integrative genomic characterization of hepatocellular carcinoma. Cell 2017;169(7):1327–41.e23.
13. Banales JM, Cardinale V, Carpino G, et al. Expert consensus document: Cholangiocarcinoma: current knowledge and future perspectives consensus statement from the European Network for the Study of Cholangiocarcinoma (ENS-CCA). Nat Rev Gastroenterol Hepatol 2016;13(5):261–80.
14. Jusakul A, Cutcutache I, Yong CH, et al. Whole-genome and epigenomic landscapes of etiologically distinct subtypes of cholangiocarcinoma. Cancer Discov 2017;7(10):1116–35.
15. Nakamura H, Arai Y, Totoki Y, et al. Genomic spectra of biliary tract cancer. Nat Genet 2015;47(9):1003–10.
16. Wang P, Dong Q, Zhang C, et al. Mutations in isocitrate dehydrogenase 1 and 2 occur frequently in intrahepatic cholangiocarcinomas and share hypermethylation targets with glioblastomas. Oncogene 2013;32(25):3091–100.
17. Saha SK, Parachoniak CA, Ghanta KS, et al. Mutant IDH inhibits HNF-4alpha to block hepatocyte differentiation and promote biliary cancer. Nature 2014; 513(7516):110–4.
18. Hedvat M, Huszar D, Herrmann A, et al. The JAK2 inhibitor AZD1480 potently blocks Stat3 signaling and oncogenesis in solid tumors. Cancer cell 2009; 16(6):487–97.

19. Wu YM, Su F, Kalyana-Sundaram S, et al. Identification of targetable FGFR gene fusions in diverse cancers. Cancer Discov 2013;3(6):636–47.

20. Sia D, Losic B, Moeini A, et al. Massive parallel sequencing uncovers actionable FGFR2-PPHLN1 fusion and ARAF mutations in intrahepatic cholangiocarcinoma. Nat Commun 2015;6:6087.

21. Graham RP, Barr Fritcher EG, Pestova E, et al. Fibroblast growth factor receptor 2 translocations in intrahepatic cholangiocarcinoma. Hum Pathol 2014;45(8): 1630–8.

22. Churi CR, Shroff R, Wang Y, et al. Mutation profiling in cholangiocarcinoma: prognostic and therapeutic implications. PLoS One 2014;9(12):e115383.

23. Fujimoto A, Furuta M, Shiraishi Y, et al. Whole-genome mutational landscape of liver cancers displaying biliary phenotype reveals hepatitis impact and molecular diversity. Nat Commun 2015;6:6120.

24. Jiao Y, Pawlik TM, Anders RA, et al. Exome sequencing identifies frequent inactivating mutations in BAP1, ARID1A and PBRM1 in intrahepatic cholangiocarcinomas. Nat Genet 2013;45(12):1470–3.

25. Luchini C, Robertson SA, Hong SM, et al. PBRM1 loss is a late event during the development of cholangiocarcinoma. Histopathology 2017;71(3):375–82.

26. Ong CK, Subimerb C, Pairojkul C, et al. Exome sequencing of liver fluke-associated cholangiocarcinoma. Nat Genet 2012;44(6):690–3.

27. Roos E, Soer EC, Klompmaker S, et al. Crossing borders: a systematic review with quantitative analysis of genetic mutations of carcinomas of the biliary tract. Crit Rev Oncol Hematol 2019;140:8–16.

28. Goeppert B, Roessler S, Renner M, et al. Mismatch repair deficiency is a rare but putative therapeutically relevant finding in non-liver fluke associated cholangiocarcinoma. Br J Cancer 2019;120(1):109–14.

29. Gingras MC, Covington KR, Chang DK, et al. Ampullary cancers harbor ELF3 tumor suppressor gene mutations and exhibit frequent WNT dysregulation. Cell Rep 2016;14(4):907–19.

30. Yachida S, Wood LD, Suzuki M, et al. Genomic sequencing identifies ELF3 as a driver of ampullary carcinoma. Cancer cell 2016;29(2):229–40.

Systemic Therapy for Primary Liver Tumors

Cholangiocarcinoma and Hepatocellular Carcinoma

Check for updates

Saeed Sadeghi, MD[a], Anthony Bejjani, MD[b], Richard S. Finn, MD[b],*

KEYWORDS

- Liver cancer • Hepatocellular carcinoma • HCC • Cholangiocarcinoma
- Targeted therapy • Immunotherapy • Systemic treatment

KEY POINTS

- In the past decade, there has been significant progress in the treatment of primary liver cancer.
- There has been increasing knowledge of the molecular alterations occurring in these tumors, which is now being translated into patient care.
- Ongoing clinical trials will further advance the therapeutic options available to patients, including the introduction of molecular targeted therapeutics and immunotherapy approaches.

INTRODUCTION

Despite their rising incidence and significant morbidity and mortality, progress in the treatment of primary liver tumors has been slow. Unlike the more common malignancies, such as lung, breast, and colon cancer, the development of novel molecular therapeutics to treat these tumors has historically been met with low enthusiasm by industry and negative clinical studies. However, that has been changing dramatically in recent years. For cholangiocarcinoma, the less common of the 2 large groups of primary liver tumors, the other being hepatocellular carcinoma (HCC), cytotoxic chemotherapy has always been the mainstay of treatment. Only recently are we seeing the impact of the years of basic research into the molecular classification of cholangiocarcinoma and understanding of the disease to have an impact in the clinic.

Saeed Sadeghi is a consultant to QED and Eisia. Anthony Bejjani has nothing to disclose. Richard Finn is a consultant to Astra Zeneca, Bayer, Bristol Myers Squibb, Eisai, Eli Lilly, Merck, Novartis, PfizerRoche/ Genentech.
[a] UCLA Oncology, 2020 Santa Monica Blvd, Suite 230, Santa Monica, CA 90404, USA; [b] UCLA Oncology, 2825 Santa Monica Blvd, Suite 200, Santa Monica, CA 90404, USA
* Corresponding author.
E-mail address: rfinn@mednet.ucla.edu

Surg Oncol Clin N Am 28 (2019) 695–715
https://doi.org/10.1016/j.soc.2019.06.015
1055-3207/19/© 2019 Elsevier Inc. All rights reserved.

There is now an unprecedented amount of activity with novel kinase inhibitors and immunotherapy agents. Treatment for advanced HCC, which is now listed as the third leading cause of cancer death globally,[1] has seen incredible progress in the past 2 years. After approval of the multitargeted kinase inhibitor sorafenib in 2007, which represented the first phase 3 study to show an improvement in overall survival (OS) with systemic therapy, there was a robust effort to improve on sorafenib and to develop agents that have activity after progression on sorafenib. In this case, it was only 10 years later, in 2017, with the approval of regorafenib after progression on sorafenib that we had the first new drug approved in the treatment of advanced HCC. However, since that time we have seen 3 additional positive phase 3 studies with new agents and the dawn of the use of immune checkpoint inhibitors in HCC. Together, this is an exciting time for our patients and researchers in the area of primary liver cancers. There are likely to be ongoing advances in the coming months and years that will continue to shape our understanding of these diseases and improve outcomes for our patients. In this article, we review the current role of medical therapy in the management of these 2 cancers in various clinical settings.

CHOLANGIOCARCINOMA

The incidence of cholangiocarcinoma (CCA), a tumor that arises from the malignant transformation of the biliary epithelium, has been increasing and currently now accounts for 3% of all gastrointestinal tumors. Clinically, CCAs can be divided into intrahepatic, hilar (Klatskin-type), and extrahepatic. CCA accounted for 135,000 deaths in 2013 based on the Global Burden of Disease study, equivalent to an age-standardized death rate of 2.3 per 100,000 per year.[2] In the United States, the incidence of intrahepatic CCA has remained stable, but overall exceeds the incidence of extrahepatic CCA (1.6 vs 1.3 per 100,000 per year).[3] Overall disease prognosis is poor, with a 5-year survival rate of 5% to 15% for all patients.[4] As most patients present in advanced stage, curative surgery is feasible in only 10% to 15% of cases.[5] Furthermore, post resection recurrence rate is high and exceeds 60%.[6] As a result, systemic therapy is necessary for most patients, either following surgery, or in locally advanced/metastatic setting. Selected clinical studies with systemic therapy in cholangiocarcinoma are in **Table 1**.

Adjuvant Therapy

Most patients who undergo surgery for CCA have disease recurrence in the liver.[7] Risk factors for recurrence include presence of multiple tumors, vascular invasion, and lymph node metastasis. Historically, there have been limited data on the role of systemic therapy after resection due to the small number of patients who are undergoing curative surgery. A meta-analysis of adjuvant therapy for biliary cancers evaluated 6712 patients from 20 studies through 2010, and demonstrated a nonsignificant improvement with adjuvant therapy compared with surgery alone (odds ratio [OR] 0.74; $P = .06$).[8] When 2 registry trials were excluded, patients who had received chemotherapy or chemoradiation had statistically significant benefit compared with radiation alone (OR 0.39, 0.61, and 0.98, respectively; $P = .02$). Furthermore, the largest benefit for adjuvant therapy was in patients with lymph node–positive disease (OR 0.49, $P = .004$) and R1 disease (OR 0.36, $P = .002$).

To date, 2 prospective phase 3 adjuvant trials for CCAs have been reported. The PRODIGE 12-ACCORD trial 18 randomized 196 patients with CCA to adjuvant gemcitabine and oxaliplatin chemotherapy versus surveillance following resection. The primary endpoint was relapse-free survival (RFS). Most patients had R0 resection

Table 1
Selected trials of targeted therapy in CCA

Target	Phase	n	ORR, %	DCR, %	PFS, mo	OS, mo	Reference
IDH1 and IDH2							
AG120	I	73	6.0	62	3.8	—	Lowery et al,[22] 2017
FGFR2							
BGJ398 (Infigratinib)	II	71	31.0	75.5	6.8	12.5	Javle et al,[26] 2018; Javle et al,[27] 2018
TAS 120	I	45	25.0	79	6.8	—	Meric-Bernstam et al,[29] 2018
INCB054828 (Pemigatinib)	II	47	40.4	85.1	9.2	—	Hollebecque et al,[30] 2018
JNJ-42756493 (Erdafinib)	I	11	27.3	55	5.1	—	Tabernero et al,[106] 2015
ARQ087 (Derazatinib)	I/II	29	20.7	82.8	5.7	—	Mazzaferro et al,[32] 2019
BRAF							
Darbafenib/Trametinib	II	35	36.0	NR	9.2	11.7	Zev et al,[38] 2019
HER2							
Trastuzumab/Pertuzumab	IIA	8	37.5	75	4.2	—	Javle et al,[43] 2017
PD-1 antibody							
Nivolumab	II	29	17.0	55	3.5	NR	Kim et al,[51] 2018

Abbreviations: CCA, cholangiocarcinoma; DCR, disease control rate; FGFR, fibroblast growth factor receptor; IDH, isocitrate dehydrogenase; NR, not reported; ORR, overall response rate; OS, overall survival; PD, programmed death; PFS, progression-free survival.

and lymph node invasion was present in 37.4% of patients receiving combination chemotherapy. With a median follow-up of 46.5 months, the median RFS was 30.4 months for the chemotherapy arm and 18.5 months for surveillance, which was not significant (hazard ratio [HR] 0.88; 95% confidence interval [CI] 0.62–1.25; $P = .48$).[9] A second trial, the BILCAP study, randomized 447 patients to oral capecitabine (1250 mg/m^2 twice daily on days 1–14 every 21 days for 8 cycles) versus observation for patients with completely resected CCA or gallbladder cancer and has established adjuvant capecitabine as standard for care for this population.[10] Of the total patient population, 30% had positive margins and 54% had node-positive disease following surgery. Intent-to-treat analysis of OS (primary outcome) was 51.1 months with capecitabine and 36.4 months with observation, resulting in a nonsignificant reduction in risk of death by approximately 20% (HR 0.81; 95% CI 0.63–1.04; $P = .097$). In a prespecified sensitivity analysis taking into consideration patient gender, nodal status, and tumor grade, the OS HR was 0.71 (95% CI 0.55–0.92; $P = .010$). Again, in a prespecified per-protocol analysis, the median OS was statistically improved with capecitabine; 53 months and 36 months, respectively, or 25% reduction in the risk of death with capecitabine (HR 0.75; 95% CI 0.58–0.97; $P = .028$). Grade 3 or 4 toxicity was less than anticipated and there was no treatment-related death. BILCAP is the first phase 3 randomized trial that has shown a benefit for adjuvant therapy in CCA. Additional adjuvant trials are ongoing, including ACTICCA-1, which is a randomized phase 3 trial comparing adjuvant gemcitabine and cisplatin with observation after resection of CCA (NCT02170090). The trial has subsequently been amended, in light of the positive BILCAP trial, to compare cisplatin and gemcitabine with capecitabine in patients with resected CCA.[11]

Locally Advanced and Metastatic Cholangiocarcinoma

Chemotherapy

Since 2010, the standard of care regimen for advanced CCA remains gemcitabine and cisplatin in the first-line setting. The ABC-02 trial was a phase 3 trial comparing gemcitabine and cisplatin with gemcitabine monotherapy; 60% of the patients had cholangiocarcinoma and 40% had gallbladder cancer. The combination of gemcitabine and cisplatin was associated with a median OS of 11.7 months compared with 8.1 months for gemcitabine (HR 0.64; $P<.001$). There was an improvement in progression-free survival (PFS) (8 vs 5 months; $P<.001$). Common adverse events, occurring in more than 10% of patients, included fatigue and increased risk of any infection that occurred at similar rate in both groups. A nonsignificant increase in neutropenia and a significant increase in liver dysfunction was seen for the cisplatin and gemcitabine combination group.[12] Several randomized phase II trials using S-1 have been done since ABC-02 in the first-line setting, with outcomes being inferior to gemcitabine and cisplatin.[13] Furthermore, efforts to incorporate biologic agents have also failed in improving survival over gemcitabine and cisplatin. Valle and colleagues[14] assessed the addition of cediranib, an oral inhibitor of vascular endothelial growth factor (VEGF) receptor 1, 2, and 3, to cisplatin and gemcitabine in a multicenter randomized phase 2 study of 124 patients. At follow-up of 12.2 months, the median PFS was 8.0 months for the cediranib and chemotherapy group and 7.4 months for the placebo and chemotherapy group (HR 0.93; $P = .72$), which was not significant. In addition, patients in the cediranib group had increase grade 3 to 4 toxicity. The potential benefit of addition of epidermal growth factor receptor (EGFR) monoclonal antibody cetuximab, was evaluated in the BINGO Trial. In this randomized, phase 2 trial, patients with unresectable or metastatic cholangiocarcinoma, gallbladder carcinoma, or ampullary carcinoma were randomized to cisplatin and gemcitabine with or without cetuximab. The trial failed to show benefit for addition of cetuximab to chemotherapy. The median PFS was 6.1 months for the cetuximab and chemotherapy arm and median PFS was 5.5 months for the chemotherapy arm alone. The median OS was 11 months and 12.4, respectively.[15]

Beyond cisplatin and gemcitabine in the first-line setting, there has been limited evidence supporting use of second-line chemotherapy for CCA.[16] The UK ABC-06 phase 3 trial evaluating oxaliplatin and 5-fluorouracil (5FU) (mFOLFOX regimen) with active symptom control (ASC) versus ASC was presented at the American Society of Clinical Oncology (ASCO) Annual Meeting 2019 and did demonstrate an improvement in OS with mFOLFOX from 5.3 months to 6.2 months and a corresponding HR of 0.69 (95% CI 0.50–0.97; $P = .031$).[17] As expected, there were more grade 3/4 toxicities with mFOLFOX but these were manageable.

Molecular targeted therapies

Recent efforts in next-generation sequencing of CCA tumors has led to a better understanding of the molecular alterations seen in this disease. Among the identified molecular alterations, mutations in isocitrate dehydrogenase genes (IDH1 and IDH2), fibroblast growth factor receptor-2 (FGFR2), KRAS pathway, as well as human epidermal growth factor receptor 2 (HER2) mutations or amplifications occur with varying frequency in both intrahepatic and extrahepatic CCA. Selective targeting of these pathways has shown early promising results.[18]

Isocitrate dehydrogenase 1 and isocitrate dehydrogenase 2 IDH1 and IDH2 are key enzymes in cellular metabolism and catalyze the oxidative decarboxylation of isocitrate to alpha-ketoglutarate in cytoplasm and mitochondria.[19] Gene profiling of CCA suggests that IDH1 and IDH2 mutations occur in 11% of CCAs and they are more frequency found in non–*Opisthorchis viverini* (liver fluke)–infected cases.[20,21] Activating mutations in IDH1 appear to be enriched in intrahepatic CCA and the mutation results in increased ability to produce 2-hydroxyglutarate (2-HG), an oncometabolite.[18] A phase 1 study of AG 120, an oral, reversible IDH1 inhibitor, evaluated 73 patients with CCA of whom 83% had intrahepatic CCA. In a treatment-refractory patient population with at least 2 prior treatments, the median PFS was 3.8 months with a 6-month PFS of 40%. Although only 6% (n = 4) of patients achieved a partial response, an additional 56% (n = 40) of patients achieved stable disease.[22] A global, phase 3, double-blind, randomized (2:1) trial evaluating AG 120 (500 mg once daily) versus matched placebo in IDH1 mutant cholangiocarcinoma with 1 or 2 prior therapies is currently ongoing (NCT02989857). A recent press release states the study met its primary endpoint of improving PFS and full data is awaited.[23] IDH2 mutations are identified less frequently in CCA. Studies with AG121, an IDH2 inhibitor (NCT02273739) and AG881, an IDH1 and 2 inhibitor (NCT02481154), in solid tumors are currently enrolling patients. Finally, preclinical work has demonstrated that IDH-mutated CCAs have a pronounced dependency on SRC signaling for cell growth and survival, and treatment of CCA xenografts with the SRC/ABL inhibitor dasatinib results in marked apoptosis and tumor regression.[24] A clinical trial of dasatinib in IDH-mutated advanced intrahepatic CCA (NCT02428855) has completed accrual and results are currently pending.

Fibroblast growth factor receptor-2 The fibroblast growth factor receptor (FGFR) is a receptor tyrosine kinase consisting of 4 related receptors (FGFR 1–4) and more than 20 ligands. Aberrant activation of FGFRs has been implicated in several malignant pathways, including angiogenesis and proliferation.[18] Molecular alterations in FGFRs, including amplification, mutations, and translocations, have been associated with bile duct tumors and vary with the site of origin. Specifically, FGFR2 translocations result in fusion proteins in 15% to 20% of intrahepatic CCAs.[18] FGFR-altered CCA tends to occur in younger patients, has a more indolent disease course, and may potentially benefit from FGFR targeted therapy.[25] The safety and efficacy of a pan-FGFR inhibitor, infigratinib (BGJ398), was evaluated in a phase 2 study of patients who harbored FGFR amplification or fusion following systemic therapy with platinum and gemcitabine. The investigators reported an overall response rate (ORR) of 14.8% in all patients and 18.8% in FGFR2 fusion patients. Disease control rate was 75.4% in all patients (83.3% in FGFR2 fusion only) with a median PFS of 5.8 months (95% CI 4.3–7.6 months).[26] Javle and colleagues[27] presented the updated results of 71 patients with FGFR2 fusions/translocations at the European Society for Medical Oncology 2018 Congress (ESMO 2018). With longer follow-up, the median duration of treatment was 5.5 months with ORR of 31% and a confirmed ORR of 26.9%. Median PFS was 6.8 (95% CI 5.3–7.6) months and median OS was 12.5 (95% CI 9.9–16.6) months. A phase 3 randomized study comparing oral infigratinib with cisplatin and gemcitabine in previously untreated patients with FGFR2 altered CCA is planned (NCT03773302).

Several other FGFR2 inhibitors are currently in clinical development. TAS-120 irreversibly inhibits mutant and wild-type FGFR2 and has shown efficacy in FGFR inhibitor resistant cell lines. Preliminary analysis of phase 1 data in a CCA cohort demonstrated a 50% partial response in the 8 patients with FGFR2 fusions. Interestingly, 1 of the 3 patients who was previously treated with an FGFR inhibitor and harboring an FGFR2 fusion also achieved a confirmed response.[28] Recent updated data of the trial were presented at ESMO 2018. Of the 45 patients with CCA, 28 had FGFR2 fusions and 7 achieved confirmed partial response (cPR) with ORR of 25%. Among the 13 patients who had received a prior FGFR inhibitor, 4 had cPR on TAS-120. The overall disease control rate was 79%.[29]

Also presented at ESMO 2018 were the interim results of the FIGHT-202 trial of INCB054828 (pemigatinib), a selective, potent oral inhibitor of FGFR1, 2, and 3 in patients with advanced CCA. The trial had 3 cohorts: FGFR translocations (cohort A, n = 100), FGF/FGFR2 genetic alterations (cohort B, n = 20) and no FGF/FGFR2 genetic alterations (cohort C). Of the 47 evaluable patients in cohort A, 94% (n = 44) had intrahepatic CCA and the ORR was 40.4% with 19 patients (40.4%) with cPR. Median duration of response (DOR) was not reached in cohort A at time of data cutoff and disease control rate (DCR) was 85.1% in cohort A with median PFS of 9.2 months.[30] A randomized, open-label phase 3 trial of pemigatinib versus cisplatin plus gemcitabine chemotherapy in first-line treatment of patients with metastatic CCA with FGFR2 rearrangement is currently recruiting patients (NCT03656536).

Another oral pan-FGFR inhibitor, erdafitinib (JNJ-42756493) demonstrated a cPR of 27.3% (95% CI 6,61) and 27.3% stable disease per response criteria in solid tumors (RECIST) 1.1 criteria with an overall DCR of 55%.[31] In another trial of 27 evaluable patients treated with FGFR inhibitor ARQ 087 (derazantinib), ORR was 20.7% with a DCR of 82.8% and PFS of 5.7 months, confirming that this compound is active as well.[32] Finally, a phase 2 trial of ponatinib in patients with FGFR fusion (NCT02265341) is currently open to accrual.[33] Future directions include evaluation of FGFR inhibitors in combination with chemotherapy, monoclonal antibodies, or immunotherapy (NCT02393248)

BRAF inhibitors Approximately 5% to 7% of all biliary cancers harbor mutations in the BRAF gene.[34] Furthermore, studies suggest that the BRAF mutations may be harbored in intrahepatic CCA.[35] The combination of BRAF and MEK inhibitors have already demonstrated efficacy in BRAF-mutated malignancies, such as melanoma[36] and non–small-cell lung cancer.[37] This has raised interest in the potential benefit of

BRAF inhibitors in treatment of other BRAF-mutated malignancies. The ROAR trial (NCT02034110) is a phase 2, open-label, multicenter trial in which patients with different BRAF-mutated cancers were treated with dabrafenib (150 mg twice a day) and trametinib (2 mg every day) until disease progression with the primary endpoint of investigator assessed ORR by RECIST v1.1, and secondary endpoints of PFS, DOR, OS, and safety. Data pertaining to the biliary tract cancer cohort have been presented. In this study, 35 patients with biliary cancers were enrolled, with 80% of the patients having received 2 or more prior systemic therapies. Results demonstrated an ORR of 36% by independent review, all of which were partial responses. The DOR at 6 months was 66%, with 7 of the 14 responders having a duration of more than 6 months and 5 having ongoing response at time of presentation. The median PFS by investigator assessment was 9.2 months and median OS was at 11.7 months.[38]

Human epidermal growth factor receptor 2 HER2 overexpression has been described in CCA, occurring at a higher rate in extrahepatic CCA (17.4%) than in intrahepatic CCA (4.8%).[39] A single-institution case series suggested that HER2-directed therapy using trastuzumab, lapatinib, or pertuzumab may result in partial response or disease stability.[40] Phase 2 trials of lapatinib in biliary cancers have been disappointing, with one trial of 17 patients with CCA and another trial of 25 patients showing no responders.[41–43] A trial of trastuzumab in patients with advanced CCA has completed accrual with results pending (NCT00478140). Finally, the combination of trastuzumab and pertuzumab was studied in HER2-positive (HER2-amplified and HER2-mutated) biliary cancers in the MyPathway study (NCT02091141). Preliminary results of the 8 HER2-amplified patients showed 3 patients with partial response with a median PFS of 4.2 months.[43] Further studies are needed to better define the appropriate therapeutic intervention for the HER2-overexpressing CCAs.

Taken together, these early results confirm that patient selection based on molecular profiling can have a positive impact on patient outcome and survival.

Immunotherapy The recent success of immunotherapy approaches as a treatment modality in other solid tumors has raised interest in potential benefit of such therapies in CCA. Specifically, the immune checkpoint inhibitors to cytotoxic T-lymphocyte-associated protein 4 (CTLA-4) and programmed death and programmed death ligand 1 (PD/PD-L1) have changed the management of several cancer types. There is growing evidence that tumor inflammation contributes to tumor development in CCA. Tumor-associated macrophages (TAM) promote tumor growth and progression.[44] In fact, patients with intrahepatic CCA with a high number of CD163+ (M2) macrophages have a poor disease-free survival,[45] Conversely, the prognosis of CCA is improved with increased levels of tumor-infiltrating CD4+ and/or cytotoxic CD8+ cells.[46] Another pathway, which is unregulated in the tumor microenvironment, is PD-L1. Binding of PD-L1 to PD-1 leads to the loss of T-cell function, anergy, and death.[47] There is evidence for increased PD-L1 expression in CCA, with more than 60% of biopsies demonstrating increased expression in the tumor or tumor microenvironment.[48] It is, however, unclear if this increased expression correlates to response to PD-1/PDL-1–directed therapeutics. Koido and colleagues[49] examined a preclinical model of intrahepatic CCA in which they demonstrated that interferon-gamma and gemcitabine exposure led to upregulation of PD-L1 blockade, suggesting that PD-L1 blockade treatment may be beneficial. Early trials of checkpoint inhibitors have included CCA cohorts. KEYNOTE 028 explored the benefit of checkpoint inhibitor pembrolizumab for refractory mismatch repair (MMR)-deficient cancers. In subset of patients with MMR-deficient CCA, the response rate was 17% with median DOR of 40 weeks. There was one complete responder and 4 patients with stable disease.[50] A phase 2 study of nivolumab in patients with advanced refractory biliary tract cancers was reported at the ESMO World Congress on Gastrointestinal Cancer 2018. The trial included patients who had progressed on at least one line of systemic therapy. In a group of 29 evaluable patients, 5 (17%) achieved partial response and 11 patients (38%) achieved stable disease with a DCR of 55%. Of note, 4 of the responders were microsatellite stable, with 2 patients with durable response of more than 12 months. The median PFS was 3.5 months and the median OS had not been reached.[51] Given these promising data, KEYNOTE 158 basket trial is ongoing, which includes 100 patients with biliary cancers. In addition, several other trials of other checkpoint inhibitors are ongoing (NCT03110328, NCT02829918, NCT01938612) as well as combination checkpoint inhibitor studies (NCT03101566).

Finally, there has been interest in combining checkpoint inhibitors with various investigational microenvironment modulating agents. In one trial, the addition of granulocyte-macrophage colony-stimulating factor to pembrolizumab (NCT02703714) was found to be safe and resulted in partial response in 5 (21%) of 24 patients. Of these 5 patients, 1 was microsatellite unstable and 4 were microsatellite stable.[52] Another trial combining interferon-alpha 2b along with checkpoint inhibitor (NCT02982720) is also ongoing. At this time, additional results from ongoing clinical trials are necessary to better define the role of immunotherapy in treatment of CCA.

HEPATOCELLULAR CARCINOMA

HCC is the most common primary liver cancer. It arises in the background of cirrhosis in ~90% of patients and presents in an early stage in only ~30% of patients in the Americas.[53] This close relationship between underlying liver disease and cancer interacts to impact the prognosis of patients. Importantly then, staging systems need to take both of these competing risks for outcome into account. The prognostic ability of the American Joint Commission on Cancer Eighth edition TNM staging system, which is used commonly in other tumor types, is limited, as it does not account for a patient's underlying liver disease. Although there are numerous other staging systems, the Barcelona Clinic Liver Cancer (BCLC) staging system has become widely used in clinical trials and is endorsed by international guidelines, and, as a result, in practice.[54] Importantly, it combines patient-level factors (performance status, Child Pugh cirrhosis stage) and tumor factors (vascular invasion, extrahepatic spread) to divide patients into 5 stages (0, A–D).[55,56] In addition, it links each stage to data-driven recommended treatment strategies (**Fig. 1**). Systemic treatments are validated and recommended for patients with "advanced HCC," meaning patients with BCLC Stage C or Stage B who are not candidates or have progressed after local-regional treatments, such as transarterial chemoembolization (TACE). Since 2007, the only systemic agent that had shown activity in advanced HCC was the multikinase inhibitor sorafenib. However, after a decade of negative studies, there has been a robust readout in positive phase 3 studies with molecularly targeted therapeutics. In addition, through accelerated approval mechanisms, 2 immune checkpoint inhibitors have been approved in the second-line setting and, still, there are numerous phase 3 studies of novel combinations ongoing. With an increasing number of active systemic agents, which are incrementally improving OS, we anticipate more patients receiving these drugs based on high levels of evidence.

Timing of the Transition to Systemic Therapy

For the ~30% of patients who present with early-stage liver cancer BCLC Stage 0 or A, they are eligible for potentially curative strategies, such as surgical resection, liver

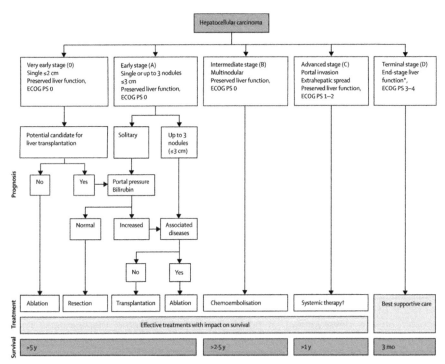

Fig. 1. The BCLC staging system. * Patients with end-stage cirrhosis due to heavily impaired liver function (Child-Pugh stage C or earlier stages with predictors of poor prognosis or high a MELD score) should be considered for liver transplantation. In these patients, hepatocellular carcinoma might become a contraindication if it exceeds enlistment criteria. † Please refer to the text for a discussion on systemic therapy in HCC. (*Reprinted with permission from* Elsevier (The Lancet, Forner A, Reig M, Bruix J. Hepatocellular carcinoma. Lancet. 2018;391(10127):1301–14.)

transplantation, or percutaneous ablative strategies. However, a number of patients will recur despite optimal management. Approximately 60% of patients have either BCLC Stage B or C disease, either as their stage on presentation or eventually migrate from Stage 0/A. BCLC Stage B includes patients eligible for local-regional treatment strategies, such as TACE, in which ablative strategies are less likely to work. BCLC Stage C includes patients who are advanced stage and have characteristics precluding locoregional therapy, such as decreased performance status/tumor symptoms, extrahepatic disease and/or macroscopic vessel invasion.

Patients with BCLC Stage B may progress on TACE or migrate to Stage C by virtue of development of extrahepatic disease or macrovascular vessel invasion, both characteristics associated with decreased benefit from TACE. TACE typically can be performed up to 3 to 4 times per year and no more frequently than every 2 months to avoid liver failure. With conventional techniques, median time to progression with TACE is >1 year.[57] Absence of response after 2 treatments or progression of previously treated lesions indicates treatment failure.[58] Some patients have a much more rapid time to progression, including those within 5 months of treatment, and likely would benefit from earlier transition to systemic therapy.[59,60] Given the potential for patients to migrate through these stages of liver cancer, a multidisciplinary team, including surgeons, interventional radiologists, hepatologists, and medical oncologists, should carefully monitor the patients throughout their treatment course. Radioembolization with yttrium-90 (Y-90) has been used increasingly in the management of BCLC B disease without high-level evidence that it is superior to TACE for improving OS. There has been interest in using Y-90 for patients who progress on TACE or for those that have BCLC C disease. This should not be done, as there have now been 3 negative phase 3 studies evaluating this concept. The SARAH and SIRveNIB studies evaluated Y-90 versus sorafenib, with both failing at their primary endpoints of superior OS compared with sorafenib (median OS of 8.8 months vs 9.9 months for SARAH, median OS of 8 months vs 10.2 months for SIRveNIB).[61,62] The SORAMIC study evaluated the combination of Y-90 and sorafenib versus sorafenib, which failed to show superior OS in the palliative cohort (12.1 months) compared with sorafenib (11.5 months, HR 1.01).[63] All 3 of these studies have been negative, and Y-90 is therefore not recommended by the EASL or American Association for the Study of Liver Diseases (AASLD) guidelines for the management of HCC after progression on TACE or with BCLC C disease.[64]

The Biologic Rationale Behind Targeted Systemic Therapies

Hepatocellular carcinoma historically has been very challenging to treat given no significant activity of cytotoxic chemotherapy. No study has demonstrated a statistically significant survival advantage in advanced HCC. As in other areas of cancer medicine, the focus of drug development in HCC has moved beyond chemotherapy and is focused on the development of novel, molecularly targeted therapeutics. There have been numerous molecular profiling studies that have highlighted the molecular heterogeneity of HCC that have spurred an intense effort to develop these drugs in patients with advanced disease.[65,66] To date, all phase 3 studies have focused on patients with Child Pugh (CP) A liver disease to minimize the risk of death from cirrhosis. Consistently it has been demonstrated that CP score is prognostic of outcome with systemic therapy, with survival decreasing with increased CP score. Other mechanisms to capture prognosis in advanced HCC are being evaluated, such as the albumin-bilirubin (ALBI) score.[67] The phase 3 studies of drugs currently approved by the US FDA are shown in **Table 2**.

First-Line Therapy: Sorafenib and Lenvatinib

Sorafenib, a multikinase inhibitor that targets vascular endothelial growth factor receptor (VEGFR) 1 to 3, platelet-derived growth factor receptor (PDGFR)-β, KIT, FLT-3, and RAF, was the first agent to demonstrate a survival advantage in advanced HCC. It gained approval from the Food and Drug Administration (FDA) in 2007 for treatment of advanced HCC (BCLC C disease or BCLC B that progressed on TACE) after demonstrating improved OS compared with placebo in 2 phase 3 trials.[68,69] One each in North America and Europe, the SHARP study demonstrated a significant improvement in OS with sorafenib (10.7 months) compared with placebo (7.9 months) with an HR of 0.69 (95% CI 0.55–0.87; $P<.001$), indicating a 31% decrease in the risk of death. The second phase 3 randomized study from Asia demonstrated the same magnitude of benefit with an HR of 0.68 (95% CI 0.50–0.93; $P = .014$), although the control arm had a poor median OS of 4.2 months that was increased to 6.5 months with sorafenib likely representing practice patterns between the West and East. Given sorafenib targets multiple kinases and given the paucity of tissue collection from trials, the exact mechanisms behind the efficacy of sorafenib remain unclear. The presence of some toxicities to sorafenib (diarrhea, hypertension, hand-foot syndrome) has been correlated with survival.[70] Increased Ras-MAPK pathway signaling is one of the drivers in the proliferation class subset of HCC, which is usually associated with

Table 2
Phase 3 studies of approved agents in advanced HCC

Trial Name	Randomization	No. Patients	Primary Endpoint	Results	Reference
SHARP	Sorafenib vs placebo 1st line	602	Overall survival	10.7 mo vs 7.9 mo (HR 0.69)	Llovet et al,[68] 2008
REFLECT	Lenvatinib vs sorafenib 1st line	954	Overall survival	13 mo vs 12.3 mo (HR 0.92–95% CI 0.79–1.06)	Kudo et al,[81] 2018
RESORCE	Regorafenib vs Placebo 2nd line	573	Overall survival	10.6 mo vs 7.8 mo (HR 0.63)	Bruix et al,[90] 2017
CELESTIAL	Cabozantinib vs placebo 2nd or 3rd line	707	Overall survival	10.2 mo vs 8 mo (HR 0.76)	Abou-Alfa et al,[95] 2018
REACH-2	Ramucirumab vs placebo 2nd line AFP >400 ng/mL	292	Overall survival	8.5 mo vs 7.3 mo (HR 0.71)	Zhu et al,[96] 2019
KEYNOTE 240	Pembrolizumab vs placebo 2nd lines	413	Overall survival and PFS (dual primary)	10.3 mo vs 13.9 mo (HR 0.781)[a]	Finn et al,[101] 2019

Abbreviations: AFP, alfa fetoprotein; CI, confidence interval; HR, hazard ratio; PFS, progression-free survival.
[a] Although a significant clinical benefit was seen with pembrolizumab in KEYNOTE 240, the study does not meet the prespecified *P* values. HR for PFS was 0.775 (0.609–0.987), *P* = .0186, and for overall survival HR was 0.781 (0.611–0.998), *P* = .0238. To be declared positive for these endpoints, the prespecified *P* values needed to be .002 and .0174 for PFS and overall survival, respectively.

hepatitis B virus (HBV) infections.[66] However, in a pooled analysis of the 2 phase 3 studies of sorafenib compared with placebo, there was a greater benefit of sorafenib in the setting of hepatitis C virus (HCV) infection as compared with HBV infection (HR 0.47, 0.32–0.69, and HR 0.78, 0.57–1.06, respectively).[71] Molecular classification schemes have helped consolidate our knowledge of tumorigenesis but have yet to be significantly translated into clinical practice.[72] Efforts to demonstrate its efficacy in earlier stage disease, such as in combination or sequence with TACE or adjuvantly after curative surgery or RFA failed to demonstrate improvements in outcomes.[73–75]

Lenvatinib is a small-molecule tyrosine kinase inhibitor that inhibits VEGFR 1 to 3, FGFR 1 to 4, PDGFRα, RET, and KIT. RET signaling is implicated in many malignancies and is essential for many cellular processes, including survival, differentiation, motility, proliferation, and growth.[76] RET mutations in HCC are rare (3%–6%) but associated with a particularly poor prognosis.[77,78] Lenvatinib demonstrated an early efficacy signal and acceptable safety in phase 1 and 2 trials, leading to a weight-based dosing paradigm for further development; 8 mg or 12 mg for less than 60 kg or $\geq$60 kg, respectively.[79,80] In the open-label phase 3 REFLECT noninferiority study, lenvatinib demonstrated an OS of 13.6 months compared with 12.3 months with sorafenib (HR 0.92; 95% CI 0.79–1.06), clearly meeting the predefined criteria for noninferiority with upper limit of CI $\leq$1.08.[81] Lenvatinib significantly improved secondary endpoints including PFS (7.4 months vs 3.7 months, HR 0.66), time to progression (8.9 months vs 3.7 months, HR 0.63), ORR by modified RECIST (mRECIST) (24.1% vs 9.2%, OR 3.13) and by RECIST independent review (18.8% vs 6.5%, OR 3.34). Subgroup analysis showed additional benefit for lenvatinib in higher-risk patients, including HBV etiology, alfa fetoprotein (AFP) greater than 200 ng/mL, and macroscopic portal vein invasion, although main portal vein invasion was excluded at entry. Compared with sorafenib, lenvatinib had less any grade hand-foot syndrome (27% vs 52%) and diarrhea (39% vs 46%) but more hypertension (42% vs 30%) and proteinuria (25% vs 11%). In the trial, lenvatinib drug interruption occurred in 190 (40%) patients and dose reduction in 176 (37%) patients, similar to sorafenib (32% dose interruption, 38% dose reduction). Both drugs also had similar discontinuation rates (9% lenvatinib, 7% sorafenib).

Why lenvatinib, after a decade of trial failures of drugs compared with sorafenib, was the first to be successful is unclear. Biomarker data from the REFLECT study suggest that lenvatinib is more potent at inhibiting antiangiogenic pathways and an unlike sorafenib, modulates FGFR signaling.[82] Perhaps most importantly, lenvatinib has a significant response rate as compared with sorafenib. In a retrospective analysis from the REFLECT study, median OS for patients who had a response to either lenvatinib or sorafenib was 22 months versus 11 months for those who did not respond.[83] These data suggest that perhaps responses do matter in HCC. Whereas in the past with sorafenib we could improve survival by slowing progression and not inducing a significant number of objective responses, lenvatinib appears more potent and able to accomplish this. Still, a predictive marker of who will respond is lacking. Based on current data, lenvatinib and sorafenib stand as the 2 front-line treatment options for advanced HCC.

Second-Line Therapy After Sorafenib Progression

Regorafenib was the first drug approved for patients who had progressed on sorafenib. Regorafenib is a multikinase inhibitor targeting VEGFR, PDGFR, RET, KIT, RAF, FGFR1, and TIE-2.[84] The addition of a fluorine atom to sorafenib yields regorafenib and, as such, it overlaps with many targets of sorafenib but with a higher potency.[84] Angiopoietin 2 (Ang2) signals via TIE-2 and high serum Ang2 levels are associated with a poor prognosis in HCC.[85] Thus, regorafenib may provide additional antiangiogenic coverage over sorafenib. Preclinical data suggest that tumors continue to rely on VEGF/VEGFR signaling and RAF/MEK/ERK signaling after progression on sorafenib, suggesting regorafenib may have activity after sorafenib.[86] The RESORCE study was a phase 3 placebo-controlled randomized trial that for the first time demonstrated an improved survival with an agent after progression on sorafenib. There had been 3 negative phase 3 trials before these results.[87–89] In RESORCE, median OS was 10.6 months with regorafenib compared with 7.8 months with placebo (HR 0.63; 95% CI 0.50–0.79; P<.0001).[90] The most significant toxicities with regorafenib include hand-foot syndrome, diarrhea, hypertension, and fatigue. These toxicities are quite similar to sorafenib and managed similarly with moisturizing lotions and keratinolytic creams (urea 40%), along with dose interruptions, being helpful for hand-foot syndrome. Importantly, for inclusion into the study, patients had to have not only documented progression on sorafenib but had to tolerate a minimal dose of 400 mg per day for at least 20 of the last 28 days. A retrospective analysis for patients on the study revealed that the median OS for patients from their start of sorafenib from death on the RESORCE trial was 26 months as compared with 19 months for patients who went from sorafenib to placebo on study. In addition, the survival benefit from regorafenib was independent of prior sorafenib dose or time on sorafenib. Although not representative of the entire advanced HCC population, because a survival of 26 months can be achieved with the sequence in properly selected patients suggests that we can change the natural history of advanced HCC.[91]

Cabozantinib, an inhibitor of VEGFR 1 to 3, RET, MET, and AXL, also appeared tailored to address resistance mechanisms to prior antiangiogenic therapy. Hepatocyte growth factor (HGF) signals through both MET and with VEGF to stimulate tumorigenesis and angiogenesis.[92] MET activation leads to signaling through the RAF/MEK/ERK pathway, suggesting that MET blockade with cabozantinib also may have overlap with RAF blockade with sorafenib/regorafenib.[93] Sorafenib-resistant HCC models showed increased HGF secretion and c-MET activation that promoted invasiveness of the cells.[94] In the phase 3 CELESTIAL trial, 707 patients were randomized 2:1 (or 1:1) to cabozantinib 60 mg versus placebo. Cabozantinib demonstrated superior OS (10.2 months) compared with placebo (8 months) after sorafenib progression (HR 0.76; 95% CI 0.63–0.92).[95] Unlike other trials in the post-sorafenib setting, the CELESTIAL trial included patients not only in the second-line but the third-line setting as well (72% and 27% of the study population, respectively). Of the 192 patients who were receiving cabozantinib in the third-line setting, only 8 patients had received regorafenib as a prior therapy and 17 patients had received anti–PD-1/PD-L1 therapy, underpowered to address what the optimal sequence of active drugs should be.

The benefit of regorafenib and cabozantinib extended to almost all subgroups in their respective phase 3 trials. Regorafenib improved both OS and PFS in commonly selected subgroups, such as macrovascular invasion, extrahepatic disease, etiology of the liver disease (HBV, HCV, alcohol use), and regardless of AFP level. Cabozantinib significantly improved OS and PFS in the HBV-infected subgroup, but not OS in the HCV subgroup.

High AFP production may represent an aggressive subtype of liver cancer, mimicking progenitor cells with proliferative gene signatures, higher microvessel densities, and a poor prognosis.[66] Typical AFP value cutoffs for high and low subgroups are either 200 or 400 ng/mL. Cabozantinib and regorafenib had benefit in their respective AFP subgroups. Ramucirumab, a monoclonal antibody directed toward VEGFR-2, was first evaluated in the phase 3 REACH trial in the second line compared with placebo. Ramucirumab failed to improve OS in the study, but in the AFP greater than 400 ng/mL subgroup, significantly prolonged OS (7.8 months) compared with placebo (4.2 months) (HR 0.67).[87] Given this significant subgroup finding, another phase 3 trial, REACH-2, was conducted, but in a population of patients all with AFP greater than 400 ng/mL. Compared with placebo in the second line, ramucirumab in this patient population significantly extended OS (8.5 months) compared with placebo (7.3 months) (HR 0.71; 95% CI 0.531–0.949).[96] Unlike the other antiangiogenic tyrosine kinase inhibitors, a significant grade $\geq$3 treatment emergent adverse event with ramucirumab included was hyponatremia (5.6%). Ramucirumab has joined regorafenib and cabozantinib as an effective antiangiogenic agent after sorafenib progression but in a biomarker-selected population of patients with AFP greater than 400 ng/mL.

Immunotherapy in the Second Line

As discussed earlier, the tumor microenvironment involves a dynamic interaction among the tumor itself, the vasculature, the stroma, and immune cells. CD8+ T cells are the main tumor effectors with prior studies showing improved OS in patients with large amounts of these tumor-infiltrating lymphocytes.[97] However, over time, these T cells lose their tumor effectiveness, termed T-cell "exhaustion," that occurs from many mechanisms, the predominant one being PD-1/PD-L1.[98] Inhibiting this axis to allow for persistent antitumor activity by the patient's own immune system has led to durable responses in many other tumors, thus leading to its exploration in HCC.

Monoclonal antibodies against PD-1, nivolumab and pembrolizumab, have both been investigated in HCC after sorafenib progression. In the CheckMate 040 phase 1/2 dose escalation/expansion trial, 262 patients were treated with nivolumab, demonstrating an ORR of 15% to 20% by RECIST 1.1.[99] Notably, the responses attained were durable, with median DOR of approximately 17 months. Most common treatment-related adverse events were rash (23%) and pruritis (19%). Treatment-emergent grade 3/4 elevations in aspartate aminotransferase were 18%, alanine aminotransferase 11%, and bilirubin 7%. Systemic steroids were required in 5% of patients. Very similar results were noted in the KEYNOTE-224 phase 2 trial evaluating pembrolizumab in the second-line setting.[100] In that trial, 169 patients were treated with pembrolizumab and had an ORR of 17%, similar DOR, and similar safety profile. Both nivolumab and pembrolizumab received accelerated approval by the FDA based on these data. Confirmatory studies with both drugs have been completed. At ASCO 2019, results of KEYNOTE-240 were presented that compared pembrolizumab to best supportive care (REFENCEXXX). This study did not meet its prespecified endpoint of a P value less than .002 for PFS and .0174 for OS despite clinically meaningful improvements in both endpoints with PFS HR of 0.775 (0.609–0.987), P = .0186 and for OS HR of 0.781 (0.611–0.998), P = .0238 and a response rate of 18% with pembrolizumab and a median DOR of more than 13 months.[101] The CHECKMATE 459 study is evaluating sorafenib versus nivolumab in the front-line setting and results are eagerly awaited (NCT02576509)

Combination Systemic Therapies

Multikinase inhibitors target angiogenesis and proliferative pathways resulting in tumor hypoxia, tumor vascular normalization, and suppressed growth and the antitumor effects seen with these drugs are likely a combination of direct kinase inhibition and effects on the tumor immune microenvironment. Antiangiogenesis is limited by tumor hypoxia inducing immune escape. Indeed, tumor hypoxia, mediated by M2 macrophages, upregulate PD-L1 via hypoxia induced factor-1 alpha (HIF-1) that allows evasion by the immune system.[102] Sorafenib treatment leads to reduced regulatory

T cells and increased PD-1 expression on Th1 cells presumably as a result of hypoxic conditions.[102] These findings suggest a possible role for combining antiangiogenic therapy with checkpoint inhibitors to target hypoxic immune evasion.

The combination of atezolizumab (anti–PD-L1) and bevacizumab (anti-VEGFA) was studied in a phase 1 trial with similar safety profiles of the individual agents together.[103] Given its safety and the high response rate, the combination received a "breakthrough therapy" designation from the FDA and the combination is being compared with sorafenib in the first-line setting in a phase 3 trial (IMBRAVE150, NCT03434379).[104] Another early-phase study trial demonstrated the safety of pembrolizumab and lenvatinib with a promising response rate of 46% by mRECIST.[105] This combination is now being studied in a phase 3 trial with lenvatinib monotherapy as the control arm (LEAP-002 study, NCT03713593). A phase 3 study of cabozantinib and atezolizumab versus sorafenib has recently been launched as well (COSMIC-312 study, NCT03755791). Combination immune therapy is also being explored in the first line with durvalumab (anti–PD-L1)/tremelimumab (anti–CTLA-4) being compared with sorafenib in the phase 3 HIMALAYA trial (NCT03298451). The phase 3 EMERALD-1 and -2 studies are evaluating durvalumab alone, the combination of durvalumab and bevacizumab, or placebo in both intermediate HCC with TACE (NCT03778957) and in the adjuvant setting post resection (NCT03847428), respectively. Similarly, the phase 3 CHECK-MATE 9DX study is evaluating nivolumab in the adjuvant setting of high-risk resected HCC (NCT03383458).

SUMMARY

In the past decade, there has been significant progress in the treatment of primary liver cancer. There has been increasing knowledge of the molecular alterations occurring in these tumors, which is now being translated into patient care. Ongoing clinical trials will further advance the therapeutic options available to patients, including the introduction of molecular targeted therapeutics and immunotherapy approaches. Critical to the success of these new drugs is the appropriate use of them in the clinic to maximize efficacy and limit toxicity.

REFERENCES

1. Bray F, Ferlay J, Soerjomataram I, et al. Global cancer statistics 2018: GLOBOCAN estimates of incidence and mortality worldwide for 36 cancers in 185 countries. CA Cancer J Clin 2018;68(6):394–424.

2. GBD 2013 Mortality and Causes of Death Collaborators. Global, regional, and national age-sex specific all-cause and cause-specific mortality for 240 causes of death, 1990-2013: a systematic analysis for the Global Burden of Disease Study 2013. Lancet 2015;385(9963):117–71.

3. Mosadeghi S, Liu B, Bhuket T, et al. Sex-specific and race/ethnicity-specific disparities in cholangiocarcinoma incidence and prevalence in the USA: an updated analysis of the 2000-2011 surveillance, epidemiology and end results registry. Hepatol Res 2016;46(7):669–77.

4. Anderson C, Kim R. Adjuvant therapy for resected extrahepatic cholangiocarcinoma: a review of the literature and future directions. Cancer Treat Rev 2009; 35(4):322–7.

5. Nathan H, Pawlik TM, Wolfgang CL, et al. Trends in survival after surgery for cholangiocarcinoma: a 30-year population-based SEER database analysis. J Gastrointest Surg 2007;11(11):1488–96 [discussion: 1496–7].

6. Endo I, Gonen M, Yopp AC, et al. Intrahepatic cholangiocarcinoma: rising frequency, improved survival, and determinants of outcome after resection. Ann Surg 2008;248(1):84–96.

7. Spolverato G, Vitale A, Cucchetti A, et al. Can hepatic resection provide a long-term cure for patients with intrahepatic cholangiocarcinoma? Cancer 2015; 121(22):3998–4006.

8. Horgan AM, Amir E, Walter T, et al. Adjuvant therapy in the treatment of biliary tract cancer: a systematic review and meta-analysis. J Clin Oncol 2012; 30(16):1934–40.

9. Edeline J, Benabdelghani M, Bertaut A, et al. Gemcitabine and oxaliplatin chemotherapy or surveillance in resected biliary tract cancer (PRODIGE 12-ACCORD 18-UNICANCER GI): a randomized phase III study. J Clin Oncol 2019;37(8):658–67.

10. Primrose JN, Fox RP, Palmer DH, et al. Capecitabine compared with observation in resected biliary tract cancer (BILCAP): a randomised, controlled, multicentre, phase 3 study. Lancet Oncol 2019;20(5):663–73.

11. Stein A, Arnold D, Bridgewater J, et al. Adjuvant chemotherapy with gemcitabine and cisplatin compared to observation after curative intent resection of cholangiocarcinoma and muscle invasive gallbladder carcinoma (ACTICCA-1 trial) - a randomized, multidisciplinary, multinational phase III trial. BMC Cancer 2015;15:564.

12. Valle J, Wasan H, Palmer DH, et al. Cisplatin plus gemcitabine versus gemcitabine for biliary tract cancer. N Engl J Med 2010;362(14):1273–81.

13. Morizane C, Ueno M, Ikeda M, et al. New developments in systemic therapy for advanced biliary tract cancer. Jpn J Clin Oncol 2018;48(8):703–11.

14. Valle JW, Wasan H, Lopes A, et al. Cediranib or placebo in combination with cisplatin and gemcitabine chemotherapy for patients with advanced biliary tract cancer (ABC-03): a randomised phase 2 trial. Lancet Oncol 2015;16(8):967–78.

15. Malka D, Cervera P, Foulon S, et al. Gemcitabine and oxaliplatin with or without cetuximab in advanced biliary-tract cancer (BINGO): a randomised, open-label, non-comparative phase 2 trial. Lancet Oncol 2014;15(8):819–28.

16. Lamarca A, Hubner RA, David Ryder W, et al. Second-line chemotherapy in advanced biliary cancer: a systematic review. Ann Oncol 2014;25(12):2328–38.

17. Lamarca A, Palmer DH, Wasan HS, et al. ABC-06 | A randomised phase III, multicentre, open-label study of active symptom control (ASC) alone or ASC with oxaliplatin/5-FU chemotherapy (ASC+mFOLFOX) for patients (pts) with locally advanced/metastatic biliary tract cancers (ABC) previously-treated with cisplatin/gemcitabine (CisGem) chemotherapy. J Clin Oncol 2019;37(15_suppl): 4003.

18. Valle JW, Lamarca A, Goyal L, et al. New horizons for precision medicine in biliary tract cancers. Cancer Discov 2017;7(9):943–62.

19. Molenaar RJ, Maciejewski JP, Wilmink JW, et al. Wild-type and mutated IDH1/2 enzymes and therapy responses. Oncogene 2018;37(15):1949–60.

20. Chan-On W, Nairismagi ML, Ong CK, et al. Exome sequencing identifies distinct mutational patterns in liver fluke-related and non-infection-related bile duct cancers. Nat Genet 2013;45(12):1474–8.

21. Farshidfar F, Zheng S, Gingras MC, et al. Integrative genomic analysis of cholangiocarcinoma identifies distinct IDH-mutant molecular profiles. Cell Rep 2017; 19(13):2878–80.

22. Lowery MA, Abou-Alfa GK, Burris HA, et al. Phase I study of AG-120, an IDH1 mutant enzyme inhibitor: Results from the cholangiocarcinoma dose escalation and expansion cohorts. Journal of Clinical Oncology 2017;35(15_suppl):4015.
23. Available at: http://investor.agios.com/news-releases/news-release-details/agios-announces-randomized-phase-3-claridhy-trial-tibsovor.
24. Saha SK, Gordan JD, Kleinstiver BP, et al. Isocitrate dehydrogenase mutations confer dasatinib hypersensitivity and SRC dependence in intrahepatic cholangiocarcinoma. Cancer Discov 2016;6(7):727–39.
25. Jain A, Borad MJ, Kelley RK, et al. Cholangiocarcinoma with FGFR genetic aberrations: a unique clinical phenotype. JCO Precision Oncology 2018;(2):1–12.
26. Javle M, Lowery M, Shroff RT, et al. Phase II study of BGJ398 in patients with FGFR-altered advanced cholangiocarcinoma. J Clin Oncol 2018;36(3):276–82.
27. M. Javle RKK, Roychowdhury S., Weiss KH, et al. Updated results from a phase II study of infigratinib (BGJ398), a selective pan-FGFR kinase inhibitor, in patients with previously treated advanced cholangiocarcinoma containing FGFR2 fusions. Proceedings from the ESMO Congress, 2018, Munich, Germany, Abstract 3652.
28. Arkenau BT H, Soria J, Bahleda R, et al. Early clinical efficacy of TAS-120, a covalently bound FGFR inhibitor, in patients with cholangiocarcinoma. Ann Oncol 2017;28:iii137–49.
29. Meric-Bernstam F, He H, Huang J, et al. O-001Efficacy of TAS-120, an irreversible fibroblast growth factor receptor (FGFR) inhibitor, in cholangiocarcinoma patients with FGFR pathway alterations who were previously treated with chemotherapy and other FGFR inhibitors. Ann Oncol 2018;29(suppl_5).
30. Hollebecque A, Lihou C, Zhen H, et al. Interim results of fight-202, a phase II, open-label, multicenter study of INCB054828 in patients (pts) with previously treated advanced/metastatic or surgically unresectable cholangiocarcinoma (CCA) with/without fibroblast growth factor (FGF)/FGF receptor (FGFR) genetic alterations. Ann Oncol 2018;29(suppl_8).
31. Soria J-C, Strickler JH, Govindan R, et al. Safety and activity of the pan-fibroblast growth factor receptor (FGFR) inhibitor erdafitinib in phase 1 study patients (Pts) with molecularly selected advanced cholangiocarcinoma (CCA) 2017;35(15_suppl):4074.
32. Mazzaferro V, El-Rayes BF, Droz Dit Busset M, et al. Derazantinib (ARQ 087) in advanced or inoperable FGFR2 gene fusion-positive intrahepatic cholangiocarcinoma. Br J Cancer 2019;120(2):165–71.
33. DeLeon T, Alberts SR, McWilliams RR, et al. A pilot study of ponatinib in cholangiocarcinoma patients with FGFR2 fusions. Journal of Clinical Oncology 2018;36(4_suppl):TPS532.
34. Ahn DH, Bekaii-Saab T. Biliary cancer: intrahepatic cholangiocarcinoma vs. extrahepatic cholangiocarcinoma vs. gallbladder cancers: classification and therapeutic implications. J Gastrointest Oncol 2017;8(2):293–301.
35. Jain A, Kwong LN, Javle M. Genomic profiling of biliary tract cancers and implications for clinical practice. Curr Treat Options Oncol 2016;17(11):58.
36. Long GV, Stroyakovskiy D, Gogas H, et al. Dabrafenib and trametinib versus dabrafenib and placebo for Val600 BRAF-mutant melanoma: a multicentre, double-blind, phase 3 randomised controlled trial. Lancet 2015;386(9992):444–51.
37. Planchard D, Kim TM, Mazieres J, et al. Dabrafenib in patients with BRAF(V600E)-positive advanced non-small-cell lung cancer: a single-arm, multicentre, open-label, phase 2 trial. Lancet Oncol 2016;17(5):642–50.

38. Zev A, Wainberg UNL, Elena Elez, et al. Efficacy and safety of dabrafenib (D) and trametinib (T) in patients (pts) with BRAF V600E–mutated biliary tract cancer (BTC): a cohort of the ROAR basket trial. J Clin Oncol 2019;37. abstr 187.

39. Galdy S, Lamarca A, McNamara MG, et al. HER2/HER3 pathway in biliary tract malignancies; systematic review and meta-analysis: a potential therapeutic target? Cancer Metastasis Rev 2017;36(1):141–57.

40. Javle M, Churi C, Kang HC, et al. HER2/neu-directed therapy for biliary tract cancer. J Hematol Oncol 2015;8:58.

41. Ramanathan RK, Belani CP, Singh DA, et al. A phase II study of lapatinib in patients with advanced biliary tree and hepatocellular cancer. Cancer Chemother Pharmacol 2009;64(4):777–83.

42. Peck J, Wei L, Zalupski M, et al. HER2/neu may not be an interesting target in biliary cancers: results of an early phase II study with lapatinib. Oncology 2012;82(3):175–9.

43. Javle MM, Hainsworth JD, Swanton C, et al. Pertuzumab + trastuzumab for HER2-positive metastatic biliary cancer: Preliminary data from MyPathway 2017;35(4_suppl):402.

44. Mantovani A, Allavena P, Sica A. Tumour-associated macrophages as a prototypic type II polarised phagocyte population: role in tumour progression. Eur J Cancer 2004;40(11):1660–7.

45. Hasita H, Komohara Y, Okabe H, et al. Significance of alternatively activated macrophages in patients with intrahepatic cholangiocarcinoma. Cancer Sci 2010;101(8):1913–9.

46. Nakakubo Y, Miyamoto M, Cho Y, et al. Clinical significance of immune cell infiltration within gallbladder cancer. Br J Cancer 2003;89(9):1736–42.

47. Chai Y. Immunotherapy of biliary tract cancer. Tumour Biol 2016;37(3):2817–21.

48. Fontugne J, Augustin J, Pujals A, et al. PD-L1 expression in perihilar and intrahepatic cholangiocarcinoma. Oncotarget 2017;8(15):24644–51.

49. Koido S, Kan S, Yoshida K, et al. Immunogenic modulation of cholangiocarcinoma cells by chemoimmunotherapy. Anticancer Res 2014;34(11):6353–61.

50. Le DT, Durham JN, Smith KN, et al. Mismatch repair deficiency predicts response of solid tumors to PD-1 blockade. Science 2017;357(6349):409–13.

51. Kim D, Zhou J, Schell M, et al. O-009A Phase II multi institutional study of nivolumab in patients with advanced refractory biliary tract cancers (BTC). Ann Oncol 2018;29(suppl_5).

52. Kelley RK, Mitchell E, Behr S, et al. Phase II trial of pembrolizumab (PEM) plus granulocyte macrophage colony stimulating factor (GM-CSF) in advanced biliary cancers (ABC). J Clin Oncol 2018;36(4_suppl):386.

53. Oliveri RS, Wetterslev J, Gluud C. Transarterial (chemo)embolisation for unresectable hepatocellular carcinoma. Cochrane Database Syst Rev 2011;(3):CD004787.

54. Forner A, Reig M, Bruix J. Hepatocellular carcinoma. Lancet 2018;391(10127):1301–14.

55. Marrero JA, Kulik LM, Sirlin CB, et al. Diagnosis, staging, and management of hepatocellular carcinoma: 2018 practice guidance by the American Association for the Study of Liver Diseases. Hepatology 2018;68(2):723–50.

56. European Association for the Study of the Liver. EASL clinical practice guidelines: management of hepatocellular carcinoma. J Hepatol 2018;69(1):182–236.

57. Ou MC, Liu YS, Chuang MT, et al. Time-to-progression following conventional compared with drug-eluting-bead transcatheter arterial chemoembolisation in patients with large hepatocellular carcinoma. Clin Radiol 2019;74(4):295–300.

58. Izumoto H, Hiraoka A, Ishimaru Y, et al. Validation of newly proposed time to transarterial chemoembolization progression in intermediate-stage hepatocellular carcinoma cases. Oncology 2017;93(Suppl 1):120–6.
59. Arizumi T, Ueshima K, Minami T, et al. Effectiveness of sorafenib in patients with transcatheter arterial chemoembolization (TACE) refractory and intermediate-stage hepatocellular carcinoma. Liver Cancer 2015;4(4):253–62.
60. Kudo M, Matsui O, Izumi N, et al. Transarterial chemoembolization failure/refractoriness: JSH-LCSGJ criteria 2014 update. Oncology 2014;87(Suppl 1):22–31.
61. Chow PKH, Gandhi M, Tan SB, et al. SIRveNIB: selective internal radiation therapy versus sorafenib in Asia-pacific patients with hepatocellular carcinoma. J Clin Oncol 2018;36(19):1913–21.
62. Vilgrain V, Pereira H, Assenat E, et al. Efficacy and safety of selective internal radiotherapy with yttrium-90 resin microspheres compared with sorafenib in locally advanced and inoperable hepatocellular carcinoma (SARAH): an open-label randomised controlled phase 3 trial. Lancet Oncol 2017;18(12):1624–36.
63. Ricke J, Sangro B, Amthauer H, et al. The impact of combining selective internal radiation therapy (SIRT) with Sorafenib on overall survival in patients with advanced hepatocellular carcinoma: The Soramic trial palliative cohort. Journal of Hepatology 2018;68:S102. Abstract LBO-005. EASL. 2018.
64. Heimbach JK, Kulik LM, Finn RS, et al. AASLD guidelines for the treatment of hepatocellular carcinoma. Hepatology 2018;67(1):358–80.
65. Cancer Genome Atlas Research Network. Electronic address wbe, Cancer Genome Atlas Research Network. Comprehensive and integrative genomic characterization of hepatocellular carcinoma. Cell 2017;169(7):1327–41.e3.
66. Llovet JM, Montal R, Sia D, et al. Molecular therapies and precision medicine for hepatocellular carcinoma. Nat Rev Clin Oncol 2018;15(10):599–616.
67. Chan AW, Kumada T, Toyoda H, et al. Integration of albumin-bilirubin (ALBI) score into Barcelona Clinic Liver Cancer (BCLC) system for hepatocellular carcinoma. J Gastroenterol Hepatol 2016;31(7):1300–6.
68. Llovet JM, Ricci S, Mazzaferro V, et al. Sorafenib in advanced hepatocellular carcinoma. N Engl J Med 2008;359(4):378–90.
69. Cheng AL, Kang YK, Chen Z, et al. Efficacy and safety of sorafenib in patients in the Asia-Pacific region with advanced hepatocellular carcinoma: a phase III randomised, double-blind, placebo-controlled trial. Lancet Oncol 2009;10(1):25–34.
70. Howell J, Pinato DJ, Ramaswami R, et al. On-target sorafenib toxicity predicts improved survival in hepatocellular carcinoma: a multi-centre, prospective study. Aliment Pharmacol Ther 2017;45(8):1146–55.
71. Bruix J, Cheng AL, Meinhardt G, et al. Prognostic factors and predictors of sorafenib benefit in patients with hepatocellular carcinoma: analysis of two phase III studies. J Hepatol 2017;67(5):999–1008.
72. Llovet JM, Zucman-Rossi J, Pikarsky E, et al. Hepatocellular carcinoma. Nat Rev Dis Primers 2016;2:16018.
73. Lencioni R, Llovet JM, Han G, et al. Sorafenib or placebo plus TACE with doxorubicin-eluting beads for intermediate stage HCC: The SPACE trial. J Hepatol 2016;64(5):1090–8.
74. Bruix J, Takayama T, Mazzaferro V, et al. Adjuvant sorafenib for hepatocellular carcinoma after resection or ablation (STORM): a phase 3, randomised, double-blind, placebo-controlled trial. Lancet Oncol 2015;16(13):1344–54.

75. Meyer T, Fox R, Ma YT, et al. Sorafenib in combination with transarterial chemo-embolisation in patients with unresectable hepatocellular carcinoma (TACE 2): a randomised placebo-controlled, double-blind, phase 3 trial. Lancet Gastroenterol Hepatol 2017;2(8):565–75.

76. Phay JE, Shah MH. Targeting RET receptor tyrosine kinase activation in cancer. Clin Cancer Res 2010;16(24):5936–41.

77. Ye S, Zhao XY, Hu XG, et al. TP53 and RET may serve as biomarkers of prognostic evaluation and targeted therapy in hepatocellular carcinoma. Oncol Rep 2017;37(4):2215–26.

78. Morishita A, Iwama H, Fujihara S, et al. Targeted sequencing of cancer-associated genes in hepatocellular carcinoma using next-generation sequencing. Oncol Lett 2018;15(1):528–32.

79. Ikeda M, Okusaka T, Mitsunaga S, et al. Safety and pharmacokinetics of lenvatinib in patients with advanced hepatocellular carcinoma. Clin Cancer Res 2016; 22(6):1385–94.

80. Ikeda K, Kudo M, Kawazoe S, et al. Phase 2 study of lenvatinib in patients with advanced hepatocellular carcinoma. J Gastroenterol 2017;52(4):512–9.

81. Kudo M, Finn RS, Qin S, et al. Lenvatinib versus sorafenib in first-line treatment of patients with unresectable hepatocellular carcinoma: a randomised phase 3 non-inferiority trial. Lancet 2018;391(10126):1163–73.

82. Finn RS. Analysis of serum biomarkers (BM) in patients (pts) from a phase 3 study of lenvatinib (LEN) vs sorafenib (SOR) as first-line treatment for unresectable hepatocellular carcinoma (uHCC). Paper presented at: ESMO. Madrid, 2017.

83. Kudo M, Finn RS, Qin S, et al. Analysis of survival and objective response (OR) in patients with hepatocellular carcinoma in a phase III study of lenvatinib (REFLECT). Paper presented at: 2019 Gastrointestinal Cancers Symposium. San Francisco, 2019.

84. Wilhelm SM, Dumas J, Adnane L, et al. Regorafenib (BAY 73-4506): a new oral multikinase inhibitor of angiogenic, stromal and oncogenic receptor tyrosine kinases with potent preclinical antitumor activity. Int J Cancer 2011;129(1): 245–55.

85. Llovet JM, Pena CE, Lathia CD, et al. Plasma biomarkers as predictors of outcome in patients with advanced hepatocellular carcinoma. Clin Cancer Res 2012;18(8):2290–300.

86. Itatani Y, Kawada K, Yamamoto T, et al. Resistance to anti-angiogenic therapy in cancer-alterations to anti-VEGF pathway. Int J Mol Sci 2018;19(4) [pii:E1232].

87. Zhu AX, Park JO, Ryoo BY, et al. Ramucirumab versus placebo as second-line treatment in patients with advanced hepatocellular carcinoma following first-line therapy with sorafenib (REACH): a randomised, double-blind, multicentre, phase 3 trial. Lancet Oncol 2015;16(7):859–70.

88. Zhu AX, Kudo M, Assenat E, et al. Effect of everolimus on survival in advanced hepatocellular carcinoma after failure of sorafenib: the EVOLVE-1 randomized clinical trial. JAMA 2014;312(1):57–67.

89. Llovet JM, Decaens T, Raoul JL, et al. Brivanib in patients with advanced hepatocellular carcinoma who were intolerant to sorafenib or for whom sorafenib failed: results from the randomized phase III BRISK-PS study. J Clin Oncol 2013;31(28):3509–16.

90. Bruix J, Qin S, Merle P, et al. Regorafenib for patients with hepatocellular carcinoma who progressed on sorafenib treatment (RESORCE): a randomised, double-blind, placebo-controlled, phase 3 trial. Lancet 2017;389(10064):56–66.

91. Finn RS, Merle P, Granito A, et al. Outcomes of sequential treatment with sorafenib followed by regorafenib for HCC: additional analyses from the phase III RESORCE trial. J Hepatol 2018;69(2):353–8.
92. Yakes FM, Chen J, Tan J, et al. Cabozantinib (XL184), a novel MET and VEGFR2 inhibitor, simultaneously suppresses metastasis, angiogenesis, and tumor growth. Mol Cancer Ther 2011;10(12):2298–308.
93. Okuma HS, Kondo S. Trends in the development of MET inhibitors for hepatocellular carcinoma. Future Oncol 2016;12(10):1275–86.
94. Firtina Karagonlar Z, Koc D, Iscan E, et al. Elevated hepatocyte growth factor expression as an autocrine c-Met activation mechanism in acquired resistance to sorafenib in hepatocellular carcinoma cells. Cancer Sci 2016;107(4):407–16.
95. Abou-Alfa GK, Meyer T, Cheng AL, et al. Cabozantinib in patients with advanced and progressing hepatocellular carcinoma. N Engl J Med 2018; 379(1):54–63.
96. Zhu AX, Kang YK, Yen CJ, et al. Ramucirumab after sorafenib in patients with advanced hepatocellular carcinoma and increased alpha-fetoprotein concentrations (REACH-2): a randomised, double-blind, placebo-controlled, phase 3 trial. Lancet Oncol 2019;20(2):282–96.
97. Ringelhan M, Pfister D, O'Connor T, et al. The immunology of hepatocellular carcinoma. Nat Immunol 2018;19(3):222–32.
98. Bejjani A, Finn RS. Current state of immunotherapy for HCC—supporting data and toxicity management. Curr Hepatol Rep 2018;17(4):434–43.
99. El-Khoueiry AB, Sangro B, Yau T, et al. Nivolumab in patients with advanced hepatocellular carcinoma (CheckMate 040): an open-label, non-comparative, phase 1/2 dose escalation and expansion trial. Lancet 2017;389(10088): 2492–502.
100. Zhu AX, Finn RS, Edeline J, et al. Pembrolizumab in patients with advanced hepatocellular carcinoma previously treated with sorafenib (KEYNOTE-224): a non-randomised, open-label phase 2 trial. Lancet Oncol 2018;19(7):940–52.
101. Finn RS, Ryoo BY, Merle P, et al. Results of KEYNOTE-240: phase 3 study of pembrolizumab (Pembro) vs best supportive care (BSC) for second line therapy in advanced hepatocellular carcinoma (HCC). J Clin Oncol 2019;37(suppl: abstr 4004).
102. Inarrairaegui M, Melero I, Sangro B. Immunotherapy of hepatocellular carcinoma: facts and hopes. Clin Cancer Res 2018;24(7):1518–24.
103. Stein S, Pishvaian MJ, Lee MS, et al. Safety and clinical activity of 1L atezolizumab + bevacizumab in a phase Ib study in hepatocellular carcinoma (HCC). J Clin Oncol 2018;36(15_suppl):4074.
104. Finn RS, Ducreux M, Qin S, et al. IMbrave150: a randomized phase III study of 1L atezolizumab plus bevacizumab vs sorafenib in locally advanced or metastatic hepatocellular carcinoma. J Clin Oncol 2018;36(15_suppl):TPS4141.
105. Ikeda M, Sung MW, Kudo M, et al. A phase 1b trial of lenvatinib (LEN) plus pembrolizumab (PEM) in patients (pts) with unresectable hepatocellular carcinoma (uHCC) 2018;36(15_suppl):4076.
106. Tabernero J, Bahleda R, Dienstmann R, et al. Phase I dose-escalation study of JNJ-42756493, an oral pan-fibroblast growth factor receptor inhibitor, in patients with advanced solid tumors. J Clin Oncol 2015;33(30):3401–8.

Regional Chemotherapy for Biliary Tract Tumors and Hepatocellular Carcinoma

Sebastian Mondaca, MD[a,1], Hooman Yarmohammadi, MD[b,1], Nancy E. Kemeny, MD[a,*]

KEYWORDS

- Cholangiocarcinoma • Hepatocellular carcinoma • Chemoembolization
- Hepatic arterial infusion chemotherapy

KEY POINTS

- Locoregional therapies have arisen as a suitable alternative for locally advanced primary liver neoplasms.
- Transarterial chemoembolization with or without drug-eluting beads is considered standard of care in intermediate stage hepatocellular carcinoma.
- Emerging evidence supports the indication of transarterial chemoembolization in intrahepatic cholangiocarcinoma.
- Hepatic arterial infusion chemotherapy combined with systemic chemotherapy is effective and safe in patients with unresectable intrahepatic cholangiocarcinoma.
- There is limited evidence comparing different locoregional modalities in hepatobiliary cancers.

INTRODUCTION

Hepatobiliary cancers comprise a spectrum of invasive carcinomas arising in the liver (hepatocellular carcinoma [HCC]), bile ducts (intrahepatic cholangiocarcinoma [ICC], and extrahepatic cholangiocarcinoma [EHC]) and the gallbladder. Although the genomic landscape of these tumors is significantly different,[1–3] they all share a dismal

Disclosure Statement: N.E. Kemeny has received research funding from Amgen. H. Yarmohammadi has received research funding from Society of Interventional Radiology, Radiological Society of North America, and The Thompson Foundation. S. Mondaca has nothing to disclose.
[a] Gastrointestinal Oncology Service, Division of Solid Tumor Oncology, Department of Medicine, Memorial Sloan Kettering Cancer Center, 1275 York Avenue, New York, NY 10065, USA;
[b] Interventional Radiology Service, Department of Radiology, Memorial Sloan Kettering Cancer Center, 1275 York Avenue, New York, NY 10065, USA
[1] These authors contributed equally to this work.
* Corresponding author. Memorial Sloan Kettering Cancer Center, 300 East 66th Street, 10th Floor, New York, NY 10065.
E-mail address: kemenyn@mskcc.org

prognosis with a high risk of recurrence after resection and poor survival in the metastatic setting.[4,5] Surgical resection, liver transplant, radiation therapy, systemic treatments, and intraarterial therapies are all potential interventions for hepatobiliary cancers in different clinical settings.[6] Therefore, treatment planning requires a multidisciplinary approach to identify patients who would benefit the most from each intervention. In patients with localized HCC, surgical resection, liver transplant, and ablation therapies are considered standard of care, whereas in biliary tract tumors surgery is the treatment of choice in patients amenable to resection. On the other end of the spectrum, in metastatic HCC, several systemic therapies have demonstrated benefit in either the first- or second-line setting, including sorafenib, lenvatinib, regorafenib, cabozantinib, ramucirumab (only in patients with elevated alpha-fetoprotein), and the checkpoint inhibitors nivolumab and pembrolizumab.[7–13] In metastatic biliary tract cancers, the available systemic options are more limited, and the only first-line therapy with evidence of benefit is the combination of gemcitabine and cisplatin.[14] There is also a group of hepatobiliary tumors characterized for unresectable locally advanced disease without metastasis. These patients benefit from locoregional therapies, which include transarterial hepatic embolization (TAE), transarterial chemoembolization (TACE), drug-eluting bead TACE (DEB-TACE), hepatic arterial infusion chemotherapy (HAI), radioembolization and stereotactic body radiation therapy (SBRT). This review focuses on the rationale, data supporting TAE, TACE, DEB-TACE, and HAI in hepatobiliary cancers, and adequate patient selection for these therapies.

RATIONALE FOR REGIONAL CHEMOTHERAPY

The healthy liver has dual blood supply receiving most of its perfusion from the portal vein (75%). Liver malignancies, particularly HCC, mainly derive their blood supply from the hepatic artery. This unique characteristic provides the rationale for the use selective intraarterial therapies. TAE, TACE, and DEB-TACE are targeted locoregional therapies in which the tumor arterial blood supply is selectively occluded with a variety of embolic agents with or without the presence of local chemotherapeutic drugs.[15]

In TAE, small particles without any chemotherapeutic agents are used to block arterial supply to the tumor, resulting in extreme hypoxia or anoxia, inducing cell death and tumor necrosis. In TACE, an emulsion of a chemotherapeutic agent and an oil-based contrast agent (most commonly Lipiodol) is locally delivered in high concentrations into the tumor. This procedure is usually followed by an injection of gel foam to slow down the blood flow and increase the bioavailability of the chemotherapy drugs.[16] In DEB-TACE, doxorubicin is loaded on microspheres and selectively injected into the tumor arterial supply. DEB-TACE allows for slow and sustained release of doxorubicin into the tumor. In addition, the injected microspheres cause ischemic injury.

HAI consists of localized delivery of chemotherapeutics to the liver through a catheter or pump (**Fig. 1**).[17] The rationale of HAI is based on the differential perfusion of liver tumors, which depends on the hepatic artery.[18] Thus, this strategy allows for selective drug delivery to the tumor, minimizing systemic toxicity of the chemotherapeutic agent, particularly if drugs with large first-pass extraction are used.[19] Drugs with a high total body clearance and short plasma half-life are usually favored. Importantly, first-pass extraction limits both toxicity and systemic benefit from chemotherapy, and therefore, HAI is often combined with systemic therapy to maintain disease control. In HCC, cisplatin and 5-fluorouracil (5-FU) have been used in HAI protocols because their half-lives are 20 and 10 minutes, respectively. The estimated increased exposure for these drugs with HAI is higher compared with systemic

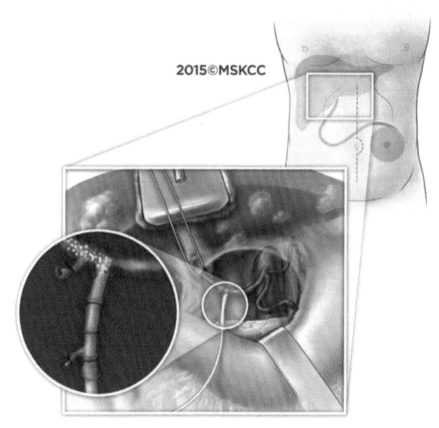

2015©MSKCC

Fig. 1. Placement of the hepatic arterial infusion pump catheter into the GDA. (*From* Qadan M, D'Angelica MI, Kemeny NE, Cercek A, Kingham TP. Robotic hepatic arterial infusion pump placement. *HPB (Oxford).* 2017;19(5):429-435 with permission.)

administration and has been estimated between 4- and 7-fold for cisplatin and 5- and 10-fold for 5-FU.[20] Floxuridine (FUDR) has been found to have numerous advantages for HAI. Between 94% and 99% of FUDR is extracted during the first pass, compared with 19% to 55% of 5-FU, and the estimated increased exposure for FUDR is between 100- and 400-fold.[21]

REGIONAL CHEMOTHERAPY IN BILIARY TRACT TUMORS
Transarterial Hepatic Embolization, Transarterial Chemoembolization, and Drug-Eluting Bead Transarterial Chemoembolization

Unresectable locally advanced ICC has a poor prognosis with median survival of 3 to 8 months without treatment.[22] Chemotherapy regimens, including the combination of gemcitabine with cisplatin, have shown a modest benefit in overall survival (OS).[14] Therefore, there has been interest in using locoregional therapies in treating these patients resulting in a substantial amount of literature validating the indication of TAE, TACE, and DEB-TACE (**Table 1**).[22–35] Patients with unresectable disease without extrahepatic disease are candidates for these locoregional therapies, which have been associated with better OS compared with historic controls.

Table 1
Summary of individual studies of transarterial hepatic embolization, transarterial chemoembolization, drug-eluting bead transarterial chemoembolization, and hepatic arterial infusion for unresectable intrahepatic cholangiocarcinoma

Author	Study Design	N	Treatment Regimen	Median OS (mo)
TAE, TACE, and DEB-TACE				
Hyder et al,[23] 2013	RS	198	TAE, TACE, and DEB-TACE	13.2
Kirchhoff et al,[24] 2005	PC	8	CCDP + Doxo (TACE)	12
Burger et al,[22] 2005	PC	17	CCDP + Doxo + MMC (TACE)	23
Herber et al,[25] 2007	RS	15	MMC (TACE)	16.3
Gusani et al,[26] 2008	RS	42	Gemcitabine-based regimen (TACE)	9.1
Kim et al,[27] 2008	RS	49	CCDP (TACE)	10
Park et al,[28] 2011	RS	72	CCDP (TACE)	12.2
Kiefer et al,[29] 2011	PC	62	MMC + Doxo + CCDP (TACE)	20
Kuhlmann et al,[30] 2012	PC	10/26	MMC (TACE)/Iri (DEB-TACE)	5.7/11.7
Halappa et al,[31] 2012	RS	29	MMC + Doxo + CCDP (TACE)	16
Vogl et al,[32] 2012	RS	115	MMC-based regimen (TACE)	13
Scheuermann et al,[33] 2013	RS	32	MMC (TACE)/Doxo (DEB-TACE)	11
Aliberti et al,[34] 2008	PC	11	Doxo (DEB-TACE)	13
Poggi et al,[35] 2009	PC	9	Oxaliplatin (DEB-TACE)	30
HAI				
Tanaka et al,[40] 2002	PC	11	5-FU-based combinations	26[a]
Jarnagin et al,[41] 2009	PC	34[c]	FUDR	29.5[b]
Kemeny et al,[42] 2011	PC	22[d]	FUDR + systemic bevacizumab	31.1
Massani et al,[43] 2015	PC	11	5-FU + oxaliplatin	17.6
Konstantinidis et al,[44] 2016	RS	78	FUDR-based regimen + sys chemo	30.8
Cercek et al,[45] 2018	PC	39	FUDR + systemic GemOx	53% (2-y OS)
Inaba et al,[46] 2011	PC	13	Gemcitabine	13
Sinn et al,[47] 2013	PC	37	5-FU + oxaliplatin	13.5
Cantore et al,[48] 2005	PC	30[e]	Epi + CCDP + sys chemo	13.2
Mambrini et al,[49] 2007	PC	20[f]	Epi + CCDP + sys chemo	18

Abbreviations: CCDP, cisplatin; Doxo, doxorubicin; Epi, epirubicin; Iri, irinotecan; MMC, mitomycin C; PC, prospective cohort; RS, retrospective study; sys chemo, systemic chemotherapy.
  [a] Mean survival.
  [b] Disease-specific survival.
  [c] Includes 8 patients with HCC.
  [d] Includes 4 patients with HCC.
  [e] Includes 5 patients with gallbladder cancer.
  [f] Includes 7 patients with gallbladder cancer.

In a multi-institutional study, TAE, TACE, DEB-TACE, and radioembolization were used to treat ICC, and their efficacy was compared.[23] TAE was used to treat 14 ICC patients and was able to prolong OS to 14.3 months. In this study, there was no significant difference in median OS between different locoregional therapies, including TACE (13.4 months), DEB-TACE (10.5 months), and radioembolization (11.3 months).

Conventional lipiodol-based TACE is the most commonly used and reported locoregional method in treating ICC with median OS ranging from 5.7 to 23 months (see **Table 1**). Unfortunately, most studies on TACE are retrospective with a small number of patients, and there is a significant amount of variability in the literature on the method and chemotherapeutic agents used. Common chemotherapy regimens for this indication include doxorubicin, mitomycin C, and cisplatin. In a large prospective study, 62 patients with ICC or adenocarcinoma of unknown origin deemed likely ICC received TACE with this combination regimen. The median OS reported in this study was 20 months, and they also found improved OS in patients receiving concomitant systemic chemotherapy versus patients who did not receive systemic chemotherapy (OS 28 months vs 16 months; $P = .02$).[29] In a metaanalysis of different transarterial chemotherapy methods, including TACE, HAI, and DEB-TACE, Ray and colleagues[36] reported an OS of 15.7 months from the time of diagnosis for all 3 treatments. They concluded that transarterial chemotherapy-based treatments for cholangiocarcinoma are safe and well tolerated and provide survival benefits of 2 to 7 months compared with systemic therapies.

Three studies on DEB-TACE have been reported in the literature.[30,34,35] Doxorubicin, oxaliplatin, and irinotecan were the 3 chemotherapeutic agents loaded on the particles. Median OS in these studies were similar to the results of TACE with the exception of the study by Kuhlmann and colleagues[30] in which the DEB-TACE group had a longer OS (11.7 vs 5.7 months).

Deciding among locoregional treatment options is challenging. Multiple studies have compared different methods; however, based on the available efficacy and safety data, it is not possible to determine which is the method of choice. Therefore, accessibility and familiarity of the interventionalist appear to be the most important factor in deciding which modality should be used.

Hepatic Arterial Infusion

HAI FUDR has been used more frequently for the treatment of colorectal cancer liver metastases, showing significant benefit as adjuvant therapy after metastasectomy and as conversion therapy in patients with initially unresectable disease.[37,38] In locally advanced ICC, the experience with this treatment modality is more limited; however, encouraging results have been reported. Initial series of ICC patients showing activity of HAI FUDR were reported more than 30 years ago.[39] Subsequently, multiple prospective and retrospective studies have shown promising results (see **Table 1**).[40–49] In a phase 2 trial, 34 unresectable patients (26 ICC; 8 HCC) received HAI FUDR. In this cohort, the objective response rate was 47%, and 1 patient with initially unresectable ICC could undergo resection. Median progression-free survival (PFS) was 7.4 months, and disease-specific survival was 29 months.[41] Similar outcomes were obtained in a succeeding study, in which 22 patients (18 ICC; 4 HCC) were treated with HAI FUDR plus the antiangiogenic monoclonal antibody bevacizumab. In this trial, median PFS and OS were 8.5 and 31.1 months, respectively. Despite these encouraging results, this study was prematurely terminated owing to increased biliary toxicity associated with bevacizumab.[42] In a retrospective review of 78 ICC patients, who underwent treatment with combined HAI FUDR and systemic chemotherapy, the OS was superior compared with patients who received systemic treatment alone (30.8 vs 18.4 months, respectively; $P<.001$).[44] PFS was also better for the combination group, although this was not statistically significant (12 vs 7 months; $P = .2$). Recently, the results of a multicenter phase 2 trial assessing the efficacy and safety of HAI FUDR combined with systemic gemcitabine and oxaliplatin (GemOx) in unresectable ICC were presented. In 39 evaluable patients, the objective response rate was 46%.

PFS and 2-year OS were 11.5 months and 53%, respectively (**Fig. 2**). Four patients (10%) had grade 4 toxicities requiring removal from the study, including portal hypertension, gastroduodenal artery (GDA) aneurysm, GDA extravasation related to HAI catheter, and hyperbilirubinemia.[45] Other chemotherapy drugs besides FUDR have been included in HAI protocols for ICC. Tanaka and colleagues[40] reported their initial experience of 11 ICC patients treated with 3 different 5-FU–based combination regimens (epirubicin, mitomycin, and cisplatin). In this study, 7 patients (64%) showed some degree of response in the liver, and 3-year survival was 20%. Two phase 2 trials, including altogether 50 patients, confirmed the activity of HAI with the combination of cisplatin and epirubicin in ICC. In these trials, concurrent systemic 5-FU or capecitabine was administered, and response rate ranged between 32% and 40%.[48,49] No safety concerns were described. More recently, the combination of intraarterial 5-FU and oxaliplatin also showed some activity in a phase 2 trial in which 37 patients with locally advanced biliary tract malignancies (32 ICC; 1 EHC; 4 gallbladder cancer) were included. In this trial, the response rate, PFS, and OS were 16%, 6.5 months, and 13.5 months, respectively.[47] Although there are no adequately powered randomized controlled trials (RCTs) comparing hepatic artery-based therapies, a recent systematic review compared HAI with TACE and radioembolization.[50] In this review, 20 studies were analyzed, and the longest median survival was obtained with HAI (22.8 months, 95% confidence interval [CI] 9.8–35.8) followed by radioembolization (13.9 months, 95% CI 9.5–18.3) and TACE (12.4 months, 95% CI 10.9–13.9).

REGIONAL CHEMOTHERAPY IN HEPATOCELLULAR CARCINOMA
Transarterial Hepatic Embolization, Transarterial Chemoembolization, and Drug-Eluting Bead Transarterial Chemoembolization

Indications for performing TAE, TACE, or DEB-TACE in HCC are based on their benefits on symptomatic control and OS, and in eligible candidates, they are also used as bridging therapy to liver transplantation.[51] Patients with unresectable disease without extrahepatic involvement and with a well-compensated liver function (Child-Pugh score A or B) are suitable candidates for locoregional therapy.

There are approximately 55 RCT comparing different catheter-directed therapies with each other and to best supportive care (BSC).[52] The 2 initial RCTs published in 2002 proved that TACE improves OS when compared with BSC.[53,54] These 2 RCTs

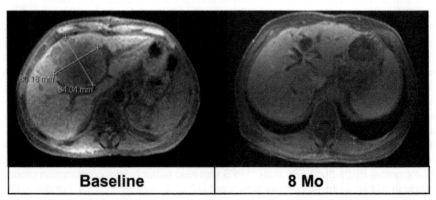

Fig. 2. Serial CT scan imaging of an unresectable ICC patient showing 76% decrease in sum of diameters of target lesions after 8 months of treatment with HAI FUDR and systemic GemOx.

Table 2
Summary of individual studies of transarterial hepatic embolization, transarterial chemoembolization, drug-eluting bead transarterial chemoembolization, and hepatic arterial infusion for unresectable hepatocellular carcinoma

Author	Study Design	N	Treatment Regimen	Control Arm	Median OS (mo)
TAE, TACE, and DEB-TACE					
Llovet et al,[53] 2002	RCT	112	TAE or TACE	BSC	25.3 vs 28.7 vs 17.9[a]
Maluccio et al,[58] 2008	RS	322	TAE	n/a	21
Malagari et al,[59] 2010	RCT	84	DEB-TACE	TAE	85% vs 86% (1-y OS) (NS)
Meyer et al,[60] 2013	RCT	86	TAE	TACE (CCDP)	16.2 vs 16 (NS)
Yu et al,[61] 2014	RCT	90	TAE	TACE (CCDP)	24.3 vs 20.1 (NS)
Brown et al,[62] 2016	RCT	101	TAE	DEB-TACE (Doxo)	19.6 vs 20.8 (NS)
Lo et al,[54] 2002	RCT	79	TACE (CCDP)	BSC	26% vs 3% (3-y OS) P = .002
Mabed et al,[63] 2009	RCT	100	TACE (Doxo and CCDP)	Sys chemo	38 vs 32 (wk) (NS)
Lammer et al,[64] 2010	RCT	201	DEB-TACE (Doxo)	TACE (Doxo)	Not evaluated (no difference in RR)
Sacco et al,[65] 2011	RCT	67	DEB-TACE (Doxo)	TACE (Doxo)	87% vs 84% (2-y OS) (NS)
van Malenstein et al,[66] 2011	RCT	30	DEB-TACE (Doxo)	TACE (Doxo)	Not evaluated (no difference in RR)
Golfieri et al,[67] 2014	RCT	177	DEB-TACE (Doxo)	TACE (Epi)	[b]29 vs 28 (NS)
Kloeckner et al,[68] 2015	RS	250	DEB-TACE (Doxo)	TACE (MMC)	12.2 vs 13.6 (NS)
HAI					
Doci et al,[70] 1998	PC	28	Doxo or 5-FU	n/a	3.5
Audisio et al,[71] 1990	PC	30	MMC	n/a	7
Atiq et al,[72] 1992	PC	10[c]	FUDR + MMC	n/a	14.5
Yamashita et al,[73] 2011	RCT	114	5-FU + CCDP	5-FU	17.6 vs 10.5 (NS)
Ueshima et al,[74] 2010	PC	52	5-FU + CCDP	n/a	15.9
Ishikawa et al,[75] 2007	PC	10	Et + Carbo + Epi + 5-FU + sys chemo	n/a	15.2
Ku et al,[76] 1998	PC	28	Doxo	n/a	16
Ku et al,[77] 2004	PC	25	Doxo + surgery	n/a	42% (5-y OS)

Abbreviations: Carbo, carboplatin; Et, etoposide; n/a, not applicable; NS, not significant; RR, response rate.
[a] Mean survival (P<.009 TACE vs control).
[b] Projected median OS.
[c] Includes 2 patients with ICC.

were further validated by 2 systematic reviews that also showed significant improvement in OS when compared with BSC.[55,56] Therefore, TACE is currently the standard of care for treating unresectable intermediate or advanced stage HCC in patients with preserved liver function. Similar to ICC, there is no standard TACE technique, and a variety of drugs, including doxorubicin, mitomycin, and cisplatin, has been used alone or in combination. A recent network metaanalysis reported a median survival of 18.1 months (95% CI, 15.6–21.6) for patients treated with TACE.[52]

TAE causes extreme ischemia in an already hypoxic cirrhotic liver, resulting in ischemic necrosis of HCC.[57] In a retrospective study on 322 HCC patients with and without limited extrahepatic disease and portal vein thrombosis who were treated with TAE, OS was 21 months, which is similar to OS in HCC patients treated with TACE and DEB-TACE.[58] **Table 2** describes studies comparing TAE with BSC, TACE, and DEB-TACE.[53,54,58–68] In a recent prospective randomized study, TAE was compared with DEB-TACE in 101 patients with HCC.[62] In this study, no significant difference between TAE and DEB-TACE was found in PFS (6.2 vs 2.8 months; $P = .11$) or OS (19.6 vs 20.8 months; $P = .64$).[62] In the Prospective Randomized Study of Doxorubicin in the Treatment of Hepatocellular Carcinoma by Drug-Eluting Bead Embolization V (PRECISION V) trial, DEB-TACE was compared with TACE in treating 201 HCC patients.[64] Again, no difference in complete response, overall response, or disease control rate was observed; however, patients in the DEB-TACE arm had fewer adverse events. Subsequently, in a study with similar design, the PRECISION Italia Study Group included 117 HCC patients and found no difference in OS between the DEB-TACE and TACE groups.[67] Finally, in a network metaanalysis, a median OS of 20.6 months in patients treated with DEB-TACE was reported that was similar to TAE and TACE with no statistically significant difference.[52]

Hepatic Arterial Infusion

Although most patients with HCC develop either hematogenous or regional metastases, many patients die from progressive intrahepatic tumor in the setting of a cirrhotic liver.[69] The underlying liver dysfunction in these patients has been an important challenge for the development of both systemic and regional therapeutic approaches. Early trials assessing the efficacy of HAI with FUDR, 5-FU, doxorubicin, or mitomycin-C in selected HCC patients showed response rates between 22% and 43%; however, responses were not durable, and catheter- or pump-related complications were common in this frail population.[70–72] Since then, multiple prospective and retrospective cohorts, most of them from Asia, have reported variable results in unresectable HCC patients in terms of efficacy and safety. Main characteristics of these trials are summarized in **Table 2**.[70–77] Complications associated with HAI have decreased as some institutions have developed experience in the main aspects of this procedure; however, as other less invasive locoregional treatment alternatives such as radioembolization and SBRT have been further developed, HAI has not gained a place in the HCC treatment algorithm.

SUMMARY

Both TACE and HAI, as locoregional therapies, have an emerging role in the treatment of locally advanced primary liver tumors. In this heterogeneous population, the development of RCTs to compare these treatments against each other or against other locoregional therapies, such as TAE, radioembolization, or SBRT, has been particularly challenging. Hence, collaborative research among centers with expertise in these techniques should be prioritized. Specifically, in ICC, TACE and HAI have demonstrated compelling activity in multiple single-arm prospective studies; thus, they can be considered for adequately selected patients in centers with experience in these procedures. In HCC, TACE has a clear indication in patients with stage B according to the Barcelona Clinic Liver Cancer staging system, and multiple studies are exploring novel combinations with systemic treatments, such as immune checkpoint inhibitors. The evidence supporting HAI in HCC at this point remains preliminary. Further research demonstrating the safety and efficacy of HAI in the context of other locoregional alternatives and novel systemic treatments is needed before its use as a standard therapy.

REFERENCES

1. Javle M, Bekaii-Saab T, Jain A, et al. Biliary cancer: utility of next-generation sequencing for clinical management. Cancer 2016;122(24):3838–47.
2. Cancer Genome Atlas Research Network, Electronic address wheeler@bcm.edu, Cancer Genome Atlas Research Network. Comprehensive and integrative genomic characterization of hepatocellular carcinoma. Cell 2017;169(7): 1327–41.e23.
3. Lowery MA, Ptashkin R, Jordan E, et al. Comprehensive molecular profiling of intrahepatic and extrahepatic cholangiocarcinomas: potential targets for intervention. Clin Cancer Res 2018;24(17):4154–61.
4. Gluer AM, Cocco N, Laurence JM, et al. Systematic review of actual 10-year survival following resection for hepatocellular carcinoma. HPB (Oxford) 2012;14(5): 285–90.
5. de Jong MC, Nathan H, Sotiropoulos GC, et al. Intrahepatic cholangiocarcinoma: an international multi-institutional analysis of prognostic factors and lymph node assessment. J Clin Oncol 2011;29(23):3140–5.
6. Habib A, Desai K, Hickey R, et al. Transarterial approaches to primary and secondary hepatic malignancies. Nat Rev Clin Oncol 2015;12(8):481–9.
7. Llovet JM, Ricci S, Mazzaferro V, et al. Sorafenib in advanced hepatocellular carcinoma. N Engl J Med 2008;359(4):378–90.
8. Kudo M, Finn RS, Qin S, et al. Lenvatinib versus sorafenib in first-line treatment of patients with unresectable hepatocellular carcinoma: a randomised phase 3 non-inferiority trial. Lancet 2018;391(10126):1163–73.
9. Bruix J, Qin S, Merle P, et al. Regorafenib for patients with hepatocellular carcinoma who progressed on sorafenib treatment (RESORCE): a randomised, double-blind, placebo-controlled, phase 3 trial. Lancet 2017;389(10064):56–66.
10. Abou-Alfa GK, Meyer T, Cheng AL, et al. Cabozantinib in patients with advanced and progressing hepatocellular carcinoma. N Engl J Med 2018;379(1):54–63.
11. Zhu AX, Kang Y-K, Yen C-J, et al. REACH-2: a randomized, double-blind, placebo-controlled phase 3 study of ramucirumab versus placebo as second-line treatment in patients with advanced hepatocellular carcinoma (HCC) and elevated baseline alpha-fetoprotein (AFP) following first-line sorafenib. J Clin Oncol 2018;36(15_suppl):4003.
12. El-Khoueiry AB, Sangro B, Yau T, et al. Nivolumab in patients with advanced hepatocellular carcinoma (CheckMate 040): an open-label, non-comparative, phase 1/2 dose escalation and expansion trial. Lancet 2017;389(10088):2492–502.
13. Zhu AX, Finn RS, Edeline J, et al. Pembrolizumab in patients with advanced hepatocellular carcinoma previously treated with sorafenib (KEYNOTE-224): a non-randomised, open-label phase 2 trial. Lancet Oncol 2018;19(7):940–52.
14. Valle J, Wasan H, Palmer DH, et al. Cisplatin plus gemcitabine versus gemcitabine for biliary tract cancer. N Engl J Med 2010;362(14):1273–81.

15. Tsochatzis EA, Fatourou E, O'Beirne J, et al. Transarterial chemoembolization and bland embolization for hepatocellular carcinoma. World J Gastroenterol 2014; 20(12):3069–77.

16. Shah RP, Brown KT, Sofocleous CT. Arterially directed therapies for hepatocellular carcinoma. AJR Am J Roentgenol 2011;197(4):W590–602.

17. Qadan M, D'Angelica MI, Kemeny NE, et al. Robotic hepatic arterial infusion pump placement. HPB (Oxford) 2017;19(5):429–35.

18. Breedis C, Young G. The blood supply of neoplasms in the liver. Am J Pathol 1954;30(5):969–77.

19. Ensminger WD, Gyves JW. Clinical pharmacology of hepatic arterial chemotherapy. Semin Oncol 1983;10(2):176–82.

20. Kemeny NE, Atiq OT. Intrahepatic chemotherapy for metastatic colorectal cancer. In: Markman eM, editor. Regional chemotherapy. Current clinical oncology. Totowa (NJ): Humana Press; 2000.

21. Ensminger WD, Rosowsky A, Raso V, et al. A clinical-pharmacological evaluation of hepatic arterial infusions of 5-fluoro-2'-deoxyuridine and 5-fluorouracil. Cancer Res 1978;38(11 Pt 1):3784–92.

22. Burger I, Hong K, Schulick R, et al. Transcatheter arterial chemoembolization in unresectable cholangiocarcinoma: initial experience in a single institution. J Vasc Interv Radiol 2005;16(3):353–61.

23. Hyder O, Marsh JW, Salem R, et al. Intra-arterial therapy for advanced intrahepatic cholangiocarcinoma: a multi-institutional analysis. Ann Surg Oncol 2013; 20(12):3779–86.

24. Kirchhoff T, Zender L, Merkesdal S, et al. Initial experience from a combination of systemic and regional chemotherapy in the treatment of patients with nonresectable cholangiocellular carcinoma in the liver. World J Gastroenterol 2005;11(8): 1091–5.

25. Herber S, Otto G, Schneider J, et al. Transarterial chemoembolization (TACE) for inoperable intrahepatic cholangiocarcinoma. Cardiovasc Intervent Radiol 2007; 30(6):1156–65.

26. Gusani NJ, Balaa FK, Steel JL, et al. Treatment of unresectable cholangiocarcinoma with gemcitabine-based transcatheter arterial chemoembolization (TACE): a single-institution experience. J Gastrointest Surg 2008;12(1):129–37.

27. Kim JH, Yoon HK, Sung KB, et al. Transcatheter arterial chemoembolization or chemoinfusion for unresectable intrahepatic cholangiocarcinoma: clinical efficacy and factors influencing outcomes. Cancer 2008;113(7):1614–22.

28. Park SY, Kim JH, Yoon HJ, et al. Transarterial chemoembolization versus supportive therapy in the palliative treatment of unresectable intrahepatic cholangiocarcinoma. Clin Radiol 2011;66(4):322–8.

29. Kiefer MV, Albert M, McNally M, et al. Chemoembolization of intrahepatic cholangiocarcinoma with cisplatinum, doxorubicin, mitomycin C, ethiodol, and polyvinyl alcohol: a 2-center study. Cancer 2011;117(7):1498–505.

30. Kuhlmann JB, Euringer W, Spangenberg HC, et al. Treatment of unresectable cholangiocarcinoma: conventional transarterial chemoembolization compared with drug eluting bead-transarterial chemoembolization and systemic chemotherapy. Eur J Gastroenterol Hepatol 2012;24(4):437–43.

31. Halappa VG, Bonekamp S, Corona-Villalobos CP, et al. Intrahepatic cholangiocarcinoma treated with local-regional therapy: quantitative volumetric apparent diffusion coefficient maps for assessment of tumor response. Radiology 2012; 264(1):285–94.

32. Vogl TJ, Naguib NN, Nour-Eldin NE, et al. Transarterial chemoembolization in the treatment of patients with unresectable cholangiocarcinoma: results and prognostic factors governing treatment success. Int J Cancer 2012;131(3):733–40.

33. Scheuermann U, Kaths JM, Heise M, et al. Comparison of resection and transarterial chemoembolisation in the treatment of advanced intrahepatic cholangiocarcinoma–a single-center experience. Eur J Surg Oncol 2013;39(6):593–600.

34. Aliberti C, Benea G, Tilli M, et al. Chemoembolization (TACE) of unresectable intrahepatic cholangiocarcinoma with slow-release doxorubicin-eluting beads: preliminary results. Cardiovasc Intervent Radiol 2008;31(5):883–8.

35. Poggi G, Amatu A, Montagna B, et al. OEM-TACE: a new therapeutic approach in unresectable intrahepatic cholangiocarcinoma. Cardiovasc Intervent Radiol 2009;32(6):1187–92.

36. Ray CE Jr, Edwards A, Smith MT, et al. Metaanalysis of survival, complications, and imaging response following chemotherapy-based transarterial therapy in patients with unresectable intrahepatic cholangiocarcinoma. J Vasc Interv Radiol 2013;24(8):1218–26.

37. Groot Koerkamp B, Sadot E, Kemeny NE, et al. Perioperative hepatic arterial infusion pump chemotherapy is associated with longer survival after resection of colorectal liver metastases: a propensity score analysis. J Clin Oncol 2017;35(17):1938–44.

38. Kemeny NE, Melendez FD, Capanu M, et al. Conversion to resectability using hepatic artery infusion plus systemic chemotherapy for the treatment of unresectable liver metastases from colorectal carcinoma. J Clin Oncol 2009;27(21):3465–71.

39. Seeger J, Woodcock TM, Blumenreich MS, et al. Hepatic perfusion with FUdR utilizing an implantable system in patients with liver primary cancer or metastatic cancer confined to the liver. Cancer Invest 1989;7(1):1–6.

40. Tanaka N, Yamakado K, Nakatsuka A, et al. Arterial chemoinfusion therapy through an implanted port system for patients with unresectable intrahepatic cholangiocarcinoma–initial experience. Eur J Radiol 2002;41(1):42–8.

41. Jarnagin WR, Schwartz LH, Gultekin DH, et al. Regional chemotherapy for unresectable primary liver cancer: results of a phase II clinical trial and assessment of DCE-MRI as a biomarker of survival. Ann Oncol 2009;20(9):1589–95.

42. Kemeny NE, Schwartz L, Gonen M, et al. Treating primary liver cancer with hepatic arterial infusion of floxuridine and dexamethasone: does the addition of systemic bevacizumab improve results? Oncology 2011;80(3–4):153–9.

43. Massani M, Nistri C, Ruffolo C, et al. Intrahepatic chemotherapy for unresectable cholangiocarcinoma: review of literature and personal experience. Updates Surg 2015;67(4):389–400.

44. Konstantinidis IT, Groot Koerkamp B, Do RK, et al. Unresectable intrahepatic cholangiocarcinoma: systemic plus hepatic arterial infusion chemotherapy is associated with longer survival in comparison with systemic chemotherapy alone. Cancer 2016;122(5):758–65.

45. Cercek A, Kemeny NE, Boerner T, et al. A bi-institutional phase II study of hepatic arterial infusion (HAI) with floxuridine (FUDR) and dexamethasone (Dex) combined with systemic gemcitabine and oxaliplatin (GemOx) for unresectable intrahepatic cholangiocarcinoma (ICC). J Clin Oncol 2018;36(15_suppl):4092.

46. Inaba Y, Arai Y, Yamaura H, et al. Phase I/II study of hepatic arterial infusion chemotherapy with gemcitabine in patients with unresectable intrahepatic cholangiocarcinoma (JIVROSG-0301). Am J Clin Oncol 2011;34(1):58–62.

47. Sinn M, Nicolaou A, Gebauer B, et al. Hepatic arterial infusion with oxaliplatin and 5-FU/folinic acid for advanced biliary tract cancer: a phase II study. Dig Dis Sci 2013;58(8):2399–405.

48. Cantore M, Mambrini A, Fiorentini G, et al. Phase II study of hepatic intraarterial epirubicin and cisplatin, with systemic 5-fluorouracil in patients with unresectable biliary tract tumors. Cancer 2005;103(7):1402–7.

49. Mambrini A, Guglielmi A, Pacetti P, et al. Capecitabine plus hepatic intra-arterial epirubicin and cisplatin in unresectable biliary cancer: a phase II study. Anticancer Res 2007;27(4C):3009–13.

50. Boehm LM, Jayakrishnan TT, Miura JT, et al. Comparative effectiveness of hepatic artery based therapies for unresectable intrahepatic cholangiocarcinoma. J Surg Oncol 2015;111(2):213–20.

51. Lei J, Wang W, Yan L. Downstaging advanced hepatocellular carcinoma to the Milan criteria may provide a comparable outcome to conventional Milan criteria. J Gastrointest Surg 2013;17(8):1440–6.

52. Katsanos K, Kitrou P, Spiliopoulos S, et al. Comparative effectiveness of different transarterial embolization therapies alone or in combination with local ablative or adjuvant systemic treatments for unresectable hepatocellular carcinoma: a network meta-analysis of randomized controlled trials. PLoS One 2017;12(9): e0184597.

53. Llovet JM, Real MI, Montana X, et al. Arterial embolisation or chemoembolisation versus symptomatic treatment in patients with unresectable hepatocellular carcinoma: a randomised controlled trial. Lancet 2002;359(9319):1734–9.

54. Lo CM, Ngan H, Tso WK, et al. Randomized controlled trial of transarterial lipiodol chemoembolization for unresectable hepatocellular carcinoma. Hepatology 2002;35(5):1164–71.

55. Camma C, Schepis F, Orlando A, et al. Transarterial chemoembolization for unresectable hepatocellular carcinoma: meta-analysis of randomized controlled trials. Radiology 2002;224(1):47–54.

56. Llovet JM, Bruix J. Systematic review of randomized trials for unresectable hepatocellular carcinoma: chemoembolization improves survival. Hepatology 2003; 37(2):429–42.

57. Lee KH, Liapi E, Vossen JA, et al. Distribution of iron oxide-containing Embosphere particles after transcatheter arterial embolization in an animal model of liver cancer: evaluation with MR imaging and implication for therapy. J Vasc Interv Radiol 2008;19(10):1490–6.

58. Maluccio MA, Covey AM, Porat LB, et al. Transcatheter arterial embolization with only particles for the treatment of unresectable hepatocellular carcinoma. J Vasc Interv Radiol 2008;19(6):862–9.

59. Malagari K, Pomoni M, Kelekis A, et al. Prospective randomized comparison of chemoembolization with doxorubicin-eluting beads and bland embolization with BeadBlock for hepatocellular carcinoma. Cardiovasc Intervent Radiol 2010; 33(3):541–51.

60. Meyer T, Kirkwood A, Roughton M, et al. A randomised phase II/III trial of 3-weekly cisplatin-based sequential transarterial chemoembolisation vs embolisation alone for hepatocellular carcinoma. Br J Cancer 2013;108(6):1252–9.

61. Yu SC, Hui JW, Hui EP, et al. Unresectable hepatocellular carcinoma: randomized controlled trial of transarterial ethanol ablation versus transcatheter arterial chemoembolization. Radiology 2014;270(2):607–20.

62. Brown KT, Do RK, Gonen M, et al. Randomized trial of hepatic artery embolization for hepatocellular carcinoma using doxorubicin-eluting microspheres compared with embolization with microspheres alone. J Clin Oncol 2016;34(17):2046–53.
63. Mabed M, Esmaeel M, El-Khodary T, et al. A randomized controlled trial of trans-catheter arterial chemoembolization with lipiodol, doxorubicin and cisplatin versus intravenous doxorubicin for patients with unresectable hepatocellular carcinoma. Eur J Cancer Care 2009;18(5):492–9.
64. Lammer J, Malagari K, Vogl T, et al. Prospective randomized study of doxorubicin-eluting-bead embolization in the treatment of hepatocellular carcinoma: results of the PRECISION V study. Cardiovasc Intervent Radiol 2010; 33(1):41–52.
65. Sacco R, Bargellini I, Bertini M, et al. Conventional versus doxorubicin-eluting bead transarterial chemoembolization for hepatocellular carcinoma. J Vasc Interv Radiol 2011;22(11):1545–52.
66. van Malenstein H, Maleux G, Vandecaveye V, et al. A randomized phase II study of drug-eluting beads versus transarterial chemoembolization for unresectable hepatocellular carcinoma. Onkologie 2011;34(7):368–76.
67. Golfieri R, Giampalma E, Renzulli M, et al. Randomised controlled trial of doxorubicin-eluting beads vs conventional chemoembolisation for hepatocellular carcinoma. Br J Cancer 2014;111(2):255–64.
68. Kloeckner R, Weinmann A, Prinz F, et al. Conventional transarterial chemoembolization versus drug-eluting bead transarterial chemoembolization for the treatment of hepatocellular carcinoma. BMC Cancer 2015;15:465.
69. Venook AP, Warren RS. Regional chemotherapy approaches for primary and metastatic liver tumors. Surg Oncol Clin N Am 1996;5(2):411–27.
70. Doci R, Bignami P, Bozzetti F, et al. Intrahepatic chemotherapy for unresectable hepatocellular carcinoma. Cancer 1988;61(10):1983–7.
71. Audisio RA, Doci R, Mazzaferro V, et al. Hepatic arterial embolization with microencapsulated mitomycin C for unresectable hepatocellular carcinoma in cirrhosis. Cancer 1990;66(2):228–36.
72. Atiq OT, Kemeny N, Niedzwiecki D, et al. Treatment of unresectable primary liver cancer with intrahepatic fluorodeoxyuridine and mitomycin C through an implantable pump. Cancer 1992;69(4):920–4.
73. Yamashita T, Arai K, Sunagozaka H, et al. Randomized, phase II study comparing interferon combined with hepatic arterial infusion of fluorouracil plus cisplatin and fluorouracil alone in patients with advanced hepatocellular carcinoma. Oncology 2011;81(5–6):281–90.
74. Ueshima K, Kudo M, Takita M, et al. Hepatic arterial infusion chemotherapy using low-dose 5-fluorouracil and cisplatin for advanced hepatocellular carcinoma. Oncology 2010;78(Suppl 1):148–53.
75. Ishikawa T, Imai M, Kamimura H, et al. Improved survival for hepatocellular carcinoma with portal vein tumor thrombosis treated by intra-arterial chemotherapy combining etoposide, carboplatin, epirubicin and pharmacokinetic modulating chemotherapy by 5-FU and enteric-coated tegafur/uracil: a pilot study. World J Gastroenterol 2007;13(41):5465–70.
76. Ku Y, Iwasaki T, Fukumoto T, et al. Induction of long-term remission in advanced hepatocellular carcinoma with percutaneous isolated liver chemoperfusion. Ann Surg 1998;227(4):519–26.
77. Ku Y, Iwasaki T, Tominaga M, et al. Reductive surgery plus percutaneous isolated hepatic perfusion for multiple advanced hepatocellular carcinoma. Ann Surg 2004;239(1):53–60.

Role of Radioembolization for Biliary Tract and Primary Liver Cancer

Amy C. Taylor, MD[a], Dilip Maddirela, PhD[b],
Sarah B. White, MD, MS, FSIR[c],*

KEYWORDS

- Hepatocellular carcinoma • Cholangiocarcinoma • Transarterial radioembolization
- ^{90}Y • Radiation segmentectomy • Radiation lobectomy
- Selective internal radiotherapy (SIRT)

KEY POINTS

- Transarterial radioembolization is an effective treatment of hepatocellular carcinoma and cholangiocarcinoma by delivering a high tumoral dose of radiation, while limiting the toxicity to the normal liver parenchyma and adjacent organs.
- Radiation segmentectomy is an alternative to percutaneous ablation in tumors that are not anatomically suited for ablation.
- Radiation lobectomy can be used as an alternative to portal vein embolization to induce future liver remnant compensatory hypertrophy and provide disease control before surgical resection.
- The limited data available on ^{90}Y radioembolization for intrahepatic cholangiocarcinoma shows promise, especially when combined with radiosensitizing chemotherapy.

INTRODUCTION

Hepatocellular carcinoma (HCC) is the sixth most common malignancy diagnosed worldwide, and is the fourth leading cause of cancer-related deaths.[1] Due to late-stage presentation, underlying cirrhosis, and limited donor availability, many patients are ineligible for surgical curative treatment with resection or liver transplant. Systemic therapy with sorafenib has only been shown to confer a 3-month survival benefit.[2] Locoregional therapies, such as percutaneous ablation, transarterial embolization (TAE), transarterial chemoembolization (TACE), and transarterial radioembolization

[a] Radiology Consultants of Little Rock, 9601 Baptist Health Drive, Suite 1100, Little Rock, AR 72205, USA; [b] Department of Radiology, Medical College of Wisconsin, 9200 West Wisconsin Avenue, Milwaukee, WI 53226, USA; [c] Department of Radiology, Division of Vascular and Interventional Radiology, Medical College of Wisconsin, 9200 West Wisconsin Avenue, Milwaukee, WI 53226, USA
* Corresponding author.
E-mail address: sbwhite@mcw.edu

Surg Oncol Clin N Am 28 (2019) 731–743
https://doi.org/10.1016/j.soc.2019.07.001
1055-3207/19/© 2019 Elsevier Inc. All rights reserved.

surgonc.theclinics.com

(TARE), have arisen as additional options for this complex patient population. In 2002, a randomized controlled trial comparing conservative therapy with conventional transarterial chemoembolization (cTACE) and TAE demonstrated a significant survival benefit of 10.8 months in the cTACE group.[3] A retrospective analysis published in 2017 demonstrated an even greater survival benefit of cTACE, with median overall survival of 20.1 months in those receiving TACE versus 4.3 months in those who were not treated with TACE.[4] Similar survival benefits have been demonstrated with TACE using drug-eluting beads (DEB-TACE) and TARE,[5–7] with TARE use becoming more widespread over the past decade.

Intrahepatic cholangiocarcinoma (ICC) is the second most common primary hepatic malignancy after HCC, with a poor prognosis, because most patients present with advanced disease that is not amenable to surgical resection. Systemic chemotherapy offers only a modest survival benefit and is limited by significant toxicities. Given the relative radiation sensitivity of ICC, yttrium-90 (^{90}Y) radioembolization shows promise as an effective locoregional treatment.[8]

TRANSARTERIAL RADIOEMBOLIZATION

Conventional external beam radiotherapy has limited usability in the treatment of hepatic malignancies given the low irradiation tolerance of the liver. TARE, also known as selective internal radiation therapy (SIRT), is a technique that delivers a high dose of radiation to a hepatic tumor, while limiting the dose to the normal liver parenchyma and adjacent organs. (**Fig. 1**) The most commonly used radionuclide is ^{90}Y bound to either glass or resin microspheres. ^{90}Y is a pure beta-emitting radionuclide with a half-life of approximately 64 hours. It can travel in tissue of up to 10 mm, with a mean distance traveled of 2.5 mm. Therefore, ^{90}Y deposits greater than 90% of its energy within 5 mm of tissue to which it was delivered in less than 11 days. The radioactivity of the ^{90}Y delivered depends on the volume of liver treated and is adjusted based on hepatopulmonary shunting, as estimated on a pretreatment mapping angiogram and ^{99}Tc-macroaggregated albumin scan.[9]

PATIENT SELECTION

Unlike other solid tumor malignancies, patients with HCC typically have underlying cirrhosis, which is important, because chronic liver disease alone is associated with a 5- to 10-fold increase in all-cause mortality.[10] Therefore, treatment algorithms must take more than tumor status into consideration. Tumor staging for HCC is often defined according to the Barcelona Clinic for Liver Cancer (BCLC) staging system, which includes liver function, tumor stage, and performance status, and provides guidelines for appropriate treatments based on stage.[11,12] More recently, the Hong Kong Combined Liver Cancer staging system was developed, with data demonstrating survival benefit with more aggressive treatment in subsets of patients with intermediate or advanced BCLC stages.[13] Both staging systems emphasize that, in addition to tumor status, performance status and hepatic reserve are critical in predicting which patients will benefit from liver-directed therapy (LDT).

Performance Status

Performance status is a global assessment of a patient's level of function and is most commonly assessed using the Eastern Cooperative Oncology Group (ECOG)/Zubrod Performance Status Scale or Karnofsky Score.[14] Performance status is used to determine a patient's eligibility for inclusion in clinical trials and to determine their level of fitness for cancer treatment. Performance status has been shown to be a predictor of

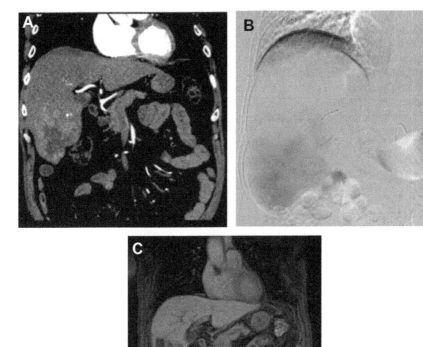

Fig. 1. TARE. (*A*) Coronal contrast enhanced CT scan in the arterial phase of a 59-year-old male with alcohol cirrhosis with multifocal HCC. Alpha-fetoprotein (AFP) at diagnosis was 7126. He was not a surgical candidate because of comorbid conditions. The multidisciplinary board decided that he should undergo liver-directed therapy. (*B*) Mapping angiography was performed, demonstrating tumor blush. The decision was made to perform radioembolization. (*C*) MRI obtained 1-year post procedure demonstrates no residual viable tumor; AFP was 156.

overall survival, with median survival ranging from 293 days in patients with ECOG 0 to 25.5 days in patients with ECOG 4 in patients with cancer.[15] However, many patients with HCC have a baseline ECOG status of 1 because of their underlying liver disease.[16] Factors that are associated with a worse ECOG score are older age, alcoholism, hypoalbuminemia, hyponatremia, hyperbilirubinemia, elevated creatinine, and prolonged partial thromboplastin time.[17] Low alpha-fetoprotein has been associated with a better ECOG score. Importantly, any change in performance status needs to be carefully evaluated, as deterioration of performance status is an independent predictor of decreased survival. Therefore, performance status should be reassessed before all LDT.

Hepatic Reserve

Hepatic reserve can be assessed by using the Child-Pugh (CP) score, albumin-bilirubin (ALBI) grade, and evaluation of serum transaminase and bilirubin levels.

The CP score includes serum albumin and total bilirubin levels, INR, and presence or absence of ascites and/or encephalopathy. It was originally developed to predict surgical mortality in patients with portal hypertension,[18,19] although now it is currently widely used to assess prognosis in all areas of chronic liver disease and need for liver transplantation. Several studies have demonstrated that the CP score has a significant impact on overall survival after locoregional therapy, with decreasing rates of survival with increasing CP classes.[20,21] The ALBI grade is a newer model that eliminates the subjective characteristics of the CP score, focusing only on serum ALBI levels. This has been tested across international populations and has been shown to provide a more refined survival stratification within CP class and BCLC stage.[22–25] However, irrespective of the CP or ALBI scores, caution should be exercised before treating patients with serum aminotransferase levels greater than 200 U/L or total bilirubin greater than 2.0 mg/dL, or any patient with an acute change in liver function.

Tumor Characteristics

Various characteristics of individual tumors have a significant impact on whether locoregional therapies are an option. Tumor burden, portal vein invasion, and presence of extrahepatic disease have all been shown to decrease survival,[21,26] but tumor location, presence of arteriovenous shunting, and extrahepatic blood supply are also important factors to consider. Central tumors with close proximity to bile ducts and vascular structures are not well suited for percutaneous ablation due to increased risk of complications and recurrence.[27] Portal vein thrombosis (PVT) can limit hepatic reserve, not only because the portal vein is the primary blood supply to the hepatic parenchyma, but also because it is also associated with significant arteriovenous shunting. However, studies have shown a survival benefit with transarterial therapies in select patients with PVT.[28,29] (**Fig. 2**) Arteriovenous shunting can limit the ability to provide an effective treatment dose of either chemotherapy or radiation to the tumor if the shun results in the agent bypassing the targeted area of liver. In one study evaluating the presence of arteriovenous shunting in 292 patients with HCC, the overall rate of arteriovenous shunting was 31%, 92% of which was arterioportal shunting, and 8% of which was hepatopulmonary shunting.[30] A higher risk of hepatopulmonary shunting was associated with an infiltrative tumor morphology, greater than 50% hepatic tumor burden, PVT/portal vein compression, presence of arterioportal shunting, and hypervascular tumors. Multiple studies have demonstrated that higher lung shunt fractions are correlated with poorer overall survival.[31,32]

Other Considerations

Any previous therapies that the patient may have received must also be reviewed, such as previous surgical resection, ablation, stereotactic body radiation therapy, or previous LDT with either radioembolization or chemoembolization, because these may alter vascular anatomy or flow dynamics. Current or previous systemic chemotherapeutic or biologic agent use is also important, as many agents increase the friability of the vessels, making them prone to catheter-induced injury during angiography,[33] and limiting the efficacy of treatment due to impaired delivery of the intra-arterial agent. It is generally recommended that offending agents be held for 4 to 6 weeks before therapy.

Other considerations for patient selection for LDT include the goals of care: transplant with either downstaging into transplant criteria or maintaining on the transplant list, versus palliative therapies to prolong survival or to improve pain. Another important factor influencing patients' decisions to pursue therapy is their overall quality of life. It has been shown that patients' quality of life scores worsen with advancing

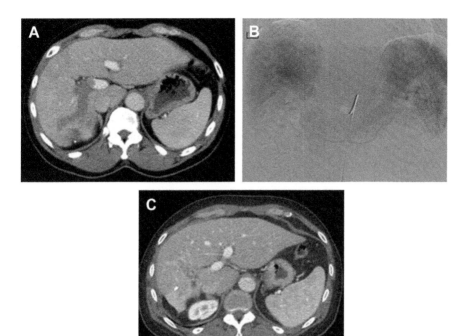

Fig. 2. TARE in the setting of portal vein invasion. (*A*) An axial image from a contrast enhanced CT scan of the abdomen in a 56-year-old woman with hepatitis C/alcohol cirrhosis, who presented with an infiltrative HCC with extensive portal vein invasion. AFP at diagnosis was 3909. The multidisciplinary board decided that she should undergo liver-directed therapy. (*B*) Mapping angiography was performed, demonstrating that the main supply to the PVT arose from the right hepatic artery. The decision was made to perform a radioembolization. (*C*) CT obtained 9-month post procedure demonstrates no residual viable tumor, and retraction of the PVT; AFP was 128.5.

stages of HCC,[34] with pain, jaundice, anorexia, and depression as common symptoms. Many patients with advanced disease would rather focus on quality of life than longevity, and for those undergoing LDT, TARE has been shown to have better quality of life outcomes compared to TACE.[35]

TRANSARTERIAL RADIOEMBOLIZATION FOR HEPATOCELLULAR CARCINOMA

There is currently no level I evidence demonstrating the superiority of TARE over the other embolotherapies (TAE, cTACE, DEB-TACE),[36] and there is significant variability in preferred methods among practicing interventional radiologists.[37] As TACE was the first embolotherapy with level I data demonstrating survival benefit, it is the standard of reference, and thus many of the TARE studies are performed in comparison with TACE. The available data supporting the use of TARE in HCC is summarized here.

One of the applications of LDT is downstaging patients with HCC into transplant criteria. A single-center comparative analysis study was performed comparing the efficacy of TACE versus TARE in downstaging patients with HCC from UNOS T3 (1 nodule >5 cm; or 2–3 nodules, with at least 1 nodule >3 cm) to T2 (1 nodule 2–5 cm; or 2–3 nodules, all <3 cm) to make them eligible for transplant.[38] Eighty-six patients were treated with either TACE (n = 43) or TARE (n = 43). Successful downstaging to T2 stage was achieved in 31% of the TACE group and 58% of the TARE group (P = .023). As liver transplant is a potentially curative treatment of HCC, the ability to create or maintain transplant eligibility for a patient can have significant impact on survival. Whereas both TACE and TARE can be used to downstage patients into transplant criteria, this study suggests that TARE is more efficacious at doing so.

A large, single-center, comparative effectiveness analysis comparing patients with HCC treated with TACE versus TARE demonstrated a significantly longer time to progression in the TARE group (13.3 vs 8.4 months, P = .046).[39] Abdominal pain and increased transaminase activity was more frequent in the TACE group ($P<.05$). Response rates were similar (69% in the TACE group vs 72% in the TARE group, P = .748) and there was no significant difference in overall survival (17.4 months in the TACE group vs 20.5 months in the TARE group, P = .232). Although there were no differences in overall survival or response rates, this study showed that progression-free survival (PFS) is better with TARE, which is advantageous for patients awaiting transplant. These data also suggests that TARE is better tolerated than TACE and should be considered in patients with poorer performance status.

The PREMIERE trial was a prospective, single-blind, randomized, phase 2, single-center trial expanding on the above data comparing ^{90}Y versus cTACE.[40] The primary endpoint was time to progression with secondary endpoints of safety and toxicity, tumor response, and overall survival. Whereas a needed sample size of 124 patients was calculated, only 45 patients were enrolled because of slow accrual and competing trials. Of these, 24 were randomized to the ^{90}Y group and 21 were randomized to the cTACE group. Patients in the ^{90}Y group had significantly longer time to progression compared with the cTACE group (>26 vs 6.8 months, P = .0012). More patients in the cTACE group experienced adverse events than those in the ^{90}Y group, including diarrhea (21% vs 0%, P = .031) or hypoalbuminemia (58% vs 4%, $P<.001$). There was, however, no difference in overall response rates (74% in the cTACE group vs 87% in the ^{90}Y group, P = .433), and no difference in the median overall survival (17.7 months in the cTACE group vs 18.6 months in the ^{90}Y group, P = .99). Because this study demonstrated no difference in response or survival rates, ^{90}Y in the palliative setting was not found to be more efficacious. However, in the transplant population, in whom PFS is critical to remaining on the transplant list, this trial showed strong evidence that ^{90}Y should be first line for patients on the transplant list or those being evaluated for transplant.

The SARAH trial was a prospective, phase 3, randomized, controlled, multicenter, national trial in France comparing SIRT with sorafenib in patients with locally advanced HCC who were not eligible for surgical resection, had failed previous TACE, or both.[41] The primary endpoint was overall survival, with secondary endpoints of safety and toxicity, quality of life, health care costs, and PFS. A total of 459 patients were enrolled, with 237 randomized to SIRT and 222 randomized to the sorafenib arm. There was no significant difference in overall survival (8.0 vs 9.9 months, P = .179) or PFS (4.1 vs 3.7 months, P = .765), although the tumor response rate was significantly higher in the SIRT group (19% vs 11.6%, P = .042). In addition, the overall quality of life was significantly higher with fewer serious adverse events in the SIRT group compared with the sorafenib group. A similar trial, the SIRveNIB trial, was a prospective, phase 3, randomized, controlled, multicenter trial comparing SIRT with sorafenib, but performed in the Asia-Pacific population.[42] The inclusion criteria and primary and secondary endpoints were the same as the SARAH trial. A total of 360 patients were enrolled, with 182 randomized to SIRT and 178 randomized to sorafenib. This study also found no significant difference in overall survival between SIRT and sorefenib (8.8 vs 10.0 months, P = .36); however, the tumor response rate in the SIRT group was significantly higher (16.5% vs 1.7% on an intent-to-treat analysis, $P<.01$). There were also significantly fewer serious adverse events in the SIRT group compared with the sorafenib group (27.7% vs 50.6% of $\geq$ grade 3 AEs, $P<.01$). The results of this trial were somewhat surprising, because the SHARP trial only demonstrated a 3 month survival benefit over best supportive care.[2] This study debunked the idea that locoregional therapy was superior to systemic therapy for HCC. The benefit of TARE, however, was the tolerance of the therapy; TARE was far better tolerated than sorafenib with minimal changes in quality of life with TARE.

Radiation segmentectomy has evolved as an alternative to percutaneous ablation, and is defined as selective radioembolization of fewer than 2 Couinaud segments using an ablative dose, considered to be >190 Gy based on pathologic necrosis[43] or greater than 205 Gy using SPECT/CT response.[44] (**Fig. 3**) A multicenter study assessing the efficacy of radiation segmentectomy in treating solitary HCC not amenable to resection or percutaneous ablation was performed using radiologic–pathologic

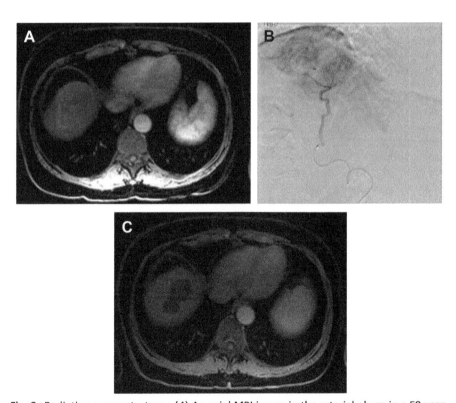

Fig. 3. Radiation segmentectomy. (*A*) An axial MRI image in the arterial phase in a 58-year-old woman with hepatitis C, who presented with a 5.0 × 7.3 × 4.1 cm mass in the dome of the liver that was, on biopsy, proven to be poorly differentiated HCC. AFP at diagnosis was 1758. She was not a surgical candidate, because her portosystemic gradient was found to be 20 mm Hg and biopsy of her liver showed stage 4 fibrosis. The multidisciplinary board decided that she should undergo liver-directed therapy. Due to the size and location, ablation was not an option. (*B*) Mapping angiography was performed, demonstrating a single segment 8 artery supplying the tumor. The decision was made to perform a radiation segmentectomy. (*C*) MRI obtained 1-month post procedure demonstrates no residual viable tumor; AFP was 24.6.

correlation.[43] Thirty-three patients underwent transplant, with 52% of the explants showing complete pathologic necrosis and 44% showing greater than 90% pathologic necrosis. More complete pathologic necrosis was observed when the irradiation dose exceeded 190 Gy (n = 14 in >190 Gy group with complete pathologic necrosis vs n = 3 in <190 Gy group, P = .03), suggesting the possibility of a threshold dose needed to achieve complete pathologic necrosis. A retrospective study was performed evaluating the long-term outcomes of radiation segmentectomy for early HCC, with the hypothesis that outcomes would be comparable with curative treatments for patients with solitary HCC ≤5 cm and preserved liver function.[45] Seventy patients were included, who all underwent radiation segmentectomy with doses greater than 190 Gy; patients who underwent subsequent liver transplant were excluded. 90% of patients showed response using EASL criteria and median time to progression was 2.4 years, with 72% having no signs of progression at 5 years. Median overall survival was 6.7 years with a 5-year survival rate of 57%. In comparison, published 5-year survival rates for radiofrequency ablation are 50% to 60%.[46] For tumors less than 3 cm in size, the 5-year survival rate was 75%. Five-year survival rates for transplant or surgical resection range from 60% to 80%. These data suggest that, in select patients, radiation segmentectomy exhibits outcomes similar to "curative" therapies, including transplant and/or ablation.

Radiation lobectomy has recently arisen as an alternative to portal vein embolization (PVE) to potentially make unresectable patients candidates for resection by inducing compensatory hypertrophy of the uninvolved contralateral lobe.[47,48] One series of 83 patients with right unilobar disease with HCC, cholangiocarcinoma, or metastatic colorectal cancer treated with right radiation lobectomy demonstrated median future liver remnant hypertrophy of 45% at 9 months with no tumor progression in the left lobe.[47] Although the volumetric changes were similar to PVE, they were slower to take effect. Another series of 45 patients with right unilobar HCC treated with right radiation lobectomy demonstrated mean future liver remnant hypertrophy of 30.8% at 6 months and 40.1% at 12 months, also with adequate local tumor control.[48] These studies show that radiation lobectomy creates a similar increase in contralateral lobe volume as PVE, while providing tumor control, which may translate to more patients being able to undergo subsequent resection.

INTRAHEPATIC CHOLANGIOCARCINOMA

ICC is a rapidly progressing malignancy with a rising incidence that frequently presents at an advanced stage. In contrast to hilar and distal bile duct cholangiocarcinoma, ICC lesions are asymptomatic but appear as mass lesions without jaundice. Patients receiving standard chemotherapy for ICC (gemcitabine and cisplatin [gem/cis]) have an overall survival of 11.7 months.[49] Because systemic therapy only offers minimal improvement in overall survival, radioembolization with ^{90}Y microspheres has become an adjuvant treatment in patients with unresectable ICC. However, the data for ^{90}Y remains limited. A systematic pooled analysis on ^{90}Y treatment of ICC indicated an overall median survival of 15.5 months.[50] Tumor response using RECIST,[8,51,52] mRECIST,[53] and other radiologic criteria[54] showed partial response rates of 28% and stable disease in 54% of patients at 3 months. The mean number of ^{90}Y treatments per patient was 1.5 with a weighted mean dose of 1.6 GBq.[50] Naive patients experienced overall median survival of 15 months[55] after treatment with ^{90}Y, compared with 11.7 months with gem/cis. These retrospective studies therefore demonstrate that overall survival may be prolonged with the addition of [90]Y.

A pilot study, as per EASL guidelines, revealed greater than 50% tumor necrosis in 77% patients on imaging follow-up.[56] In addition, prolonged overall survival was observed in patients with objective response based on mRECIST and EASL criteria ($P<.005$, $P = .001$, respectively) at 3 months without correlating RECIST[57] and downstaged to curative resection.[8] In addition, retrospective studies have shown ^{90}Y in patients with ICC is well tolerated, as demonstrated by a study demonstrating an improvement in performance status after therapy.[58] Recently, a small phase 1b prospective trial was performed looking at the effects of combining gemcitabine and [90]Y.[59] The study included 14 patients with ICC or pancreas cancer, who underwent induction with gemcitabine, a potent radiosensitizer, followed by ^{90}Y, then additional gemcitabine dosing after [90]Y. The cohort included 5 patients with ICC and the hepatic PFS for these patients was 20.7 months. All patients experienced grade 1 or 2 toxicities, and all patients maintained or had improvement in their performance status.

There is currently an ongoing prospective multicenter randomized controlled evaluating gem/cis alone versus gem/cis with the addition of ^{90}Y for first line therapy in patients with ICC (SIRCCA). The primary endpoint of this study is survival at 18 months, with secondary endpoints including liver-specific PFS, PFS at any site, overall response rate, overall survival, adverse events, and ability of patients to be downstaged to resection and/or ablation. The results of the trial are anticipated to be forthcoming in 2021.[60]

COMPLICATIONS

Perhaps one of the greatest benefits of TARE is that the overall incidence of complications following radioembolization is low, with significant adverse events occurring in less than 9% of patients.[61] The most common complication is the post radioembolization syndrome (PRS), which occurs in 20% to 55% of patients. PRS consists of fatigue, nausea, vomiting, anorexia, fever, and abdominal discomfort, but is less severe than the postembolization syndromes seen with other embolic therapies. The remaining complications are related to the nontarget deposition of radioactive spheres, including radiation-induced liver disease, gastrointestinal ulceration, cholecystitis, hepatic abscess, and radiation pneumonitis. Initial management is conservative, although surgery is rarely required in refractory cases.[62]

SUMMARY

In conclusion, although ^{90}Y has not been proven superior in oncologic outcomes compared with other embolotherapies or systemic therapy; however, it does confer some advantages in select patients and should be part of the treatment algorithm for HCC and ICC. For patients with poorer performance status, TARE is preferred, because it is better tolerated. It should be considered as the first line as a bridge to transplant, because it offers a significantly longer time to progression. It is also the preferred therapy in patients with PVT. For small tumors, TARE can be considered as a potentially curative alternative to tumors that are not amenable to percutaneous ablation using a radiation segmentectomy technique. In addition, radiation lobectomy can be used as an alternative to PVE to induce future liver remnant compensatory hypertrophy, while allowing for interim disease control. However, in patients with poor hepatic reserve, TARE is not recommended given the increased risk of hepatotoxicity. Tumors with high hepatopulmonary shunting may also not be good candidates for ^{90}Y if a treatment dose cannot be effectively delivered to the liver.

In recent years, immunotherapy has proven beneficial for HCC. Many ongoing trials are currently evaluating the efficacy of combination therapy (immunotherapy plus

LDT), which takes advantage of some of the immunologic side effects of locoregional therapy. There have been promising results in animal models, and results should be coming out soon evaluating TARE in combination with various immunologic agents.[63]

In regards to ICC, with the growing global importance of the disease and lack of any other effective treatment of unresectable ICC, ^{90}Y radioembolization should be considered in the treatment algorithm for ICC. Further studies are necessary to understand where ^{90}Y best fits into therapy.

REFERENCES

1. Bray F, Ferlay J, Soerjomataram I, et al. Global cancer statistics 2018: GLOBO-CAN estimates of incidence and mortality worldwide for 36 cancers in 185 countries. CA Cancer J Clin 2018;68:394–424.
2. Llovet JM, Ricci S, Mazzaferro V, et al. Sorafenib in advanced hepatocellular carcinoma. N Engl J Med 2008;359:378–90.
3. Llovet JM, Real MI, Montana X, et al. Arterial embolisation or chemoembolisation versus symptomatic treatment in patients with unresectable hepatocellular carcinoma: a randomized controlled trial. Lancet 2002;359(9319):1734–9.
4. Gray SH, White JA, Li P, et al. A SEER database analysis of the survival advantage of transarterial chemoembolization for hepatocellular carcinoma: an underutilized therapy. J Vasc Interv Radiol 2017;28(2):231–7.
5. Lammer J, Malagari K, Vogl T, et al. Prospective randomized study of doxorubicin-eluting-bead embolization in the treatment of hepatocellular carcinoma: results of the PRECISION V study. Cardiovasc Intervent Radiol 2010; 33(1):41–52.
6. Salem R, Lewandowski RJ, Mulcahy M, et al. Radioembolization for hepatocellular carcinoma using yttrium-90 microspheres: a comprehensive report of long-term outcomes. Gastroenterology 2010;138(1):52–64.
7. Hilgard P, Hamami M, Fouly AE, et al. Radioembolization with yttrium-90 glass microspheres in hepatocellular carcinoma: European experience on safety and long-term survival. Hepatology 2010;52(5):1741–9.
8. Mouli S, Memon K, Baker T, et al. Yttrium-90 radioembolization for intrahepatic cholangiocarcinoma: safety, response, and survival analysis. J Vasc Interv Radiol 2013;24(8):1227–34.
9. Lencioni R, Liapi E, Geschwind JFH. Hepatocellular carcinoma: ablative therapies, intra-arterial therapies. In: Geschwind JFH, Dake MD, editors. Abrams' angiography: interventional radiology. 3rd edition. Philadelphia: Lippincott Williams & Wilkins; 2014. p. 61–86.
10. Musso G, Gambino R, Cassader M, et al. Meta-analysis: natural history of non-alcoholic fatty liver disease (NAFLD) and diagnostic accuracy of non-invasive tests for liver disease severity. Ann Med 2011;43(8):617–49.
11. Llovet JM, Bru C, Bruix J. Prognosis of hepatocellular carcinoma: the BCLC staging classification. Semin Liver Dis 1999;19(3):329–38.
12. Forner A, Reig ME, Rodriguez de Lope C, et al. Current strategy for staging and treatment: the BCLC update and future prospects. Semin Liver Dis 2010;30(1): 61–74.
13. Yau T, Tang VYF, Yao TJ, et al. Development of Hong Kong Liver Cancer staging system with treatment stratification for patients with hepatocellular carcinoma. Gastroenterology 2014;146(7):1691–700.
14. Oken MM, Creech RH, Tormey DC, et al. Toxicity and response criteria of the Eastern Cooperative Oncology Group. Am J Clin Oncol 1982;5(6):649–56.

15. Jang RW, Caraiscos VB, Swami N, et al. Simple prognostic model for patients with advanced cancer based on performance status. J Oncol Pract 2014;10(5): e335–41.
16. Orman ES, Ghabril M, Chalasani N. Poor performance status is associated with increased mortality in patients with cirrhosis. Clin Gastroenterol Hepatol 2016; 14:1189–95.
17. Hsu CY, Lee YH, Hsia CY, et al. Performance status in patients with hepatocellular carcinoma: determinants, prognostic impact, and ability to improve the Barcelona Clinic Liver Cancer system. Hepatology 2013;57(1):112–9.
18. Child CG, Turcotte JG. Surgery and portal hypertension. In: Child CG, editor. The liver and portal hypertension. Philadelphia: Saunders; 1964. p. 50–8.
19. Pugh RN, Murray-Lyon IM, Dawson JL, et al. Transection of the oesophagus for bleeding oesophageal varices. Br J Surg 1973;60:646–9.
20. Yan K, Chen MH, Yang W, et al. Radiofrequency ablation of hepatocellular carcinoma: long-term outcome and prognostic factors. Eur J Radiol 2008;67(2): 336–47.
21. Greten TF, Papendorf F, Bleck JS, et al. Survival rate in patients with hepatocellular carcinoma: a retrospective analysis of 389 patients. Br J Cancer 2005;92: 1862–8.
22. Johnson PJ, Berhane S, Kagebayashi C, et al. Assessment of liver function in patients with hepatocellular carcinoma: a new evidence-based approach—the ALBI grade. J Clin Oncol 2015;33(6):550–8.
23. Hansmann J, Evers MJ, Bui JT, et al. Albumin-bilirubin and platelet-albumin-bilirubin grades accurately predict overall survival in high-risk patients undergoing conventional transarterial chemoembolization for hepatocellular carcinoma. J Vasc Interv Radiol 2017;28(9):1224–31.
24. Hickey R, Mouli S, Kulik L, et al. Independent analysis of albumin-bilirubin grade in a 765-patient cohort treated with transarterial locoregional therapy for hepatocellular carcinoma. J Vasc Interv Radiol 2016;27(6):795–802.
25. Pinato DJ, Sharma R, Allara E, et al. The ALBI grade provides objective hepatic reserve estimation across each BCLC stage of hepatocellular carcinoma. J Hepatol 2017;66(2):338–46.
26. Schutte K, Schulz C, Poranzke J, et al. Characterization and prognosis of patients with hepatocellular carcinoma (HCC) in the non-cirrhotic liver. BMC Gastroenterol 2014;14:117.
27. Kang TW, Lim HK, Lee MW, et al. Aggressive intrasegmental recurrence of hepatocellular carcinoma after radiofrequency ablation: risk factors and clinical significance. Radiology 2015;276(1):274–85.
28. Luo J, Guo RP, Lai ECH, et al. Transarterial chemoembolization for unresectable hepatocellular carcinoma with portal vein tumor thrombosis: a prospective comparative study. Ann Surg Oncol 2011;18(2):413–20.
29. Garin E, Rolland Y, Edeline J, et al. Personlized dosimetry with intensification using ^{90}Y-loaded glass microsphere radioembolization induces prolonged overall survival in hepatocellular carcinoma patients with portal vein thrombosis. J Nucl Med 2015;56(3):339–46.
30. Ngan H, Peh WCG. Arteriovenous shunting in hepatocellular carcinoma: its prevalence and clinical significance. Clin Radiol 1997;52(1):36–40.
31. Xing M, Lahti S, Kokabi N, et al. [90]Y radioembolization lung shunt fraction in primary and metastatic liver cancer as a biomarker for survival. Clin Nucl Med 2016; 41(1):21–7.

32. Gaba RC, Zivin SP, Dikopf MS, et al. Characteristics of primary and secondary hepatic malignancies associated with hepatopulmonary shunting. Radiology 2014;271(2):602–12.

33. Liu DM, Salem R, Bui JT, et al. Angiographic considerations in patients undergoing liver-directed therapy. J Vasc Interv Radiol 2005;16(7):911–35.

34. Qiao CX, Zhai XF, Ling CQ, et al. Health-related quality of life evaluated by tumor node metastasis staging system in patients with hepatocellular carcinoma. World J Gastroenterol 2012;18(21):2689–94.

35. Salem R, Gilbertsen M, Butt Z, et al. Increased quality of life among hepatocellular carcinoma patients treated with radioembolization, compared with chemoembolization. Clin Gastroenterol Hepatol 2013;11(10):1358–65.

36. Qi X, Zhao Y, Li H, et al. Management of hepatocellular carcinoma: an overview of major findings from meta-analyses. Oncotarget 2016;7(23):34703–51.

37. Gaba RC. Chemoembolization practice patterns and technical methods among interventional radiologists: results of an online survey. AJR Am J Roentgenol 2012;198(3):692–9.

38. Lewandowski RJ, Kulik LM, Riaz A, et al. A comparative analysis of transarterial downstaging for hepatocellular carcinoma: chemoembolization versus radioembolization. Am J Transplant 2009;9(8):1920–8.

39. Salem R, Lewandowski RJ, Kulik L, et al. Radioembolization results in longer time-to-progression and reduced toxicity compared with chemoembolization in patients with hepatocellular carcinoma. Gastroenterology 2011;140(2):497–507.

40. Salem R, Gordon AC, Mouli S, et al. Y90 radioembolization significantly prolongs time to progression compared with chemoembolization in patients with hepatocellular carcinoma. Gastroenterology 2016;151(6):1155–63.

41. Vilgrain V, Pereira H, Assenat E, et al. Efficacy and safety of selective internal radiotherapy with yttrium-90 resin microspheres compared with sorafenib in locally advanced and inoperable hepatocellular carcinoma (SARAH): an open-label randomized controlled phase 3 trial. Lancet Oncol 2017;18(12):1624–36.

42. Chow PKH, Gandhi M, Tan SB, et al. SIRveNIB: selective internal radiation therapy versus sorafenib in Asia-Pacific patients with hepatocellular carcinoma. J Clin Oncol 2018;36(19):1913–21.

43. Vouche M, Habib A, Ward TJ, et al. Unresectable solitary hepatocellular carcinoma not amenable to radiofrequency ablation: multicenter radiology-pathology correlation and survival of radiation segmentectomy. Hepatology 2014;60(1):192–201.

44. Garin E, Lenoir L, Rolland Y, et al. Dosimetry based on ^{99m}Tc-macroaggergated albumin SPECT/CT accurately predicts tumor response and survival in hepatocellular carcinoma patients treated with ^{90}Y-loaded glass microspheres: preliminary results. J Nucl Med 2012;53(2):255–63.

45. Lewandowski RJ, Gabr A, Abouchaleh N, et al. Radiation segmentectomy: potential curative therapy for early hepatocellular carcinoma. Radiology 2018;287(3):1050–8.

46. Lencioni R, Cioni D, Crocetti L, et al. Early-stage hepatocellular carcinoma in patients with cirrhosis: long-term results of percutaneous image-guided radiofrequency ablation. Radiology 2005;234(3):961–7.

47. Vouche M, Lewandowski RJ, Atassi R, et al. Radiation lobectomy: time-dependent analysis of future liver remnant volume in unresectable liver cancer as a bridge to resection. J Hepatol 2013;59(5):1029–36.

48. Theysohn JM, Ertle J, Muller S, et al. Hepatic volume changes after lobar selective internal radiation therapy (SIRT) of hepatocellular carcinoma. Clin Radiol 2014;69(2):172–8.
49. Valle J, Wasan H, Palmer DH, et al. Cisplatin plus gemcitabine versus gemcitabine for biliary tract cancer. N Engl J Med 2010;362:1273–81.
50. Al-Adra DP, Gill RS, Axford SJ, et al. Treatment of unresectable intrahepatic cholangiocarcinoma with yttrium-90 radioembolization: a systematic review and pooled analysis. Eur J Surg Oncol 2015;41(1):120–7.
51. Hoffmann RT, Paprottka PM, Schon A, et al. Transarterial hepatic yttrium 90 radioembolization in patients with unresectable intrahepatic cholangiocarcinoma: factors associated with prolonged survival. Cardiovasc Intervent Radiol 2012;35(1):105–16.
52. Saxena A, Bester L, Chua TC, et al. Yttrium-90 radiotherapy for unresectable intrahepatic cholangiocarcinoma: a preliminary assessment of this novel treatment option. Ann Surg Oncol 2010;17(2):484–91.
53. Chaiteerakij R, Schmit GD, Mettler TA. Comparison of transarterial radioembolization (TARE) and transarterial chemoembolization (TACE) for the treatment of unresectable intrahepatic cholangiocarcinoma. Gastroenterology 2011;140(5):S920–1.
54. Bower G, Little A. Experience with selective internal radiotherapy for patients with intrahepatic cholangiocarcinoma. Intern Med J 2013;43:5.
55. Reimer P, Virarkar MK, Binnenhei M, et al. Prognostic factors in overall survival of patients with unresectable intrahepatic cholangiocarcinoma treated by means of yttrium-90 radioembolization: results in therapy-naïve patients. Cardiovasc Intervent Radiol 2018;41(5):744–52.
56. Ibrahim SM, Mulcahy MF, Lewandowski RJ, et al. Treatment of unresectable cholangiocarcinoma using yttrium-90 microspheres: results from a pilot study. Cancer 2008;113(8):2119–28.
57. Camacho JC, Kokabi N, Xing M, et al. Modified response evaluation criteria in solid tumors and European Association for The Study of the Liver criteria using delayed-phase imaging at an early time point predict survival in patients with unresectable intrahepatic cholangiocarcinoma following yttrium-90 radioembolization. J Vasc Interv Radiol 2014;25(2):256–65.
58. Rafi S, Piduru SM, El-Rayes B, et al. Yttrium-90 radioembolization for unresectable standard-chemorefractory intrahepatic cholangiocarcinoma: survival, efficacy, and safety study. Cardiovasc Intervent Radiol 2013;36(2):440–8.
59. Nezami N, Camacho JC, Kokabi N, et al. Phase Ib trial of gemcitabine with yttrium-90 in patients with hepatic metastasis of pancreatobiliary origin. J Gastrointest Oncol 2019. https://doi.org/10.21037/jgo.2019.05.10.
60. SIRT followed by CIS-GEM chemotherapy versus CIS-GEM chemotherapy alone as 1st line treatment of patients with unresectable intrahepatic cholangiocarcinoma (SIRCCA). 2016. Available at: https://clinicaltrials.gov/ct2/show/NCT02807181. Accessed June 26, 2019.
61. Riaz A, Awais R, Salem R. Side effects of yttrium-90 radioembolization. Front Oncol 2014;4:198.
62. Riaz A, Lewandowski RJ, Kulik L, et al. Complications following radioembolization with yttrium-90 microspheres: a comprehensive literature review. J Vasc Interv Radiol 2009;20(9):1121–30.
63. Greten TF, Mauda-Havakuk M, Heinrich B, et al. Combined locoregional-immunotherapy for liver cancer. J Hepatol 2019;70(5):999–1007.

Inoperable Biliary Tract and Primary Liver Tumors

Palliative Treatment Options

Sophia K. McKinley, MD, EdM[a], Akhil Chawla, MD[b],
Cristina R. Ferrone, MD[b],*

KEYWORDS

- Hepatocellular carcinoma • Cholangiocarcinoma • Palliation • Chemoembolization
- Ablative therapy • Targeted therapies

KEY POINTS

- Hepatocellular carcinoma and intrahepatic cholangiocarcinoma often present at a late, inoperable stage.
- Patients who present with unresectable hepatocellular carcinoma and intrahepatic cholangiocarcinoma may benefit from noncurative or palliative treatment options, which span ablative therapies, biliary decompression, radiotherapy, and systemic therapies.
- Palliation may involve solo or combination therapies to improve both patient survival and quality of life.
- Selection of nonoperative treatment depends on patient and tumor factors as well as institutional resources and expertise.

INTRODUCTION

Hepatocellular carcinoma (HCC) and intrahepatic cholangiocarcinoma (ICC) account for most primary liver tumors. In the United States, approximately 90% of primary liver tumors are HCC, whereas the remaining 10% are ICC.[1,2] Importantly, the incidence of HCC has been increasing in the United States for the past several decades, with more than 24,000 cases of HCC diagnosed on an annual basis.[3,4] This increase is attributed to hepatitis C virus (HCV), obesity, metabolic syndrome, diabetes, and longer survival after the diagnosis of cirrhosis. Although rarer than HCC, the incidence of ICC also seems to be increasing both in the United States and worldwide over the past several decades.[5–7] This increase in incidence is accompanied by a concomitant increase in

Disclosures: No disclosures.
[a] Department of Surgery, Massachusetts General Hospital, Harvard Medical School, 55 Fruit Street, GRB-425, Boston, MA 02114, USA; [b] Department of Surgery, Massachusetts General Hospital, Harvard Medical School, 55 Fruit Street, WAC 4-460, Boston, MA 02114, USA
* Corresponding author.
E-mail address: cferrone@mgh.harvard.edu

Surg Oncol Clin N Am 28 (2019) 745–762
https://doi.org/10.1016/j.soc.2019.06.009
1055-3207/19/© 2019 Elsevier Inc. All rights reserved.

ICC mortality, because the disease portends a poor prognosis.[5,8,9] The relationship between cholangiocarcinoma (CCA) and primary sclerosing cholangitis and liver fluke infection is well established. Other potential risk factors include male gender, smoking, diabetes, cirrhosis, and HCV.[7,10]

For both HCC and ICC, surgical resection or transplant offers the only chance for cure. However, primary liver tumors often present beyond the point of resectability. A Surveillance, Epidemiology, and End Results–Medicare data set–based study showed that less than 10% of patients with HCC underwent attempted resection.[11] For ICC, attempted resection rates vary widely from less than 20% to up to 70%, but most studies report that fewer than half of patients with ICC are resectable at the time of presentation.[7,12–16] Resection of both HCC and ICC is limited by a variety of factors, including number and location of the cancers intrahepatically and extrahepatically, proximity or invasion of vascular and/or biliary structures, and an adequate functional liver remnant.[16–22] The prognosis for inoperable tumors is extremely poor. For HCC, the natural history of patients who cannot undergo surgical resection shows a median overall survival of less than 6 months.[23] In ICC, inoperable disease is associated with a median overall survival of less than 12 months.[7,15,16]

Given the frequency with which these tumors present beyond resectability and the associated poor prognosis, it is important for hepatobiliary surgeons to understand the nonoperative and palliative treatment options for primary liver tumors. This article reviews a broad range of treatment options for inoperable HCC and ICC.

At present, treatment selection depends on several key factors, including individual patient and tumor factors, such as degree of liver disease and the ability to tolerate a major operation; institutional preference and provider expertise, including the availability of clinical trials; and guidelines such as those published by the Barcelona Clinic, National Comprehensive Cancer Network (NCCN), and European Association for the Study of the Liver–European Organization for Research and Treatment of Cancer (EASL-EORTC).[24]

Ablative Therapies

Several ablative therapies are available for inoperable HCC and ICC. Ablative therapies lead to the focal destruction of tissue using radiofrequency ablation (RFA), microwave ablation (MWA), cryoablation (CRA), and percutaneous ethanol injection (PEI). Other less commonly used ablative techniques include high-intensity focused ultrasonography, laser ablation, and irreversible electroporation (IRE), all of which are currently being used as experimental treatment options. At present, MWA and RFA continue to be the most commonly used ablation treatments.[25]

Radiofrequency ablation

RFA allows radio waves to generate heat resulting in focal areas of tissue destruction. In HCC, RFA is used with a curative and palliative intent, as well as a bridge to transplant. For very-early-stage HCC as determined by the Barcelona Clinic Liver Cancer (BCLC) staging system, randomized controlled trials have shown equivalent local control rates and overall survival for lesions less than 3 cm.[26,27] Ablation is associated with less morbidity than an operation, which is of benefit in patients who have underlying hepatic dysfunction that is prohibitive for operative resection.[26,28] Although at least 1 group has shown the effectiveness of RFA for tumors up to 5.0 cm, it is generally accepted that RFA is best for tumors less than 3.0 cm.[28] A 2017 Cochrane Review showed no difference in all-cause mortality in patients with early-stage HCC treated with RFA versus surgical resection.[29] Importantly, this review showed a lower cancer death rate in surgically resected patients; however, the rate of serious adverse events was also higher in this group.

For ICC, small patient series show that RFA may be effective in treating inoperable cholangiocarcinomas less than 5.0 cm, resulting in a median overall survival of 38.5 months.[30] Another series of 20 patients with ICC treated with RFA showed a median disease-free survival of 8.2 months and median overall survival of 23.6 months.[31] However, a National Cancer Database analysis of patients with ICC treated nonsurgically showed that the use of RFA was associated with a significant survival benefit compared with no local therapy only in stage I disease, suggesting that its benefit may be outweighed in patients with aggressive tumor biology.[32]

RFA does have its limitations. The therapeutic efficacy of RFA is inversely associated with the size of the lesion treated. Unlike small tumors with high rates of complete necrosis that may rival the outcomes of surgical resection, tumors larger than this have complete necrosis rates nearing only 50%, thus limiting use of RFA for tumors greater than 3 cm.[33] RFA is limited not only by size but also by location of the lesion, particularly for those tumors that are in close proximity to large vessels and the biliary tree. Large portal and hepatic vein branches can result in a heat-sink effect, which results in an inability to reach maximal ablation temperatures and incomplete cell death. Furthermore, the biliary system is more vulnerable to thermal damage than the arterial or venous systems, resulting in anatomically restrictive use in both HCC and ICC.

Microwave ablation

MWA, similar to RFA, generates high temperatures within lesions, resulting in coagulation necrosis. Compared with RFA, high temperatures are generated more quickly. Because of the higher peak temperatures, shorter ablation times, as well as the lack of a heat-sink effect, MWA may be better suited for larger lesions.[34] A 2016 meta-analysis comparing RFA and MWA showed that although both treatments are safe for HCC, MWA may be more effective in the treatment of larger tumors with respect to long-term progression of disease.[35] Retrospective comparison of RFA and MWA with regard to ablation rate, local recurrence rate, disease-free survival, cumulative survival, and major complications in approximately 200 patients failed to show major differences in clinical effectiveness.[36] MWA has been associated with few complications and low mortality, although, like RFA, the effectiveness of MWA in achieving complete ablation declines with tumor size.[37,38] A retrospective review of 72 patients undergoing MWA for liver tumors of varied histology showed a local recurrence rate of 8% and a median recurrence-free survival of 18 months.[39] For ICC, there is limited information available in the literature regarding the use of MWA. A 2018 study examining treatment outcomes of 6 ICC tumors treated with MWA compared long-term progression with ICCs treated with RFA found no difference.[31]

Cryoablation

CRA leads to the destruction of focal areas of tissue by generating freezing temperatures leading to cell death. Formation of ice crystals within cells and blood vessels leads to necrosis through cell membrane disruption and ischemia.[40] In HCC, RFA and MWA are generally considered superior, with early comparative studies showing lower rates of recurrence and complications in patients compared with CRA.[41,42] More recently, there is evidence that CRA achieves lower rates of complete tumor ablation than RFA.[43] In a meta-analysis of 433 patients with HCC, RFA was superior in local recurrence in addition to complication rates.[44] However, there are individual studies that have shown superior outcomes with CRA compared with RFA, in particular regarding local tumor progression rates in tumors greater than 3.0 cm (7.7% in CRA vs 18.2% in RFA).[45] Some investigators advocate increasing the use of cryotherapy, because the ice ball formation can be visualized on computed tomography.

In addition, CRA has the advantage of being performed under local anesthesia as opposed to general anesthesia for RFA.[46] There is a lack of literature on the use of CRA for ICC.

Percutaneous ethanol injection

PEI is the method of ablation with the lowest cost, but it is a less effective method for ablation, often requiring repeated procedures. PEI is a form of chemical ablation that results in focal liver tissue destruction using ethanol, which induces tumor necrosis through protein denaturation, cellular dehydration, and small vessel thrombosis. It is more effective in smaller lesions and its effects can be limited by tumor septa as well as tumor nodules beyond the periphery of a larger dominant lesion.[47] Complete necrosis with PEI is more likely in tumors less than 2.0 cm.[48] In a series of more than 700 patients, PEI was shown to have few complications and the benefits of repeatability and low cost, making it a potentially appealing ablative therapy for patients with inoperable liver tumors.[49] PEI was the standard percutaneous treatment of small, nonsurgical HCC before the widespread use of RFA.[22,50] Compared as solo treatments, studies generally show better outcomes with RFA than with PEI. For example, in a series of 82 patients, fewer sessions of RFA were required for ablation and complete tumor necrosis than when treating with PEI.[51] In addition, all-cause mortality has been shown to be higher in patients treated with PEI than with RFA.[29] A 2013 Cochrane Review concluded that RFA is superior to PEI in terms of overall survival.[52] Another meta-analysis included 6 studies encompassing 396 patients treated with RFA and 391 patients treated with PEI and showed that a survival advantage for patients treated with RFA was present at 1 year and increased with time.[53] Although RFA may be better than PEI when used as monotherapy, combination therapy may be more effective than either alone.[54] As in other forms of ablative therapy, there is limited information on PEI in ICC.

Intra-arterial Therapies

The underlying rationale behind the use of intra-arterial therapies is that liver tumors derive their blood supply primarily from the hepatic artery. In contrast, normal hepatocytes depend primarily on the portal vein. This difference in vascular supply affords an opportunity to administer therapy in a precise manner by embolizing the vessel or vessels that selectively feed the tumor, leading to ischemic necrosis. Intra-arterial therapies have been used in both HCC and intrahepatic CCA.[55,56]

Transarterial chemoembolization

Transarterial chemoembolization (TACE) is the most widely used treatment of unresectable HCC and is currently recommended for intermediate BCLC-staged tumors according to the EASL-EORTC.[22] TACE administers chemotherapy as a bolus along with lipiodol followed by arterial embolization. Lipiodol allows an increased treatment time and tumor concentration of cytotoxic agents. The addition of arterial embolization leads to ischemic necrosis of the tumor.[57] Early work describing transcatheter arterial embolization confirmed the benefit of arterial embolization through evidence of tumor necrosis and subsequent increased survival in early-stage HCC.[58] A variety of reports have shown that TACE leads to significantly prolonged survival relative to natural history in unresectable HCC.[59,60] Meta-analysis of 7 randomized controlled trials including 516 patients showed a survival benefit of TACE relative to control groups who were conservatively managed.[61] An area of active investigation has been identifying the relative contribution of mechanical embolization compared with the use of regional chemotherapy alone.[62–64] A randomized phase III trial has shown that embolization does not add survival benefit to transarterial chemotherapy without embolization for patients with unresectable HCC.[65] Given the available data, there is no strong evidence to support the use of embolization in addition to regional chemotherapy.

In theory, the use of TACE may be limited in ICC because many of these tumors do not have angiographic hypervascularity in the arterial phase of contrast injection and no blush of a feeding artery. However, there is mounting evidence that TACE may also be effective in ICC. In a study of 155 patients with unresectable ICC, patients undergoing TACE had a median survival of 12.2 months compared with 3.3 months for patients undergoing supportive therapy.[66] Current efforts focus on the optimal chemotherapy agent for TACE in ICC. In a retrospective study of 42 patients with unresectable ICC, TACE using combination gemcitabine and cisplatin resulted in an improved overall survival compared with TACE with gemcitabine alone (13.8 months vs 6.3 months).[67]

Drug eluting beads (DEBs) have both chemotherapeutic and embolic function and can be loaded with a variety of cytotoxic agents, including oxaliplatin, doxorubicin, and irinotecan.[68–70] DEB-TACE has now become a commonly used therapy for both HCC and ICC. Huang and colleagues[68] performed a meta-analysis including more than 700 patients evaluating the efficacy of DEB-TACE versus conventional TACE. Superior objective tumor response rates and survival were shown in patients receiving DEB-TACE compared with conventional therapy. In patients with unresectable ICC, irinotecan DEBs have been shown to improve overall survival compared with conventional TACE with mitomycin C.[69] Adding oxaliplatin DEB-TACE to systemic chemotherapy in unresectable ICC was superior to systemic chemotherapy alone (30 vs 12.7 months).[70]

Transarterial radioembolization

Transarterial radioembolization (TARE) is an intra-arterial therapy using a radioactive isotope to target the liver tumor. Liver parenchyma is highly sensitive to radiation. Therefore, intra-arterial radioembolization is a way to take advantage of the cytotoxic effects of radiation while minimizing collateral damage to the nonmalignant liver parenchyma. Sparing the noncancerous liver is especially important in HCC and ICC because patients with varying degrees of liver dysfunction and cirrhosis are limited in terms of treatment options because of the lack of functional hepatic reserve. One potential benefit of TARE relative to TACE is in the setting of HCC with portal vein thrombosis, because the effects from radiation may have better efficacy for these patients compared with arterial embolization–induced ischemic necrosis.[71]

Both iodine-131 and yttrium-90 are being used in the treatment of HCC. I-131 has been shown to have a survival benefit in patients with advanced HCC, with a median survival of 32 weeks compared with 8 weeks for untreated patients.[72] In a report of patients with HCC treated with Y-90, the response rate was 42% and time to progression was 7.9 months.[73] The benefits of TARE are modulated by the severity of the underlying liver disease and HCC stage, with patients with more advanced liver disease and more advanced BCLC stage showing a shorter survival after radioembolization.[74] At present, given the lack of level-1 evidence, TACE persists as the recommended intra-arterial treatment of HCC, although some groups are calling for wider use of TARE given that it may have a better toxicity profile and is associated with longer time to disease progression.[75] A 2016 Cochrane Review reported limited data availability to complete systematic review on Y-90 in unresectable HCC.[76] The results of several large-scale prospective randomized controlled trials examining the efficacy of Y-90 in HCC will be reported in the coming years.[77]

In ICC, Y-90 is commonly used as a treatment modality at specialized centers. It has evidence to support its use, including the potential for initially unresectable tumors to be downstaged to the point of resectability.[78,79] A 2015 systematic review calculated a median survival of 15.5 months after the use of TARE in patients with unresectable ICC, which is higher than historical survival rates in this disease subset, and similar to that of TACE with systemic chemotherapy, suggesting that TARE may be a treatment option for patients with advanced ICC.[80]

Hepatic artery infusion

Hepatic artery infusion (HAI) is a type of intra-arterial treatment in which chemotherapy is administered as a continuous infusion, rather than a bolus. An infusion catheter is generally placed within the gastroduodenal artery with its pump implanted subcutaneously.[81] HAI may be most beneficial in patients with large or multiple tumors, or tumors with limited ablative options given their anatomic location. Like TACE, HAI leads to high tumor chemotherapy concentrations with lower systemic effect of cytotoxic drugs.[81] In 34 patients with either unresectable HCC (n = 8) or ICC (n = 26), HAI was associated with partial responses in 47% of patients, a prolonged time to progression of 7.4 months, and a median overall survival of 29.5 months.[82]

Recent efforts have focused on understanding whether the addition of HAI to systemic chemotherapy leads to added survival benefit. The addition of HAI to gemcitabine-based regimens was found to improve overall survival in a retrospective analysis of 525 patients. Patients treated with HAI plus systemic chemotherapy achieved a median overall survival of 30.8 months versus 18.4 months in patients treated with systemic chemotherapy alone.[83] The same group also showed that some patients with unresectable ICC treated with floxuridine HAI achieved long-term survival of 3 years, and even 5 years. In this study, patients treated with the combination of floxuridine and bevacizumab showed no survival benefit compared with floxuridine alone.[84] In line with this, a comparison of patients with ICC or HCC treated with floxuridine/dexamethasone HAI with or without systemic bevacizumab showed that the addition of bevacizumab was associated with increased biliary toxicity without an outcome improvement, further suggesting that combination therapy with systemic chemotherapy and HAI may have the disadvantage of a difficult-to-manage toxicity profile with only modest improvements in survival.[85] Further supporting the use of HAI, a 2015 meta-analysis also confirmed that HAI may be associated with longer survival in unresectable ICC; however, there was an increased rate of greater than or equal to grade 3 toxicities associated with HAI compared with other intra-arterial therapies, such as TACE and TARE.[86]

External Beam Radiotherapy

Radiation therapy for primary, inoperable liver tumors has historically been limited by the low tolerance of liver to radiation.[87–89] This intolerance to radiation is particularly challenging given that primary liver tumors frequently occur in the background of chronic liver disease and cirrhosis. Contemporary radiotherapy techniques enhance the capability to effectively target tumors, while limiting damage to the surrounding liver parenchyma. Therefore, there is an increasing interest in role of radiation as a treatment modality for unresectable HCC.[90,91]

Stereotactic body radiotherapy (SBRT) is an area of particular interest because of its ability to deliver dose-dense radiation in an anatomically precise manner. A 2012 study by Ibarra and colleagues[92] showed promising results for SBRT because of its ability to increase time to local progression in both HCC and ICC. In 21 patients with HCC and 11 patients with ICC, the median time to local progression was 6.3 months, with 1-year and 2- year survival rates of 85% and 55% respectively. Approximately 40% of patients developed nausea and fatigue as low-grade toxicity. Other groups have shown that radiation doses to the HCC or ICC may be escalated with the use of SBRT while maintaining an acceptable toxicity profile.[93] For HCC, radiotherapy is appealing because work on HCC metastases shows that these tumors are highly radiosensitive.[94,95] In patients with HCC not suitable for other locoregional therapies, SBRT was evaluated prospectively in a phase I/II trial showing a median overall survival time of 17.0 months.[96] In another study, 42 patients with HCC tumors ineligible for local ablation or surgical resection underwent SBRT and were found to have promising overall survival rates of 93% and 59% at 1 and 3 years, respectively.[97] Consistent with these early reports, the NCCN guidelines now support use of SBRT as an option for HCC.[98]

SBRT has also been used in ICC, with several studies showing improved local disease control and overall survival. In a series of 34 patients, SBRT was associated with a local control rate of 79% and median overall survival of 17 months.[99] In another series of 79 patients with inoperable ICC, radiotherapy was administered after systemic chemotherapy and was associated with median overall survival of 30 months with a 3-year overall survival rate of 44%.[100] This study showed a dose response, with higher radiation doses correlating with improved local control rates and longer survival. Radiotherapy should be considered part of the arsenal of treatment options for inoperable ICC.

Recently, proton beam therapy has been explored for unresectable HCC, with clinical trials underway.[101–103] The use of proton therapy offers an attractive opportunity for patients with unresectable liver malignancies in the setting of underlying liver disease. Protons deliver no exit dose and thus have the potential to deliver higher doses of radiation to large tumors while minimizing radiation to uninvolved liver.[104] In a single-arm, multi-institutional, phase II trial evaluating 92 patients with unresectable HCC or ICC, patients treated with high-dose proton therapy delivered in 15 fractions (median dose 58 Gy) achieved local control rates of more than 94% at 2 years, with 2-year overall survival reaching 63.2% for patients with HCC and 46.5% for patients with ICC. Only 4 patients experienced grade-3 radiation-related toxicity, showing both the safety and the efficacy of this strategy.[101]

Biliary Decompression

Biliary decompression is an important component in the management of inoperable liver tumors, particularly for ICC, which is more likely to cause biliary obstruction leading to jaundice, pruritus, cholangitis, and hepatic failure. Nonsurgical options include endoscopic retrograde pancreatoscopy (ERCP) or percutaneous transhepatic cholangiography (PTC) with stent placement.

Cholangiography allows delineation of the extent of the tumor in terms of proximal biliary involvement, which can have important implications for defining resectability. In addition, biliary decompression allows improved hepatic function, which includes ameliorating coagulopathy and renal function, while at the same time palliating pruritus. At least 1 study has shown increased survival after biliary drainage in the context of inoperable HCC, with patients undergoing effective biliary drainage procedures living 5 times as long as patients who did not achieve effective biliary drainage (247 days vs 44 days).[105]

Controversy exists with respect to the superiority of ERCP or percutaneous transhepatic biliary drainage. Both ERCP and transhepatic drainage allow for biliary brushings, which may aid in the diagnosis of a biliary stricture or obstruction. Although ERCP has a lower bleeding risk, it has a risk of pancreatitis. Proponents of percutaneous transhepatic biliary drainage cite that it may allow more reliable drainage of the biliary tree, particularly for more proximal obstructions, and the catheter can be flushed if cholangitis develops. However, patients with transhepatic catheters that drain externally may have significant issues with dehydration and metabolic derangements caused by the loss of bile. Nevertheless, the use of these methods are generally favored rather than surgical options for biliary decompression, including choledochojejunostomy, choledochoduodenostomy, hepaticojejunostomy. Endoscopic biliary decompression has been shown to be effective, with a superior safety profile compared with surgical biliary decompression.[106]

In general practice, the use of PTC may be useful in situations in which biliary obstruction cannot be primarily treated with ERCP and stenting. PTC may be less desirable because of the inconvenience of an external catheter and the loss of bile and electrolytes potentially resulting in serious metabolic derangements. In situations in which ERCP is unsuccessful in gaining access to the biliary tree, establishing percutaneous access can later be combined with a rendezvous procedure in which percutaneous access and passage of a guidewire allows endoscopic guidance. Note that practice patterns with respect to preference for ERCP or PTC for biliary decompression vary widely based on the institution and country.

For patients with hilar cholangiocarcinoma who present with obstruction of both the right and the left ductal systems, there has been interest in understanding whether single versus double stenting is superior. A randomized controlled trial of patients with malignant hilar obstruction showed that, on an intention-to-treat analysis, unilateral hepatic duct drainage had a higher rate of success and lower complication rate without any difference in median survival. This study suggests that insertion of more than 1 stent does not necessarily derive benefit for the patient.[107]

In general, metal stents have been found to have longer patency with less need for reintervention compared with plastic stents.[108,109] Thus, self-expanding metal stents have been recommended for patients with inoperable biliary tumors who are not likely to undergo surgical resection in order to maximize stent patency. Some clinicians have argued that plastic stents may not need to be changed for metal stents in patients with an expected survival of less than 4 months, given the lower likelihood of biliary stent occlusion.[110]

In terms of metal stents, debate often revolves around the use of covered versus uncovered metal stents. In a review of 749 patients treated with metal stents for malignant biliary strictures, there was no significant difference in terms of survival outcomes. Covered metal stents were much less likely to be complicated by secondary tumor ingrowth and recurrent obstruction compared with uncovered metal stents (9% vs 76%, $P<.001$). However, patients who received covered metal stents were more often afflicted with stent migration and pancreatitis.[111] In another study evaluating 645 patients with malignant biliary strictures treated with metal stent placement, covered stents led to a 6-fold greater risk of developing acute cholecystitis in those patients who still had an intact gallbladder. The use of covered stents was found to be an independent predictor of stent migration.[112] Taken together, covered stents, which are often more costly, may have better patency and lower risk of tumor ingrowth causing recurrent obstruction, but may have morbidity in terms of jailing the cystic duct or pancreatic duct, and have a greater chance of stent migration, which may lead to additional procedures and cost.

Adjuncts to mechanical decompression include photodynamic therapy (PDT), intraluminal brachytherapy (ILBT), irreversible electroporation, and endoscopic radiofrequency ablation. The goal for all of these adjunctive therapies is to prolong metal stent patency. In PDT, the patient receives a photosensitizer that accumulates in tumor cells 48 to 96 hours before the therapy session. When these cells are exposed to particular wavelengths of light, the photosensitizer is activated and leads to cellular destruction. A randomized prospective study of 39 patients undergoing PDT with drainage versus drainage alone showed that addition of PDT was associated with increased survival in inoperable ICC (493 days vs 98 days). Biliary drainage and quality of life were also improved in the PDT plus drainage group.[113] These findings were replicated in another randomized study of 32 patients.[114] A study of 184 patients with ICC confirmed that only surgical resection leads to long-term survival with ICC, but that palliative PDT plus stenting is comparable in survival benefit to an R1 or R2 resection.[115] Intraluminal brachytherapy is also thought to improve outcomes with stenting, because both a single-institution study and meta-analysis suggests improved survival and less frequent stent occlusion when stenting is accompanied by ILBT.[116,117] Irreversible electroporation (IRE) has shown promise in the treatment of obstructive jaundice in the setting of advanced ICC. In a group of 26 patients who underwent IRE after percutaneous transhepatic biliary drainage, median time to drain removal was 122 days, with 305 days of catheter-free time before drain replacement.[118] These findings suggest that IRE provides durable biliary decompression and may improve patient quality of life by permitting patients to live with external drainage catheters for months at a time. In recent years, several groups have also reported on the role of endoscopic radiofrequency ablation in the treatment of malignant biliary strictures.[119–122]

Systemic Therapies

Systemic therapy for inoperable liver tumors includes traditional chemotherapy, immunotherapy, and targeted molecular therapies. The treatment options for both HCC and cholangiocarcinoma are often limited by underlying liver dysfunction and cirrhosis. HCC is generally considered a chemoresistant tumor.[57] Sorafenib, an oral tyrosine kinase inhibitor, represented a major breakthrough in the treatment of HCC and is currently the standard of care for systemic treatment of advanced, unresectable HCC.[22,123] In 2008, a multicenter randomized, double-blind, placebo controlled study known as the Sorafenib Hepatocellular Carcinoma Assessment Randomized Protocol (SHARP) showed the benefits of sorafenib in 600 patients with advanced HCC.[124] Treatment with sorafenib was associated with a median overall survival time of 10.7 months compared with 7.9 months in the placebo group, and a median time to radiologic progression of 5.5 months compared with 2.8 months. A survival benefit was also identified in another prospective phase III randomized trial enrolling more than 200 patients in Asia.[125] Work is ongoing to determine whether sorafenib plus combination therapy with systemic chemotherapy or locoregional therapies such as TACE can augment the survival benefit.[56,126]

Until recently, no effective therapies had been identified, with a large number of trials showing marginal responses using a variety of small molecules.[127–129] However, the combination of immune therapy using the programmed death-ligand 1 (PD-L1) inhibitor, atezolizumab, and a vascular endothelial growth factor inhibitor, bevacizumab, has recently shown great promise in terms of antitumor activity for patients with advanced HCC. Patients in a phase I trial treated with the combination were found to have an exceptional objective response rate of 65%, a partial response rate of 61%, and a complete response rate of 4% with an acceptable safety profile, leading to the US Food and Drug Administration (FDA) granting atezolizumab breakthrough designation for use in combination with bevacizumab. At present, an ongoing phase III randomized trial is comparing this combination with sorafenib for the primary treatment of advanced HCC.[130,131]

Unlike in HCC, traditional chemotherapy has been more effective in the setting of unresectable ICC. The ABC (Advanced Biliary Cancer) trial compared gemcitabine plus cisplatin with gemcitabine alone in 410 patients with locally advanced or metastatic biliary cancer. Gemcitabine plus cisplatin resulted in an increased median overall survival compared with gemcitabine alone (11.7 vs 8.1 months).[132] Time to progression and rates of 6-month disease-free survival were also improved with gemcitabine/cisplatin.[133] The BILCAP trial further supports the use of chemotherapy for ICC. This landmark trial randomized 447 patients to adjuvant capecitabine or observation in patients with surgically resected biliary tract malignancies, in which nearly half of patients had intrahepatic or hilar cholangiocarcinoma. Capecitabine was superior to observation in terms of median overall survival (51 months vs 36 months), establishing it as the standard of care for cholangiocarcinoma in the adjuvant setting.[134]

Despite the improved survival with chemotherapy in ICC, the prognosis for unresectable disease remains poor, and work is ongoing to develop novel strategies to prolong survival.[16,135] Work is being done to identify patients with specific gene expression alterations that have prevalence in cholangiocarcinoma in order to use specific mutational profiles for targeted therapy. For example, TP53 and ERBB2 gene amplifications, programmed cell death protein 1 and PD-L1 expression levels, epigenetic mutations in isocitrate dehydrogenase-1, and fibroblast growth factor receptor fusions are all mutational pathways in which targeted therapies may benefit a specific population of patients with cholangiocarcinoma.[136] Trials investigating these agents with enriched target-positive populations are necessary.

SUMMARY

Primary liver tumors are most commonly HCC and ICC. Although surgical resection offers a chance for cure, these tumors generally present at a late, inoperable stage, necessitating an understanding of noncurative and palliative treatment options. These options include ablative therapies, including radiofrequency ablation; intra-arterial therapies, including transcatheter chemoembolization; biliary decompression; radiotherapy; systemic therapies, including traditional chemotherapeutic agents; immune modulators; and molecular therapies. Recommending nonoperative treatment to patients with primary liver tumors depends on patient and tumor factors, as well as institutional resources and expertise.

REFERENCES

1. London WT, Petrick JL, McGlynn K. Liver cancer. In: Thun MJ, Linet MS, Cerhan JR, et al, editors. Schottenfeld and fraumeni cancer epidemiology and prevention. 4th edition. New York: Oxford university press; 2018. p. 635–60.
2. Altekruse SF, Devesa SS, Dickie LA, et al. Histological classification of liver and intrahepatic bile duct cancers in SEER registries. J Registry Manag 2011;38(4): 201–5.
3. White DL, Thrift AP, Kanwal F, et al. Incidence of hepatocellular carcinoma in all 50 United States, from 2000 through 2012. Gastroenterology 2017;152(4): 812–20.e5.
4. El-Serag HB, Mason AC. Rising incidence of hepatocellular carcinoma in the United States. N Engl J Med 1999;340(10):745–50.
5. Khan SA, Taylor-Robinson SD, Toledano MB, et al. Changing international trends in mortality rates for liver, biliary and pancreatic tumours. J Hepatol 2002;37(6): 806–13.

6. Antwi SO, Mousa OY, Patel T. Racial, ethnic, and age disparities in incidence and survival of intrahepatic cholangiocarcinoma in the United States; 1995-2014. Ann Hepatol 2018;17(4):604–14.

7. Endo I, Gonen M, Yopp AC, et al. Intrahepatic cholangiocarcinoma: rising frequency, improved survival, and determinants of outcome after resection. Ann Surg 2008;248(1):84–96.

8. Bertuccio P, Bosetti C, Levi F, et al. A comparison of trends in mortality from primary liver cancer and intrahepatic cholangiocarcinoma in Europe. Ann Oncol 2013;24(6):1667–74.

9. Patel T. Increasing incidence and mortality of primary intrahepatic cholangiocarcinoma in the United States. Hepatology 2001;33(6):1353–7.

10. Welzel TM, Graubard BI, El-Serag HB, et al. Risk factors for intrahepatic and extrahepatic cholangiocarcinoma in the United States: a population-based case-control study. Clin Gastroenterol Hepatol 2007;5(10):1221–8.

11. El-Serag HB, Siegel AB, Davila JA, et al. Treatment and outcomes of treating of hepatocellular carcinoma among Medicare recipients in the United States: a population-based study. J Hepatol 2006;44(1):158–66.

12. Morise Z, Sugioka A, Tokoro T, et al. Surgery and chemotherapy for intrahepatic cholangiocarcinoma. World J Hepatol 2010;2(2):58–64.

13. Dhanasekaran R, Hemming AW, Zendejas I, et al. Treatment outcomes and prognostic factors of intrahepatic cholangiocarcinoma. Oncol Rep 2013;29(4):1259–67.

14. DeOliveira ML, Cunningham SC, Cameron JL, et al. Cholangiocarcinoma: thirty-one-year experience with 564 patients at a single institution. Ann Surg 2007;245(5):755–62.

15. Tan JCC, Coburn NG, Baxter NN, et al. Surgical management of intrahepatic cholangiocarcinoma–a population-based study. Ann Surg Oncol 2008;15(2):600–8.

16. Bridgewater J, Galle PR, Khan SA, et al. Guidelines for the diagnosis and management of intrahepatic cholangiocarcinoma. J Hepatol 2014;60(6):1268–89.

17. Fan ST, Lo CM, Liu CL, et al. Hepatectomy for hepatocellular carcinoma: toward zero hospital deaths. Ann Surg 1999;229(3):322–30.

18. Fong Y, Sun RL, Jarnagin W, et al. An analysis of 412 cases of hepatocellular carcinoma at a Western center. Ann Surg 1999;229(6):790–9 [discussion: 799–800].

19. Forner A, Llovet JM, Bruix J. Hepatocellular carcinoma. Lancet 2012;379(9822):1245–55.

20. Colella G, Bottelli R, De Carlis L, et al. Hepatocellular carcinoma: comparison between liver transplantation, resective surgery, ethanol injection, and chemo-embolization. Transpl Int 1998;11(Suppl 1):S193–6.

21. Brown KM, Parmar AD, Geller DA. Intrahepatic cholangiocarcinoma. Surg Oncol Clin N Am 2014;23(2):231–46.

22. European Association For The Study Of The Liver, European Organisation For Research And Treatment Of Cancer. EASL-EORTC clinical practice guidelines: management of hepatocellular carcinoma. J Hepatol 2012;56(4):908–43.

23. Yeung YP, Lo CM, Liu CL, et al. Natural history of untreated nonsurgical hepatocellular carcinoma. Am J Gastroenterol 2005;100(9):1995–2004.

24. Fong ZV, Tanabe KK. The clinical management of hepatocellular carcinoma in the United States, Europe, and Asia: a comprehensive and evidence-based comparison and review. Cancer 2014;120(18):2824–38.

25. Facciorusso A, Serviddio G, Muscatiello N. Local ablative treatments for hepatocellular carcinoma: an updated review. World J Gastrointest Pharmacol Ther 2016;7(4):477–89.

26. Chen M-S, Li J-Q, Zheng Y, et al. A prospective randomized trial comparing percutaneous local ablative therapy and partial hepatectomy for small hepatocellular carcinoma. Ann Surg 2006;243(3):321–8.

27. Lü M, Kuang M, Liang L-J, et al. Surgical resection versus percutaneous thermal ablation for early-stage hepatocellular carcinoma: a randomized clinical trial. Zhonghua Yi Xue Za Zhi 2006;86(12):801–5 [in Chinese].

28. Livraghi T, Meloni F, Di Stasi M, et al. Sustained complete response and complications rates after radiofrequency ablation of very early hepatocellular carcinoma in cirrhosis: is resection still the treatment of choice? Hepatology 2008; 47(1):82–9.

29. Majumdar A, Roccarina D, Thorburn D, et al. Management of people with early- or very early-stage hepatocellular carcinoma: an attempted network meta-analysis. Cochrane Database Syst Rev 2017;(3):CD011650.

30. Kim JH, Won HJ, Shin YM, et al. Radiofrequency ablation for the treatment of primary intrahepatic cholangiocarcinoma. AJR Am J Roentgenol 2011;196(2): W205–9.

31. Takahashi EA, Kinsman KA, Schmit GD, et al. Thermal ablation of intrahepatic cholangiocarcinoma: safety, efficacy, and factors affecting local tumor progression. Abdom Radiol (NY) 2018. https://doi.org/10.1007/s00261-018-1656-3.

32. Kolarich AR, Shah JL, George TJ Jr, et al. Non-surgical management of patients with intrahepatic cholangiocarcinoma in the United States, 2004-2015: an NCDB analysis. J Gastrointest Oncol 2018;9(3):536–45.

33. Livraghi T, Goldberg SN, Lazzaroni S, et al. Hepatocellular carcinoma: radiofrequency ablation of medium and large lesions. Radiology 2000;214(3):761–8.

34. Lubner MG, Brace CL, Ziemlewicz TJ, et al. Microwave ablation of hepatic malignancy. Semin Intervent Radiol 2013;30(1):56–66.

35. Chinnaratha MA, Chuang M-YA, Fraser RJL, et al. Percutaneous thermal ablation for primary hepatocellular carcinoma: a systematic review and meta-analysis. J Gastroenterol Hepatol 2016;31(2):294–301.

36. Ding J, Jing X, Liu J, et al. Comparison of two different thermal techniques for the treatment of hepatocellular carcinoma. Eur J Radiol 2013;82(9):1379–84.

37. Sun A-X, Cheng Z-L, Wu P-P, et al. Clinical outcome of medium-sized hepatocellular carcinoma treated with microwave ablation. World J Gastroenterol 2015; 21(10):2997–3004.

38. Ziemlewicz TJ, Hinshaw JL, Lubner MG, et al. Percutaneous microwave ablation of hepatocellular carcinoma with a gas-cooled system: initial clinical results with 107 tumors. J Vasc Interv Radiol 2015;26(1):62–8.

39. Groeschl RT, Wong RK, Quebbeman EJ, et al. Recurrence after microwave ablation of liver malignancies: a single institution experience. HPB (Oxford) 2013;15(5):365–71.

40. Baust JG, Gage AA. The molecular basis of cryosurgery. BJU Int 2005;95(9): 1187–91.

41. Pearson AS, Izzo F, Fleming RY, et al. Intraoperative radiofrequency ablation or cryoablation for hepatic malignancies. Am J Surg 1999;178(6):592–9.

42. Adam R, Hagopian EJ, Linhares M, et al. A comparison of percutaneous cryosurgery and percutaneous radiofrequency for unresectable hepatic malignancies. Arch Surg 2002;137(12):1332–9 [discussion: 1340].

43. Luo W, Zhang Y, He G, et al. Effects of radiofrequency ablation versus other ablating techniques on hepatocellular carcinomas: a systematic review and meta-analysis. World J Surg Oncol 2017;15(1):126.

44. Huang Y-Z, Zhou S-C, Zhou H, et al. Radiofrequency ablation versus cryosurgery ablation for hepatocellular carcinoma: a meta-analysis. Hepatogastroenterology 2013;60(125):1131–5.

45. Wang C, Wang H, Yang W, et al. Multicenter randomized controlled trial of percutaneous cryoablation versus radiofrequency ablation in hepatocellular carcinoma. Hepatology 2015;61(5):1579–90.

46. Hu K-Q. Advances in clinical application of cryoablation therapy for hepatocellular carcinoma and metastatic liver tumor. J Clin Gastroenterol 2014;48(10): 830–6.

47. Shiina S, Tagawa K, Unuma T, et al. Percutaneous ethanol injection therapy for hepatocellular carcinoma. A histopathologic study. Cancer 1991;68(7): 1524–30.

48. Vilana R, Bruix J, Bru C, et al. Tumor size determines the efficacy of percutaneous ethanol injection for the treatment of small hepatocellular carcinoma. Hepatology 1992;16(2):353–7.

49. Livraghi T, Giorgio A, Marin G, et al. Hepatocellular carcinoma and cirrhosis in 746 patients: long-term results of percutaneous ethanol injection. Radiology 1995;197(1):101–8.

50. Nault J-C, Sutter O, Nahon P, et al. Percutaneous treatment of hepatocellular carcinoma: state of the art and innovations. J Hepatol 2017. https://doi.org/10.1016/j.jhep.2017.10.004.

51. Livraghi T, Goldberg SN, Lazzaroni S, et al. Small hepatocellular carcinoma: treatment with radio-frequency ablation versus ethanol injection. Radiology 1999;210(3):655–61.

52. Weis S, Franke A, Mössner J, et al. Radiofrequency (thermal) ablation versus no intervention or other interventions for hepatocellular carcinoma. Cochrane Database Syst Rev 2013;(12):CD003046.

53. Bouza C, López-Cuadrado T, Alcázar R, et al. Meta-analysis of percutaneous radiofrequency ablation versus ethanol injection in hepatocellular carcinoma. BMC Gastroenterol 2009;9:31.

54. Tiong L, Maddern GJ. Systematic review and meta-analysis of survival and disease recurrence after radiofrequency ablation for hepatocellular carcinoma. Br J Surg 2011;98(9):1210–24.

55. Hyder O, Marsh JW, Salem R, et al. Intra-arterial therapy for advanced intrahepatic cholangiocarcinoma: a multi-institutional analysis. Ann Surg Oncol 2013; 20(12):3779–86.

56. Gbolahan OB, Schacht MA, Beckley EW, et al. Locoregional and systemic therapy for hepatocellular carcinoma. J Gastrointest Oncol 2017;8(2):215–28.

57. Cunningham SC, Choti MA, Bellavance EC, et al. Palliation of hepatic tumors. Surg Oncol 2007;16(4):277–91.

58. Matsui O, Kadoya M, Yoshikawa J, et al. Subsegmental transcatheter arterial embolization for small hepatocellular carcinomas: local therapeutic effect and 5-year survival rate. Cancer Chemother Pharmacol 1994;33(Suppl):S84–8.

59. Llovet JM, Real MI, Montaña X, et al. Arterial embolisation or chemoembolisation versus symptomatic treatment in patients with unresectable hepatocellular carcinoma: a randomised controlled trial. Lancet 2002;359(9319):1734–9.

60. Lo C-M, Ngan H, Tso W-K, et al. Randomized controlled trial of transarterial lipiodol chemoembolization for unresectable hepatocellular carcinoma. Hepatology 2002;35(5):1164–71.

61. Llovet JM, Bruix J. Systematic review of randomized trials for unresectable hepatocellular carcinoma: Chemoembolization improves survival. Hepatology 2003;37(2):429–42.

62. Ma T-C, Shao H-B, Xu Y, et al. Three treatment methods via the hepatic artery for hepatocellular carcinoma - a retrospective study. Asian Pac J Cancer Prev 2013; 14(4):2491–4.

63. Sumie S, Yamashita F, Ando E, et al. Interventional radiology for advanced hepatocellular carcinoma: comparison of hepatic artery infusion chemotherapy and transcatheter arterial lipiodol chemoembolization. AJR Am J Roentgenol 2003;181(5):1327–34.

64. Hatanaka Y, Yamashita Y, Takahashi M, et al. Unresectable hepatocellular carcinoma: analysis of prognostic factors in transcatheter management. Radiology 1995;195(3):747–52.

65. Okusaka T, Kasugai H, Shioyama Y, et al. Transarterial chemotherapy alone versus transarterial chemoembolization for hepatocellular carcinoma: a randomized phase III trial. J Hepatol 2009;51(6):1030–6.

66. Park S-Y, Kim JH, Yoon H-J, et al. Transarterial chemoembolization versus supportive therapy in the palliative treatment of unresectable intrahepatic cholangiocarcinoma. Clin Radiol 2011;66(4):322–8.

67. Gusani NJ, Balaa FK, Steel JL, et al. Treatment of unresectable cholangiocarcinoma with gemcitabine-based transcatheter arterial chemoembolization (TACE): a single-institution experience. J Gastrointest Surg 2008;12(1):129–37.

68. Huang K, Zhou Q, Wang R, et al. Doxorubicin-eluting beads versus conventional transarterial chemoembolization for the treatment of hepatocellular carcinoma. J Gastroenterol Hepatol 2014;29(5):920–5.

69. Kuhlmann JB, Euringer W, Spangenberg HC, et al. Treatment of unresectable cholangiocarcinoma: conventional transarterial chemoembolization compared with drug eluting bead-transarterial chemoembolization and systemic chemotherapy. Eur J Gastroenterol Hepatol 2012;24(4):437–43.

70. Poggi G, Amatu A, Montagna B, et al. OEM-TACE: a new therapeutic approach in unresectable intrahepatic cholangiocarcinoma. Cardiovasc Intervent Radiol 2009;32(6):1187–92.

71. Kulik LM, Carr BI, Mulcahy MF, et al. Safety and efficacy of 90Y radiotherapy for hepatocellular carcinoma with and without portal vein thrombosis. Hepatology 2008;47(1):71–81.

72. Lintia-Gaultier A, Perret C, Ansquer C, et al. Intra-arterial injection of 131I-labeled Lipiodol for advanced hepatocellular carcinoma: a 7 years' experience. Nucl Med Commun 2013;34(7):674–81.

73. Salem R, Lewandowski RJ, Mulcahy MF, et al. Radioembolization for hepatocellular carcinoma using Yttrium-90 microspheres: a comprehensive report of long-term outcomes. Gastroenterology 2010;138(1):52–64.

74. Sangro B, Carpanese L, Cianni R, et al. Survival after yttrium-90 resin microsphere radioembolization of hepatocellular carcinoma across Barcelona clinic liver cancer stages: a European evaluation. Hepatology 2011;54(3):868–78.

75. Salem R, Lewandowski RJ, Kulik L, et al. Radioembolization results in longer time-to-progression and reduced toxicity compared with chemoembolization in patients with hepatocellular carcinoma. Gastroenterology 2011;140(2):497–507.e2.

76. Abdel-Rahman OM, Elsayed Z. Yttrium-90 microsphere radioembolisation for unresectable hepatocellular carcinoma. Cochrane Database Syst Rev 2016;(2):CD011313.

77. Salem R, Mazzaferro V, Sangro B. Yttrium 90 radioembolization for the treatment of hepatocellular carcinoma: biological lessons, current challenges, and clinical perspectives. Hepatology 2013;58(6):2188–97.

78. Mouli S, Memon K, Baker T, et al. Yttrium-90 radioembolization for intrahepatic cholangiocarcinoma: safety, response, and survival analysis. J Vasc Interv Radiol 2013;24(8):1227–34.

79. Rayar M, Sulpice L, Edeline J, et al. Intra-arterial yttrium-90 radioembolization combined with systemic chemotherapy is a promising method for downstaging unresectable huge intrahepatic cholangiocarcinoma to surgical treatment. Ann Surg Oncol 2015;22(9):3102–8.

80. Al-Adra DP, Gill RS, Axford SJ, et al. Treatment of unresectable intrahepatic cholangiocarcinoma with yttrium-90 radioembolization: a systematic review and pooled analysis. Eur J Surg Oncol 2015;41(1):120–7.

81. Leal JN, Kingham TP. Hepatic artery infusion chemotherapy for liver malignancy. Surg Oncol Clin N Am 2015;24(1):121–48.

82. Jarnagin WR, Schwartz LH, Gultekin DH, et al. Regional chemotherapy for unresectable primary liver cancer: results of a phase II clinical trial and assessment of DCE-MRI as a biomarker of survival. Ann Oncol 2009;20(9):1589–95.

83. Konstantinidis IT, Groot Koerkamp B, Do RKG, et al. Unresectable intrahepatic cholangiocarcinoma: systemic plus hepatic arterial infusion chemotherapy is associated with longer survival in comparison with systemic chemotherapy alone. Cancer 2016;122(5):758–65.

84. Konstantinidis IT, Do RKG, Gultekin DH, et al. Regional chemotherapy for unresectable intrahepatic cholangiocarcinoma: a potential role for dynamic magnetic resonance imaging as an imaging biomarker and a survival update from two prospective clinical trials. Ann Surg Oncol 2014;21(8):2675–83.

85. Kemeny NE, Schwartz L, Gönen M, et al. Treating primary liver cancer with hepatic arterial infusion of floxuridine and dexamethasone: does the addition of systemic bevacizumab improve results? Oncology 2011;80(3–4):153–9.

86. Boehm LM, Jayakrishnan TT, Miura JT, et al. Comparative effectiveness of hepatic artery based therapies for unresectable intrahepatic cholangiocarcinoma. J Surg Oncol 2015;111(2):213–20.

87. Lawrence TS, Robertson JM, Anscher MS, et al. Hepatic toxicity resulting from cancer treatment. Int J Radiat Oncol Biol Phys 1995;31(5):1237–48.

88. Ingold JA, Reed GB, Kaplan HS, et al. Radiation hepatitis. Am J Roentgenol Radium Ther Nucl Med 1965;93:200–8.

89. Russell AH, Clyde C, Wasserman TH, et al. Accelerated hyperfractionated hepatic irradiation in the management of patients with liver metastases: results of the RTOG dose escalating protocol. Int J Radiat Oncol Biol Phys 1993;27(1):117–23.

90. Schaub SK, Hartvigson PE, Lock MI, et al. Stereotactic body radiation therapy for hepatocellular carcinoma: current trends and controversies. Technol Cancer Res Treat 2018;17. 1533033818790217.

91. Wo JY, Dawson LA, Zhu AX, et al. An emerging role for radiation therapy in the treatment of hepatocellular carcinoma and intrahepatic cholangiocarcinoma. Surg Oncol Clin N Am 2014;23(2):353–68.

92. Ibarra RA, Rojas D, Snyder L, et al. Multicenter results of stereotactic body radiotherapy (SBRT) for non-resectable primary liver tumors. Acta Oncol 2012;51(5):575–83.
93. Tse RV, Hawkins M, Lockwood G, et al. Phase I study of individualized stereotactic body radiotherapy for hepatocellular carcinoma and intrahepatic cholangiocarcinoma. J Clin Oncol 2008;26(4):657–64.
94. Zeng Z-C, Tang Z-Y, Fan J, et al. Radiation therapy for adrenal gland metastases from hepatocellular carcinoma. Jpn J Clin Oncol 2005;35(2):61–7.
95. Kaizu T, Karasawa K, Tanaka Y, et al. Radiotherapy for osseous metastases from hepatocellular carcinoma: a retrospective study of 57 patients. Am J Gastroenterol 1998;93(11):2167–71.
96. Bujold A, Massey CA, Kim JJ, et al. Sequential phase I and II trials of stereotactic body radiotherapy for locally advanced hepatocellular carcinoma. J Clin Oncol 2013;31(13):1631–9.
97. Kwon JH, Bae SH, Kim JY, et al. Long-term effect of stereotactic body radiation therapy for primary hepatocellular carcinoma ineligible for local ablation therapy or surgical resection. Stereotactic radiotherapy for liver cancer. BMC Cancer 2010;10:475.
98. National Comprehensive Cancer Network. Hepatobiliary cancers (Version 1.2019). Available at: https://www.nccn.org/professionals/physician_gls/pdf/hepatobiliary.pdf. Accessed January 17, 2019.
99. Mahadevan A, Dagoglu N, Mancias J, et al. Stereotactic Body Radiotherapy (SBRT) for intrahepatic and hilar cholangiocarcinoma. J Cancer 2015;6(11):1099–104.
100. Tao R, Krishnan S, Bhosale PR, et al. Ablative radiotherapy doses lead to a substantial prolongation of survival in patients with inoperable intrahepatic cholangiocarcinoma: a retrospective dose response analysis. J Clin Oncol 2016;34(3):219–26.
101. Hong TS, Wo JY, Yeap BY, et al. Multi-institutional Phase II study of high-dose hypofractionated proton beam therapy in patients with localized, unresectable hepatocellular carcinoma and intrahepatic cholangiocarcinoma. J Clin Oncol 2016;34(5):460–8.
102. Bush DA, Smith JC, Slater JD, et al. Randomized clinical trial comparing proton beam radiation therapy with transarterial chemoembolization for hepatocellular carcinoma: results of an interim analysis. Int J Radiat Oncol Biol Phys 2016;95(1):477–82.
103. Qi W-X, Fu S, Zhang Q, et al. Charged particle therapy versus photon therapy for patients with hepatocellular carcinoma: a systematic review and meta-analysis. Radiother Oncol 2015;114(3):289–95.
104. Badiyan SN, Hallemeier CL, Lin SH, et al. Proton beam therapy for gastrointestinal cancers: past, present, and future. J Gastrointest Oncol 2018;9(5):962–71.
105. Cho HC, Lee JK, Lee KH, et al. Are endoscopic or percutaneous biliary drainage effective for obstructive jaundice caused by hepatocellular carcinoma? Eur J Gastroenterol Hepatol 2011;23(3):224–31.
106. Smith AC, Dowsett JF, Russell RC, et al. Randomised trial of endoscopic stenting versus surgical bypass in malignant low bileduct obstruction. Lancet 1994;344(8938):1655–60.
107. De Palma GD, Galloro G, Siciliano S, et al. Unilateral versus bilateral endoscopic hepatic duct drainage in patients with malignant hilar biliary obstruction: results of a prospective, randomized, and controlled study. Gastrointest Endosc 2001;53(6):547–53.

108. Raju RP, Jaganmohan SR, Ross WA, et al. Optimum palliation of inoperable hilar cholangiocarcinoma: comparative assessment of the efficacy of plastic and self-expanding metal stents. Dig Dis Sci 2011;56(5):1557–64.

109. Sawas T, Al Halabi S, Parsi MA, et al. Self-expandable metal stents versus plastic stents for malignant biliary obstruction: a meta-analysis. Gastrointest Endosc 2015;82(2):256–67.e7.

110. Boulay BR, Birg A. Malignant biliary obstruction: From palliation to treatment. World J Gastrointest Oncol 2016;8(6):498–508.

111. Lee JH, Krishna SG, Singh A, et al. Comparison of the utility of covered metal stents versus uncovered metal stents in the management of malignant biliary strictures in 749 patients. Gastrointest Endosc 2013;78(2):312–24.

112. Jang S, Stevens T, Parsi M, et al. Association of covered metallic stents with cholecystitis and stent migration in malignant biliary stricture. Gastrointest Endosc 2018;87(4):1061–70.

113. Ortner MEJ, Caca K, Berr F, et al. Successful photodynamic therapy for nonresectable cholangiocarcinoma: a randomized prospective study. Gastroenterology 2003;125(5):1355–63.

114. Zoepf T, Jakobs R, Arnold JC, et al. Palliation of nonresectable bile duct cancer: improved survival after photodynamic therapy. Am J Gastroenterol 2005; 100(11):2426–30.

115. Witzigmann H, Berr F, Ringel U, et al. Surgical and palliative management and outcome in 184 patients with hilar cholangiocarcinoma: palliative photodynamic therapy plus stenting is comparable to r1/r2 resection. Ann Surg 2006;244(2): 230–9.

116. Xu X, Li J, Wu J, et al. A systematic review and meta-analysis of intraluminal brachytherapy versus stent alone in the treatment of malignant obstructive jaundice. Cardiovasc Intervent Radiol 2018;41(2):206–17.

117. Chen Y, Wang X-L, Yan Z-P, et al. HDR-192Ir intraluminal brachytherapy in treatment of malignant obstructive jaundice. World J Gastroenterol 2004;10(23): 3506–10.

118. Martin EK, Bhutiani N, Egger ME, et al. Safety and efficacy of irreversible electroporation in the treatment of obstructive jaundice in advanced hilar cholangiocarcinoma. HPB (Oxford) 2018;20(11):1092–7.

119. Sharaiha RZ, Sethi A, Weaver KR, et al. Impact of radiofrequency ablation on malignant biliary strictures: results of a collaborative registry. Dig Dis Sci 2015;60(7):2164–9.

120. Dolak W, Schreiber F, Schwaighofer H, et al. Endoscopic radiofrequency ablation for malignant biliary obstruction: a nationwide retrospective study of 84 consecutive applications. Surg Endosc 2014;28(3):854–60.

121. Zheng X, Bo ZY, Wan W, et al. Endoscopic radiofrequency ablation may be preferable in the management of malignant biliary obstruction: a systematic review and meta-analysis. J Dig Dis 2016;17(11):716–24.

122. Patel J, Rizk N, Kahaleh M. Role of photodynamic therapy and intraductal radiofrequency ablation in cholangiocarcinoma. Best Pract Res Clin Gastroenterol 2015;29(2):309–18.

123. Kudo M, Ueshima K. Positioning of a molecular-targeted agent, sorafenib, in the treatment algorithm for hepatocellular carcinoma and implication of many complete remission cases in Japan. Oncology 2010;78(Suppl 1):154–66.

124. Llovet JM, Ricci S, Mazzaferro V, et al. Sorafenib in advanced hepatocellular carcinoma. N Engl J Med 2008;359(4):378–90.

125. Cheng A-L, Kang Y-K, Chen Z, et al. Efficacy and safety of sorafenib in patients in the Asia-Pacific region with advanced hepatocellular carcinoma: a phase III randomised, double-blind, placebo-controlled trial. Lancet Oncol 2009;10(1): 25–34.

126. Li L, Zhao W, Wang M, et al. Transarterial chemoembolization plus sorafenib for the management of unresectable hepatocellular carcinoma: a systematic review and meta-analysis. BMC Gastroenterol 2018;18(1):138.

127. Zhu AX, Kudo M, Assenat E, et al. Effect of everolimus on survival in advanced hepatocellular carcinoma after failure of sorafenib: the EVOLVE-1 randomized clinical trial. JAMA 2014;312(1):57–67.

128. Zhu AX, Park JO, Ryoo B-Y, et al. Ramucirumab versus placebo as second-line treatment in patients with advanced hepatocellular carcinoma following first-line therapy with sorafenib (REACH): a randomised, double-blind, multicentre, phase 3 trial. Lancet Oncol 2015;16(7):859–70.

129. Rimassa L, Assenat E, Peck-Radosavljevic M, et al. Tivantinib for second-line treatment of MET-high, advanced hepatocellular carcinoma (METIV-HCC): a final analysis of a phase 3, randomised, placebo-controlled study. Lancet Oncol 2018;19(5):682–93.

130. Stein S, Pishvaian MJ, Lee MS, et al. Safety and clinical activity of 1L atezolizumab + bevacizumab in a phase Ib study in hepatocellular carcinoma (HCC). J Clin Oncol 2018;36(15_suppl):4074.

131. FDA grants atezolizumab combo breakthrough designation for frontline HCC. OncLive. Available at: https://www.onclive.com/web-exclusives/fda-grants-atezolizumab-breakthrough-designation-for-frontline-hcc. Accessed January 15, 2019.

132. Valle J, Wasan H, Palmer DH, et al. Cisplatin plus gemcitabine versus gemcitabine for biliary tract cancer. N Engl J Med 2010;362(14):1273–81.

133. Valle JW, Wasan H, Johnson P, et al. Gemcitabine alone or in combination with cisplatin in patients with advanced or metastatic cholangiocarcinomas or other biliary tract tumours: a multicentre randomised phase II study - The UK ABC-01 Study. Br J Cancer 2009;101(4):621–7.

134. Primrose JN, Fox R, Palmer DH, et al. Adjuvant capecitabine for biliary tract cancer: The BILCAP randomized study. J Clin Oncol 2017;35(15_suppl):4006.

135. Fiteni F, Jary M, Monnien F, et al. Advanced biliary tract carcinomas: a retrospective multicenter analysis of first and second-line chemotherapy. BMC Gastroenterol 2014;14:143.

136. Jusakul A, Cutcutache I, Yong CH, et al. Whole-genome and epigenomic landscapes of etiologically distinct subtypes of cholangiocarcinoma. Cancer Discov 2017;7(10):1116–35.

Expanding the Surgical Pool for Hepatic Resection to Treat Biliary and Primary Liver Tumors

Tiffany C. Lee, MD, Mackenzie C. Morris, MD,
Sameer H. Patel, MD, Shimul A. Shah, MD, MHCM*

KEYWORDS

- Hepatocellular carcinoma • Cholangiocarcinoma • Portal vein embolization
- Transarterial radioembolization
- Associating liver partition and portal vein ligation (ALPPS) • Liver transplantation

KEY POINTS

- Advanced age and liver disease are no longer a contraindication for hepatic resection. Instead, emphasis has been placed on rigorous preoperative evaluation and appropriate patient selection.
- Sorafenib has long been the only accepted chemotherapy for advanced, unresectable hepatocellular carcinoma. Recent advances not only have expanded treatment options for advanced HCC but also broadened application of multikinase inhibitors in the adjuvant as well as neoadjuvant setting.
- Techniques to increase posthepatectomy future liver remnant include portal vein embolization, transarterial embolization, and associating liver partition and portal vein ligation.
- Liver transplantation is an established treatment modality in select patients with hepatocellular carcinoma and hilar cholangiocarcinoma, with criteria continuing to be challenged and expanded.

INTRODUCTION

Primary liver and biliary tract tumors are often managed with multimodal regimens, including chemotherapy, locoregional therapies, and surgery. Surgical resection

Disclosure Statement: The authors have no disclosures of any relationship with a commercial company that has a direct financial interest in the subject matter or materials discussed in this article or with a company making a competing product.
Cincinnati Research on Outcomes and Safety in Surgery (CROSS), Department of Surgery, University of Cincinnati College of Medicine, 231 Albert Sabin Way, ML 0558, Cincinnati, OH 45267-0558, USA
* Corresponding author. University of Cincinnati College of Medicine, 231 Albert Sabin Way, ML 0558, MSB 2006C, Cincinnati, OH 45267-0558.
E-mail address: shahsu@UCMAIL.UC.EDU

remains the optimal curative therapy in these, like many other malignancies, although many patients present with traditionally unresectable disease. Fortunately, expansion of patient selection criteria, advances in each of the multimodal therapies, and select utilization of liver transplantation (LT) have led to increased rates of surgical resection and subsequent improved outcomes. In this issue, hepatocellular carcinoma (HCC), hilar (hCCA), and intrahepatic cholangiocarcinoma (iCCA) will be specifically examined.

PATIENT SELECTION
Surgery in the Elderly

Historically, older patients have been considered less suitable surgical candidates given concern for significant comorbidities, decreased functional reserve, and more limited life expectancy. However, in recent years, this assumption has been challenged because surgical procedures have been demonstrated to be safe and effective in patients older than the traditional threshold of 65 years of age. Hepatic resection has been of particular interest, especially in Asia, where longer life expectancy and the higher incidence of viral hepatitis have resulted in an increased proportion of elderly patients with HCC. This older patient population has led to a worldwide increased interest in performing hepatic resection in selective elderly patients.

Application of prognostic tools may help stratify patients based on risk of postoperative complications or survival. In Japan as well as the United States, there is routine utilization of a frailty index, which includes domains on activities of daily living (ADL), independent ADLs, physical strength, nutrition, oral function, isolation, memory, and mood.[1,2] The presence of frailty based on this tool was associated with age-related postoperative events, including major cardiopulmonary complications, delirium, transfer to a rehabilitation facility, and dependency.[1] Cheng and colleagues[3] developed nomograms predictive of long-term survival after partial hepatectomy for HCC, with the preoperative nomogram consisting of age greater than 75, Charlson-Deyo score, hepatitis B virus DNA, alpha-fetoprotein (AFP) greater than 400, and tumor size. The postoperative nomogram included these 5 factors as well as nonanatomic hepatectomy, incomplete tumor capsule, and microvascular invasion.[3] Regardless of what tools are used, a global assessment of an individual patient's health should be made to determine whether surgical intervention is an appropriate option.

Studies of elderly patients undergoing hepatic resection have shown that although elderly patients may have higher rates of certain postoperative complications, their hospital length of stay, mortality, and overall survival are similar to younger patients. Complications more common in the elderly include pneumonia, cardiovascular events, and delirium.[4,5] However, other studies have shown no differences in postoperative complications based on age.[6–8] In addition, short-term mortality[5,6,8] and long-term survival[8,9] are comparable between elderly and younger patients.

LT in the elderly has also become more common, because it has been shown to be safe and effective. A previous study of the Scientific Registry of Transplant Recipients comparing recipients younger than 70 versus older than 70 demonstrated similar short-term mortality, hospital lengths of stay, and 30-day readmission rates as well as similar long-term patient and graft survival.[10] Another study showed comparable quality-of-life metrics in elderly versus younger transplant recipients; therefore, elderly patients appear to derive similar benefits from transplantation.[11]

Advanced age alone is no longer a contraindication for hepatic resection or transplantation. Instead, emphasis has been placed on rigorous preoperative evaluation and appropriate patient selection. In addition to the standard cardiovascular and pulmonary workup, there may be further benefit to incorporating psychiatric evaluations to identify patients more susceptible to postoperative delirium.[2,5] An open discussion regarding potential risks of complications, including discharge to a rehabilitation facility, should be undertaken for each patient in order to determine appropriateness of surgical intervention and goals of care.

Preoperative Evaluation in the Patient with Cirrhosis

Hepatic resection in patients with underlying liver disease carries significant morbidity and mortality.[12] A thorough preoperative risk evaluation is required to minimize risk and optimize patient outcomes. No scoring system has been made specifically for liver resection in patients with cirrhosis, but several are used to help predict preoperative risk in this patient population. The 3 most commonly used scoring systems are the American Society of Anesthesiologists score (ASA score), Child-Turcotte-Pugh (CTP) score, and the model for end-stage liver disease (MELD) score. The ASA score has been shown to reliably predict 7-day mortality following abdominal surgery.[12] The CTP is another scoring system that is used to predict outcomes following surgery and takes into account variables associated with liver function. Mortalities were observed to be 10%, 30%, and 80% for CTP A, B, and C, respectively, and the CTP score is commonly used for patient surgical risk stratification.[13] Advancements in surgical technique and postoperative care have allowed for improved outcomes in patients with CTP A and B cirrhosis who would otherwise be at higher risk of perioperative mortality.[14,15]

In addition, using the MELD scoring system, predicted mortality after abdominal surgery is 5% to 10% for MELD ≤ 11, 25% to 54% for MELD 12% to 25%, and 55% to 80% for MELD ≥ 26.[16] A MELD score of 9 has been described as the "cutoff" because of a study that demonstrated a mortality of 0% below 9, but a mortality of 26% in patients with a MELD score of 9 or greater.[15]

These scoring systems assist in risk-benefit analyses when deciding the best management for patients with HCC or cholangiocarcinoma and underlying liver disease. They provide granular data when estimating perioperative morbidity and mortality following hepatectomy, but ultimate decision-making should be individualized for each patient.

The preoperative workup for a patient with liver disease starts with a detailed history and physical examination. The history should focus on risk factors and sequela of liver disease. Clinical evaluation and blood tests are the most commonly used screening test, but may miss some patients.[17] Several other tests, including indocyanine green (ICG) clearance test, aminopyrine breath test, galactosyl elimination capacity, and 99m-Tc-galactosyl-human serum albumin scintigraphy, have been proposed as possible screening tests. The ICG clearance test is a noninvasive dynamic test to evaluate hepatic function that consists of injecting ICG into a peripheral vein and measuring the retention and clearance via pulse spectrophotometry. It is the most widely used test, particularly in Asia, and shows that CTP A patients with an ICG retention rate of less than 14% are eligible for large resections.[18]

Severe portal hypertension is a known contraindication for liver resection and requires preoperative evaluation. The gold-standard measurement of portal hypertension is by using a catheter to measure the hepatic venous pressure gradient. Bruix and colleagues[19] showed that a gradient higher than 10 mm Hg was associated with increased morbidity and reduced survival following hepatic resection. However, the invasiveness of the procedure has moved most centers to evaluate portal hypertension with platelet count, spleen measurement by imaging studies, and endoscopy to assess for the presence of esophageal varices.[20] The combination of the proper diagnostic workup and the multiple risk calculators discussed earlier will assist surgeons in proper patient selection and result in better outcomes.

Management Guidelines for the Patient with Cirrhosis and Hepatocellular Carcinoma

Multiple guidelines exist to assist in the management of HCC in the patient with cirrhosis. The European Association for the Study of the Liver and American Association for the Study of the Liver guidelines restrict hepatic resection to patients with small, single tumors, normal bilirubin, and the absence of portal hypertension.[21] The Barcelona Clinic Liver Cancer (BCLC) classification further recommends curative liver resection in patients with HCC and cirrhosis for early-stage tumors and in CTP A cirrhosis without portal hypertension.[22] The BCLC classification identifies patients with HCC and liver disease to classify them from early stage (A) to end stage (D). The classifications consist of stage A (CTP A or B and a single nodule or 3 nodules <3 cm); stage B (CTP A or B with multinodular disease); stage C (CTP A or B and vascular invasion or extrahepatic spread); and stage D (CTP C with HCC). However, several specialized centers around the world have shown that hepatectomy in patients with portal hypertension can be performed safely.[14] Although nonsurgical local therapies, such as transarterial chemoembolization (TACE), are effective for HCC patients with cirrhosis, studies still show better long-term survival in patients undergoing resection.[23]

The Milan criteria were proposed in 1996 by the National Cancer Institute in Milan, Italy and define the characteristics of tumors amenable to LT. The criteria include a single tumor less than 5 cm in diameter or no more than 3 tumor nodules with each being 3 cm or less, absence of major vascular invasion, and no extrahepatic spread. Despite the criteria's limits for LT, a randomized controlled trial demonstrated improved survival in patients outside of the Milan criteria who underwent resection compared with ablation.[24]

A study evaluating the use of the BCLC criteria in 10 high-volume centers showed that only 50% of resections were within the criteria, including stage 0 (single tumor <2 cm) or A. Patients in both stage B and C also underwent resection in the study. The 5-year overall survival rates after HCC resections in BCLC A, B, and C cirrhosis were 61%, 57%, and 38% and 5-year disease-free survival rates were 21%, 27%, and 18%.[25] These studies demonstrate that patients outside of the classic criteria may be appropriate for resection and are discussed in further detail elsewhere in this article. However, patients who are not eligible for LT may still benefit from resection, despite higher perioperative risk, in order to improve oncologic outcomes.

Insufficient liver volume after resection places patients at higher risk of developing posthepatectomy liver failure. In cirrhotic livers, the future liver remnant (FLR) volume should be greater than 40% to reduce that risk, in comparison to 20% for patients with normal livers.[26] Performing nonanatomic liver resections provides an opportunity to increase the volume of liver left behind compared with anatomic resections. Despite conflicting data regarding the oncologic outcomes in anatomic versus nonanatomic resections, as long as negative margins can be achieved, the use of nonanatomic resections may convert otherwise inoperable CTP B patients to candidates for resection.[27,28]

These criteria and guidelines can help assist the surgeon in the evaluation of a patient with cirrhosis who needs a hepatic resection. However, the continued improvement in surgical technique and postoperative management allows the ability for patients with worse cirrhosis to be considered for resection.

PERIOPERATIVE CHEMOTHERAPY IN HEPATOCELLULAR CARCINOMA

Patients with HCC and BCLC stage C have been considered the optimal patients for systemic therapy. The recent concentration in systemic therapy has focused on targeted molecular antagonists of pathways thought to be critical to the pathogenesis of this disease. Sorafenib is a small molecular inhibitor that abrogates phosphorylation and activation of tyrosine kinase domains of the vascular endothelial growth factor receptor, platelet-derived growth factor, c-kit, and flt1.[29] The SHARP and Asia-Pacific trials showed a survival advantage in the use of sorafenib versus placebo in advanced HCC.[30,31] Almost all of the patients were CTP class A with only 5% of patients being CTP class B. A similar study by Cheng and colleagues[32] with mostly BCLC stage C patients also showed an increase in survival with the use of sorafenib. However, when sorafenib was used in the adjuvant setting for patients after resection, the same improvements in survival were not seen.[33]

There has been little progress in drug development since the approval of sorafenib. Sunitinib, another oral multityrosine kinase inhibitor, showed significantly worse median overall survival when compared with sunitinib in advanced HCC.[34] Multiple trials over the next few years comparing other drugs to sorafenib in advanced HCC failed to show good or similar outcomes.[35–37] These studies exemplify the chemotherapy-resistant nature of HCC and the ongoing search to find effective treatment regimens.

In 2017, a phase 3 noninferiority study in patients with advanced HCC, a multiple kinase inhibitor lenvatinib was found to have similar median overall survival versus sorafenib (12.3 months vs 13.6 months, P = NS).[38] They also showed improvements in progression-free survival and time to progression in the group receiving lenvatinib. Furthermore, they were found to have similar treatment-related adverse events grade 3 or higher (57% lenvatinib vs 49% sorafenib). This recent publication has made lenvatinib another first-line agent for patients with advanced HCC. However, the efficacy of lenvatinib in the adjuvant setting is unknown and remains to be elucidated.

Local recurrence following resection in patients with HCC remains a significant problem, with no currently existing effective neoadjuvant therapy to address this issue. A recent study compared the impact of neoadjuvant radiotherapy versus adjuvant radiotherapy on survival using the Surveillance, Epidemiology and End Results database. They found that 3-year cancer-specific survival in the neoadjuvant radiotherapy group was higher than the adjuvant group (75.2% vs 32.8%).[39] The use of TACE in the neoadjuvant setting was previously shown to have improved 5-year disease-free (31.8% vs 16.5%) and overall survival (46.2% vs 31.7%).[40]

Immunotherapy has shown potential as a treatment option for HCC. At the University of Texas MD Anderson Cancer Center, investigators used a perioperative immunotherapy regimen of nivolumab and ipilimumab for resectable HCC and found an astounding pathologic complete response rate of 37.5%. Although these are only preliminary findings in a small cohort of patients, these data suggest a potential role for immunotherapy in HCC.[41] These recent clinical trials suggest that HCC is responsive to immunotherapy, and by finding the optimal regimen, use in the neoadjuvant setting may lead to expansion of the surgical pool.

TECHNIQUES TO INCREASE FUTURE LIVER REMNANT
Portal Vein Embolization

Preoperative portal vein embolization (PVE) to increase postoperative FLR was first introduced in the 1980s.[42] This technique, typically performed by an interventional radiologist, involves occlusion of portal flow to a selected portion of the liver, resulting in hepatic atrophy and subsequent hypertrophy of the remaining perfused liver (**Fig. 1**). It is indicated in situations wherein hepatic resection would result in an anticipated liver remnant volume in general less than 20% to 25% (in those with normal livers) or less than 30% to 40% (in those with compromised liver function).[43] With liver remnants less than these thresholds, the risk of postoperative liver failure is high and often precludes surgical resection. PVE has been shown to reduce the risk of liver failure as well as increase the number of patients undergoing resection who otherwise would not be candidates.[44]

A meta-analysis including 1088 patients from 37 studies assessing outcomes of PVE concluded that it was a safe and effective procedure.[45] Morbidity rate after PVE was 2.2%, with the most common complications including abdominal discomfort, fever, nausea or emesis, and ileus. There was no mortality associated with the procedure. Four to six weeks after PVE, the expected increase in FLR ranges from 8% to 13%, with degree of hypertrophy (DH = post-FLR/postfunctional liver volume − pre-FLR/prefunctional liver volume) and growth rate (GR = DH/wk since PVE) shown to be predictors of posthepatectomy liver failure.[46] A reduced risk of liver failure is associated with a DH greater than 5% in a normal liver and greater than 10% in a cirrhotic liver.[47,48]

Portal Vein Embolization in Hepatocellular Carcinoma

One of the reasons HCC is often unresectable is due to underlying chronic liver disease requiring a larger anticipated FLR. The application of PVE in HCC is well established, allowing resection in traditionally unresectable (stage III or IV) patients.[49]

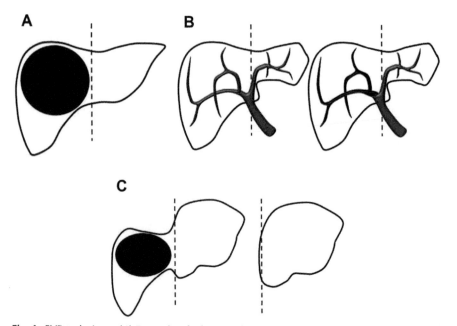

Fig. 1. PVE technique. (*A*) Example of a large right-sided primary liver tumor. Estimated FLR is insufficient if a hepatectomy is performed. (*B*) PVE can be used in this scenario to increase the FLR of the left liver (right-sided PVE is performed). (*C*) After an increase in the size of the FLR, an anatomic resection of the liver can be performed safely, reducing the risk of posthepatectomy liver failure.

This technique results in improved perioperative mortality and similar or better long-term survival.[49–51]

Another strategy to increase FLR in HCC patients is to use sequential TACE followed by PVE.[52] PVE following TACE has been shown to result in a larger increase in FLR than PVE alone.[53,54] In addition, the TACE + PVE group compared with PVE alone had a higher incidence of complete tumor necrosis as well as recurrence-free and overall survival, suggesting this may be a more effective oncologic therapy.

Portal Vein Embolization in Biliary Cancer

PVE in biliary cancer has been increasingly used, with FLR hypertrophy similar to those with HCC.[55] However, completion of hepatectomy after PVE appears to be lower in patients with biliary cancer owing to disease progression, with unresectability rates of 17% in cholangiocarcinoma.[56] Those who successfully underwent resection after PVE had a 5-year overall survival of 39% in cholangiocarcinoma. However, despite the lower resection rate, the additional time helps identify patients with better tumor biology.

Transarterial Radioembolization

Transarterial radioembolization with ^{90}Y-labeled microspheres, also known as selective internal radiotherapy, has developed into another technique to increase anticipated FLR in patients with unresectable hepatobiliary tumors. This technique has the additional benefit of treating the tumor and is particularly useful as a bridge to resection.[57,58] Some studies have shown contralateral hepatic hypertrophy comparable to PVE, although a direct matched comparison showed mean FLR increase of 29% with radioembolization versus 61.5% with PVE.[58–60] Radioembolization may provide an additional option for greater DH compared with PVE alone.

Associating Liver Partition and Portal Vein Ligation

The associating liver partition and portal vein ligation (ALPPS) procedure is an alternate technique to increase FLR, involving 2-staged hepatectomy. The first stage consists of an open right portal vein ligation and in situ parenchymal transection in the right trisectionectomy plane, with the second stage involving the right trisectionectomy.[61] Compared with PVE, ALPPS produces more hepatic hypertrophy, which may lead to higher rates of complete resection.[62,63] Given the additional operative risks, however, it is not surprising that ALPPS leads to higher morbidity and mortality compared with PVE.[62,64] Noted complications related to hepatic insufficiency include ascites, cholestasis, and sepsis, which are likely attributed to the short interval between stages.[65] Additional concerns include limited data on long-term oncologic outcomes as well as the lost opportunity to allow interval exclusion of patients who have early progression of disease, representing poor tumor biology, and are less likely to gain significant oncologic benefit from the second stage hepatectomy.[65]

The use of ALPPS specifically in the setting of HCC or cholangiocarcinoma remains controversial. Small single-center series have demonstrated that, although FLR may be lower in HCC patients, the procedure was feasible and had promising overall survival compared with HCC patients undergoing TACE or 1-stage liver resection.[66–69] However, a multicenter study using the ALPPS Registry revealed significantly higher 90-day mortality in patients with HCC versus colorectal metastases (47% vs 76%).[70] A similar study of the ALPPS Registry showed a 90-day mortality of 48% (n = 14/29) in patients with perihilar cholangiocarcinoma, although others have called into question the learning curve and prolonged operating times in this study, which have previously been associated with increased morbidity and mortality.[71,72] More evidence is needed before ALPPS can be recommended for HCC or cholangiocarcinoma.

ALPPS may be most appropriate in patients who still have insufficient FLR after PVE, or in patients with colorectal metastases who require staged resection, with ALPPS combined with initial resection of primary. At this time, however, it is not recommended for patients with HCC or cholangiocarcinoma. Indeed, the first international expert meeting on ALPPS in 2016 recommended that colorectal metastases remain the indication of choice, whereas caution should be used when considering use of ALPPS for HCC or biliary cancers.[73]

LIVER TRANSPLANTATION FOR HEPATOCELLULAR CARCINOMA

Regardless of advances in nonsurgical therapies for HCC, the best potential for curative treatment remains hepatic resection or LT. Many studies have shown the feasibility and efficacy of LT over resection, with generally superior outcomes in disease-free survival, although differences in overall survival remain unclear (**Table 1**). The range of overall survival outcomes may be due to variations in selection criteria, which have been explored since the initial use of LT for HCC.

In 1996, Mazzaferro and colleagues[74] published their landmark "Milan Criteria" for LT in patients with HCC. In a median follow-up of 26 months, they demonstrated an overall survival rate of 85% and a recurrence-free survival of 92%. Eligibility required a single tumor less than 5 cm in diameter and no more than 3 tumor nodules with each ≤3 cm, absence of major vascular invasion, and no extrahepatic spread. The patients who did not meet the criteria were found to have an overall survival and recurrence-free survival of 50% and 59%, respectively.[74] The Milan criteria have been validated in other studies, and they are currently used by the United Network for Organ Sharing (UNOS) as a basis for selection of patients with early stage HCC.

A substantial number of patients are excluded from the Milan criteria. Therefore, multiple studies have examined expanded criteria (**Table 2**) and have shown similar outcomes compared with the accepted Milan criteria. In 2000, Marsh and colleagues[75] proposed a staging system that accounted for depth of vascular invasion, lobar distribution, lymph node status, and largest tumor size, all shown to be independent predictors of recurrence-free survival. Interestingly, the number of tumors was not found to be significant on multivariate analysis. However, these modified criteria (also known as the Pittsburgh criteria) have limited applicability because of lymph node metastasis and vascular invasion being diagnosed at the time of surgery.

Subsequently, the University of California, San Francisco (UCSF) developed another set of criteria to help expand the surgical pool beyond the original Milan criteria. The UCSF criteria included either a solitary tumor ≤6.5 cm or ≤3 nodules with the largest lesion ≤0.5 cm and total tumor diameter ≤8 cm. In their study, they had a 90% and 75.2% survival at 1 and 5 years, respectively.[76] These criteria were externally validated by the University of California, Los Angeles. They reported 5-year survival of 79% and 64% in patients meeting the Milan and UCSF criteria, respectively.[77] These studies showed that reasonable outcomes could be obtained outside of the Milan criteria.

In a multicenter study, Mazzaferro and colleagues[78] demonstrated a 5-year overall survival of 71.2% when patients fell within their "up-to-7" criteria, defined as the sum of the tumor number and the size of the largest tumor (in centimeters) not larger than 7. In 2007, the University of Tokyo proposed the 5 to 5 rule, which was defined as no tumors larger than 5 cm and no more than 5 tumors. This study was the first to assess

Table 1 Hepatic resection versus liver transplantation for hepatocellular carcinoma									
Author	Tumor Burden	CTP Class	ITT	SR (n)	LT (n)	5-y OS SR	5-y OS LT	5-y DFS SR	5-y DFS LT
Squires et al,[111] 2014	Milan	A, B, C	No	45	131	44	66	23	85
Koniaris et al,[112] 2011	Milan	NA	Yes	26	73	63	41	52	46
Lee et al,[113] 2010	Milan + beyond	A, B	No	82	48	58	78	57	89
Facciuto et al,[114] 2009	Milan + beyond	A, B, C	Yes	51	106	57	53	NA	NA
Baccarani et al,[115] 2008	Milan	A, B, C	Yes	38	48	27	72	37	98
Bellavance et al,[116] 2008	Milan	A	No	245	134	46	66	40	82
Del Gaudio et al,[117] 2008	Milan	A, B, C	Yes	80	293	66	58	41	54
Cillo et al,[118] 2007	Milan + beyond	A, B, C	Yes	131	40	31	63	24	91
Shah et al,[119] 2007	Milan	A, B	Yes	121	140	56	64	56	60
Poon et al,[120] 2007	Milan	A, B, C	Yes	204	43	60	44	44	84
Margarit et al,[121] 2005	Milan	A	No	37	36	70	65	39	56
Bigourdan et al,[122] 2003	Milan	A	Yes	20	17	36	71	40	80
Adam et al,[123] 2003	Milan + beyond	A, B, C	Yes	98	195	50	61	18	58
Shabahang et al,[124] 2002	Milan + beyond	A, B, C	No	44	65	37	66	36	66
De Carlis et al,[125] 2001	Milan + beyond	A, B, C	No	154	121	40	60	38	74
Figueras et al,[126] 2000	Milan + beyond	A, B, C	No	35	85	51	60	31	60
Llovet et al,[127] 1999	Milan	A, B, C	Yes	77	87	51	69	NA	NA

Abbreviations: DFS, disease-free survival; ITT, intention-to-treat analysis; NA, not applicable; OS, overall survival; SR, surgical resection.

patients undergoing living donor LT for HCC. The study showed a recurrence-free survival of 94% for those meeting criteria and 50% for the patients who were outside the criteria.[79] A Chinese study developed the Hangzhou criteria, which included a total tumor diameter ≤8 cm or a total tumor diameter greater than 8 cm, with a histopathologic grade of I or II and a preoperative AFP level ≤400 ng/mL. The 5-year survival rate was 72.3%.[80] A subsequent study found that the Hangzhou criteria expanded the patient pool by 51.5% when compared with the use of the Milan criteria.[81] Multiple other studies have also shown expanded criteria with survival outcomes similar to the Milan criteria. The continued expansion of the Milan criteria will allow for more patients to undergo transplantation with improved long-term survival.

Table 2
Different proposed liver transplantation criteria for hepatocellular carcinoma

Criteria	Criteria Description	Overall Survival, %	Recurrence-Free Survival, %
Milan[74]	One tumor ≤5 cm, or ≤3 tumors with the largest ≤3 cm	75 (at 4 y)	83 (at 4 y)
UCSF[76]	One tumor ≤6.5 cm, or ≤3 tumors with the largest ≤4.5 cm and total tumor diameter ≤8 cm	75.2 (at 5 y)	NA
Up-to-7[78]	Total number of tumors and size of largest tumor (in cm) ≤7	71.2 (at 5 y)	9.1 (incidence of recurrence)
Tokyo[79]	≤5 tumors and each ≤5 cm	75 (at 5 y)	90 (at 5 y)
Hangzhou[80]	One of the following: total tumor diameter ≤8 cm, total tumor diameter >8 cm with histologic grade I or II, and AFP ≤400 ng/mL	72.3 (at 5 y)	NA

Another possibility to increase the population that can undergo LT is the use of locoregional therapy to downstage them. These therapies include TACE and radiofrequency ablation (RFA). Lei and Yan[82] and Yao and colleagues[83] showed that patients with advanced HCC who can be downstaged to Milan or UCSF criteria have similar outcomes than those who underwent a surgery-first approach. TACE originally showed conflicting outcomes.[84,85] However, further studies showed good outcomes following downstaging to Milan criteria. Chapman and colleagues[86] demonstrated a 94.1% survival at a median follow-up of 19.6 months. Another study demonstrated a downstaging rate of 77% to within the Milan criteria after TACE.[87] RFA when combined with other locoregional therapies has been shown to have a good survival rate in patients with HCC that were originally outside the Milan criteria.[88] A large systematic review and pooled analysis showed a pooled downstaging success rate of 48% and a recurrence rate of 16%.[89] They also showed that TACE and transarterial radioembolization had similar success with downstaging and recurrence rates.[89] Some studies have shown that patients who undergo downstaging are deemed high risk for recurrence, but these patients actually have similar survival compared with the patients who are within Milan criteria without locoregional therapy.[90,91] These data support an aggressive downstaging approach for patients who are outside the classical criteria and would otherwise be deemed unresectable.

These criteria outside of the Milan criteria and locoregional therapies will continue to allow the expansion of the surgical pool in patients with HCC. Further trials and studies will allow for patients who were once considered ineligible for resection to undergo surgery and have good long-term survival.

LIVER TRANSPLANT FOR CHOLANGIOCARCINOMA

Given the well-established efficacy of LT in HCC, there has been substantial interest in investigation of LT for cholangiocarcinoma, the second most common primary malignancy arising in the liver. Because the prognosis of cholangiocarcinoma is associated with its location as well as the ability to achieve margin-negative (R0) complete resection, LT represents an enticing potential opportunity in the setting of intrahepatic or hilar cholangiocarcinoma.[92] Because of limited supply of donor organs, it is necessary to identify appropriate patient selection criteria as well as establish sufficient efficacy and impact on survival before widely accepting a new indication for LT.

Liver Transplant for Hilar Cholangiocarcinoma

hCCA often presents with unresectable disease, owing to either technical consider-ations or underlying liver disease. In those with unresectable disease, LT remains the only method of attaining not only resection of the primary tumor but also the widest possible negative margin, which has been shown to be significantly associated with prognosis.[93,94] Even in patients with resectable disease, survival after hepatic resec-tion remains poor, with 5-year survival less than 40% and median survival of 40 months.[95,96] This poor prognosis is due in large part to significant recurrence rates, up to 40% even after R0 resection, with almost half of those involving locoregional recurrences.[95]

LT for cholangiocarcinoma was first attempted in the 1990s, although small series were discouraging, likely because of lack of standardized neoadjuvant or adjuvant therapies.[97] In 2000, more promising preliminary results were reported from the Mayo Clinic protocol of neoadjuvant therapy followed by LT.[98] The neoadjuvant protocol included chemoradiation with 5-fluorouracil and external beam radiation, followed by transluminal brachytherapy (**Table 3**). A follow-up study demonstrated that in select patients with stage I or II hCCA, with no disease progression after neo-adjuvant therapy, 5-year survival reached 82% after LT.[99] Various other studies have been conducted to further investigate these results (**Table 4**). Another study comparing LT for unresectable hCCA to hepatic resection for resectable tumors found that patients undergoing LT had significantly improved 5-year survival (82% vs 21%) as well as recurrence rates (13% vs 27%).[100] A subsequent 12-center prospective study showed a 5-year recurrence-free survival of 65% after undergoing the Mayo Clinic protocol.[101] Another multicenter study confirmed superior 5-year survival for hCCA patients undergoing LT versus resection (64% vs 18%).[102]

Whether an hCCA arises within a setting of primary sclerosing cholangitis (PSC) or as a de novo tumor impacts the indications for LT as well. Patients with PSC have

Table 3
Mayo Clinic protocol for neoadjuvant therapy and liver transplantation for hilar cholangiocarcinoma

Protocol Components	Description
Inclusion criteria	• Unresectable hCCA, or • HCCA in the setting of PSC
Diagnosis	• Intraluminal brush cytology or biopsy • Radiographic malignant-appearing stricture and Ca 19.9 >100 ng/mL • Radiographic malignant-appearing stricture and aneuploidy at fluorescence in situ hybridization
Staging	• Computerized tomography (CT) of abdomen • CT chest • Bone scan • Endoscopic ultrasound
Protocol steps	• External beam radiotherapy + intravenous fluorouracil • Transcatheter Iridium-192 brachytherapy • Staging operation (exploratory laparotomy with biopsy of hilar lymph nodes) • Listing for LT • Capecitabine orally (2 out of every 3 wk) while on the waiting list • LT

Table 4
Studies of liver transplantation for hilar cholangiocarcinoma

Institution	Reference	Patients Enrolled	Dropout Rate, %	Patients Transplanted	Patient Survival
Mayo Clinic Rochester	Rea et al,[100] *Ann Surg* 2005;242:451–461	71	34	38	82% at 5 y
University of Michigan	Welling et al,[128] *Liver Transpl* 2014;20:81–88	12	42	6	83% at 1 y
Mayo Clinic Jacksonville	Panjala et al,[129] *Liver Transpl* 2012;18:594–601	NA	NA	22	63% at 3 y
Dublin, Ireland	Duignan et al,[130] *HPB* 2014;16:91–98	27	26	20	51% at 4 y
US Multicenter	Darwish Murad et al,[101] *Gastroenterology* 2012;143:88–98	287	25	214	65% at 5 y

multifocal hepatic sites of strictures and periductal fibrosis, limiting resection options. These patients benefit more from LT, which can result in 5-year survivals between 55% and 65%.[103] Those with de novo hCCA, however, may not see as much of a survival benefit with LT compared with resection.[100,101] Therefore, an expert consensus statement recommended LT as standard of care for unresectable hCCA as well as hCCA arising in the setting of PSC regardless of respectability.[103]

Given the survival benefit seen with the Mayo Clinic protocol, UNOS has established MELD exception criteria for hCCA.[104] These criteria include the establishment of appropriate neoadjuvant therapy protocols at the given institution, along with diagnosis of hCCA based on cholangiography and biopsy or cytology, radial diameter of the mass less than 3 cm, no intrahepatic or extrahepatic metastases, and unresectability of the tumor based on technical factors or underlying liver disease.[104]

Liver Transplant for Intrahepatic Cholangiocarcinoma

iCCA is not currently an established indication for LT. Select centers have investigated this application, with overall poor outcomes, although these studies have been criticized for combining hCCA and iCCA as well as both cirrhotic and noncirrhotic patients, with no standardized neoadjuvant or adjuvant therapies administered.[92,105–107] However, a multicenter retrospective Spanish study investigating outcomes of incidentally found iCCA on explant pathology for LT performed for HCC or for cirrhosis found that "very early" iCCA (single tumor <2 cm) showed significantly better 5-year recurrence rate (18% vs 61%) and 5-year survival (65% vs 45%) compared with "advanced" iCCA (single tumor >2 cm or multifocal disease).[108] Another single-center retrospective study of early iCCA versus HCC on explant showed higher recurrence as well as worse survival for the iCCA patients.[109] A single-center prospective study found that neoadjuvant chemotherapy followed by LT for locally advanced iCCA resulted in promising overall survival (83.3% at 5 years), although recurrence-free survival was only 50%.[110] These studies have raised interest in the potential use of LT in early iCCA, although prospective trials are needed to investigate specific selection criteria as well as need for neoadjuvant or adjuvant therapies.

SUMMARY

Surgical management of primary liver and biliary tract tumors has evolved over the past few decades, resulting in improved outcomes in these malignancies with historically poor prognoses. Expansion of patient selection criteria, progress in neoadjuvant and adjuvant therapies, development of techniques to increase FLR, and the select utilization of LT have all contributed to increasing the patient pool for surgical intervention. Ongoing and future studies need to focus on improving multimodality treatment regimens and further refining the selection criteria for transplantation in order to optimize utilization of limited organ resources.

REFERENCES

1. Tanaka S, Ueno M, Iida H, et al. Preoperative assessment of frailty predicts age-related events after hepatic resection: a prospective multicenter study. J Hepatobiliary Pancreat Sci 2018;25(8):377–87.
2. Gani F, Cerullo M, Amini N, et al. Frailty as a risk predictor of morbidity and mortality following liver surgery. J Gastrointest Surg 2017;21(5):822–30.
3. Cheng Z, Yang P, Lei Z, et al. Nomograms for prediction of long-term survival in elderly patients after partial hepatectomy for hepatocellular carcinoma. Surgery 2017;162(6):1231–40.
4. Andert A, Lodewick T, Ulmer TF, et al. Liver resection in the elderly: a retrospective cohort study of 460 patients–feasible and safe. Int J Surg 2016;28:126–30.
5. Nozawa A, Kubo S, Takemura S, et al. Hepatic resection for hepatocellular carcinoma in super-elderly patients aged 80 years and older in the first decade of the 21st century. Surg Today 2015;45(7):851–7.
6. Cho SW, Steel J, Tsung A, et al. Safety of liver resection in the elderly: how important is age? Ann Surg Oncol 2011;18(4):1088–95.
7. Kondo K, Chijiiwa K, Funagayama M, et al. Hepatic resection is justified for elderly patients with hepatocellular carcinoma. World J Surg 2008;32(10):2223–9.
8. Huang J, Li BK, Chen GH, et al. Long-term outcomes and prognostic factors of elderly patients with hepatocellular carcinoma undergoing hepatectomy. J Gastrointest Surg 2009;13(9):1627–35.
9. Oishi K, Itamoto T, Kobayashi T, et al. Hepatectomy for hepatocellular carcinoma in elderly patients aged 75 years or more. J Gastrointest Surg 2009;13(4):695–701.
10. Wilson GC, Quillin RC 3rd, Wima K, et al. Is liver transplantation safe and effective in elderly ($\geq$70 years) recipients? A case-controlled analysis. HPB (Oxford) 2014;16(12):1088–94.
11. Krenzien F, Krezdorn N, Morgul MH, et al. The elderly liver transplant recipients: anxiety, depression, fatigue and life satisfaction. Z Gastroenterol 2017;55(6):557–63.
12. Teh SH, Nagorney DM, Stevens SR, et al. Risk factors for mortality after surgery in patients with cirrhosis. Gastroenterology 2007;132(4):1261–9.
13. Mansour A, Watson W, Shayani V, et al. Abdominal operations in patients with cirrhosis: still a major surgical challenge. Surgery 1997;122(4):730–5 [discussion: 735–6].
14. Ishizawa T, Hasegawa K, Aoki T, et al. Neither multiple tumors nor portal hypertension are surgical contraindications for hepatocellular carcinoma. Gastroenterology 2008;134(7):1908–16.
15. Teh SH, Christein J, Donohue J, et al. Hepatic resection of hepatocellular carcinoma in patients with cirrhosis: model of end-stage liver disease (MELD) score predicts perioperative mortality. J Gastrointest Surg 2005;9(9):1207–15 [discussion: 1215].

16. Friedman LS. Surgery in the patient with liver disease. Trans Am Clin Climatol Assoc 2010;121:192–204 [discussion: 205].

17. Emond JC, Samstein B, Renz JF. A critical evaluation of hepatic resection in cirrhosis: optimizing patient selection and outcomes. World J Surg 2005; 29(2):124–30.

18. Poon RT, Fan ST, Lo CM, et al. Extended hepatic resection for hepatocellular carcinoma in patients with cirrhosis: is it justified? Ann Surg 2002;236(5): 602–11.

19. Bruix J, Castells A, Bosch J, et al. Surgical resection of hepatocellular carcinoma in cirrhotic patients: prognostic value of preoperative portal pressure. Gastroenterology 1996;111(4):1018–22.

20. McCormack L, Petrowsky H, Clavien PA. Surgical therapy of hepatocellular carcinoma. Eur J Gastroenterol Hepatol 2005;17(5):497–503.

21. Berzigotti A, Reig M, Abraldes JG, et al. Portal hypertension and the outcome of surgery for hepatocellular carcinoma in compensated cirrhosis: a systematic review and meta-analysis. Hepatology 2015;61(2):526–36.

22. Llovet JM, Bru C, Bruix J. Prognosis of hepatocellular carcinoma: the BCLC staging classification. Semin Liver Dis 1999;19(3):329–38.

23. Vitale A, Burra P, Frigo AC, et al. Survival benefit of liver resection for patients with hepatocellular carcinoma across different Barcelona Clinic Liver Cancer stages: a multicentre study. J Hepatol 2015;62(3):617–24.

24. Yin L, Li H, Li AJ, et al. Partial hepatectomy vs. transcatheter arterial chemoembolization for resectable multiple hepatocellular carcinoma beyond Milan Criteria: a RCT. J Hepatol 2014;61(1):82–8.

25. Torzilli G, Belghiti J, Kokudo N, et al. A snapshot of the effective indications and results of surgery for hepatocellular carcinoma in tertiary referral centers: is it adherent to the EASL/AASLD recommendations?: an observational study of the HCC East-West study group. Ann Surg 2013;257(5):929–37.

26. Vauthey JN, Chaoui A, Do KA, et al. Standardized measurement of the future liver remnant prior to extended liver resection: methodology and clinical associations. Surgery 2000;127(5):512–9.

27. Cucchetti A, Cescon M, Ercolani G, et al. A comprehensive meta-regression analysis on outcome of anatomic resection versus nonanatomic resection for hepatocellular carcinoma. Ann Surg Oncol 2012;19(12):3697–705.

28. Tang YH, Wen TF, Chen X. Anatomic versus non-anatomic liver resection for hepatocellular carcinoma: a systematic review. Hepatogastroenterology 2013; 60(128):2019–25.

29. Wilhelm SM, Carter C, Tang L, et al. BAY 43-9006 exhibits broad spectrum oral antitumor activity and targets the RAF/MEK/ERK pathway and receptor tyrosine kinases involved in tumor progression and angiogenesis. Cancer Res 2004; 64(19):7099–109.

30. Llovet JM, Ricci S, Mazzaferro V, et al. Sorafenib in advanced hepatocellular carcinoma. N Engl J Med 2008;359(4):378–90.

31. Cheng AL, Kang YK, Chen Z, et al. Efficacy and safety of sorafenib in patients in the Asia-Pacific region with advanced hepatocellular carcinoma: a phase III randomised, double-blind, placebo-controlled trial. Lancet Oncol 2009;10(1): 25–34.

32. Cheng S, Wei X, Wu M. Effective ways to improve the prognosis of advanced stage (BCLC stage C) hepatocellular carcinoma. Zhonghua Wai Ke Za Zhi 2015;53(5):324–7 [in Chinese].

33. Bruix J, Takayama T, Mazzaferro V, et al. Adjuvant sorafenib for hepatocellular carcinoma after resection or ablation (STORM): a phase 3, randomised, double-blind, placebo-controlled trial. Lancet Oncol 2015;16(13):1344–54.

34. Cheng AL, Kang YK, Lin DY, et al. Sunitinib versus sorafenib in advanced hepatocellular cancer: results of a randomized phase III trial. J Clin Oncol 2013; 31(32):4067–75.

35. Johnson PJ, Qin S, Park JW, et al. Brivanib versus sorafenib as first-line therapy in patients with unresectable, advanced hepatocellular carcinoma: results from the randomized phase III BRISK-FL study. J Clin Oncol 2013;31(28):3517–24.

36. Llovet JM, Decaens T, Raoul JL, et al. Brivanib in patients with advanced hepatocellular carcinoma who were intolerant to sorafenib or for whom sorafenib failed: results from the randomized phase III BRISK-PS study. J Clin Oncol 2013;31(28):3509–16.

37. Cainap C, Qin S, Huang WT, et al. Linifanib versus Sorafenib in patients with advanced hepatocellular carcinoma: results of a randomized phase III trial. J Clin Oncol 2015;33(2):172–9.

38. Kudo M, Finn RS, Qin S, et al. Lenvatinib versus sorafenib in first-line treatment of patients with unresectable hepatocellular carcinoma: a randomised phase 3 non-inferiority trial. Lancet 2018;391(10126):1163–73.

39. Lin H, Li X, Liu Y, et al. Neoadjuvant radiotherapy provided survival benefit compared to adjuvant radiotherapy for hepatocellular carcinoma. ANZ J Surg 2018;88(10):E718–24.

40. Chen XP, Hu DY, Zhang ZW, et al. Role of mesohepatectomy with or without transcatheter arterial chemoembolization for large centrally located hepatocellular carcinoma. Dig Surg 2007;24(3):208–13.

41. Kaseb AOP RC, Vence LM, Blando JM, et al. Randomized, open-label, perioperative phase II study evaluating nivolumab alone versus nivolumab plus ipilimumab in patients with resectable HCC. J Clin Oncol 2019;37 [abstract: 185].

42. Kinoshita H, Sakai K, Hirohashi K, et al. Preoperative portal vein embolization for hepatocellular carcinoma. World J Surg 1986;10(5):803–8.

43. Abdalla EK, Hicks ME, Vauthey JN. Portal vein embolization: rationale, technique and future prospects. Br J Surg 2001;88(2):165–75.

44. Abdalla EK, Barnett CC, Doherty D, et al. Extended hepatectomy in patients with hepatobiliary malignances with and without preoperative portal vein embolization. Arch Surg 2002;137(6):675–80 [discussion: 680–1].

45. Abulkhir A, Limongelli P, Healey AJ, et al. Preoperative portal vein embolization for major liver resection: a meta-analysis. Ann Surg 2008;247(1):49–57.

46. Leung U, Simpson AL, Araujo RL, et al. Remnant growth rate after portal vein embolization is a good early predictor of post-hepatectomy liver failure. J Am Coll Surg 2014;219(4):620–30.

47. Ribero D, Abdalla EK, Madoff DC, et al. Portal vein embolization before major hepatectomy and its effects on regeneration, resectability and outcome. Br J Surg 2007;94(11):1386–94.

48. Shindoh J, D Tzeng CW, Vauthey JN. Portal vein embolization for hepatocellular carcinoma. Liver Cancer 2012;1(3–4):159–67.

49. Wakabayashi H, Ishimura K, Okano K, et al. Is preoperative portal vein embolization effective in improving prognosis after major hepatic resection in patients with advanced-stage hepatocellular carcinoma? Cancer 2001;92(9):2384–90.

50. Palavecino M, Chun YS, Madoff DC, et al. Major hepatic resection for hepatocellular carcinoma with or without portal vein embolization: Perioperative outcome and survival. Surgery 2009;145(4):399–405.

51. Tanaka H, Hirohashi K, Kubo S, et al. Preoperative portal vein embolization improves prognosis after right hepatectomy for hepatocellular carcinoma in patients with impaired hepatic function. Br J Surg 2000;87(7):879–82.

52. Aoki T, Imamura H, Hasegawa K, et al. Sequential preoperative arterial and portal venous embolizations in patients with hepatocellular carcinoma. Arch Surg 2004;139(7):766–74.

53. Yoo H, Kim JH, Ko GY, et al. Sequential transcatheter arterial chemoembolization and portal vein embolization versus portal vein embolization only before major hepatectomy for patients with hepatocellular carcinoma. Ann Surg Oncol 2011;18(5):1251–7.

54. Ogata S, Belghiti J, Farges O, et al. Sequential arterial and portal vein embolizations before right hepatectomy in patients with cirrhosis and hepatocellular carcinoma. Br J Surg 2006;93(9):1091–8.

55. Yamashita S, Sakamoto Y, Yamamoto S, et al. Efficacy of preoperative portal vein embolization among patients with hepatocellular carcinoma, biliary tract cancer, and colorectal liver metastases: a comparative study based on single-center experience of 319 cases. Ann Surg Oncol 2017;24(6):1557–68.

56. Ebata T, Yokoyama Y, Igami T, et al. Portal vein embolization before extended hepatectomy for biliary cancer: current technique and review of 494 consecutive embolizations. Dig Surg 2012;29(1):23–9.

57. Sangro B, Inarrairaegui M, Bilbao JI. Radioembolization for hepatocellular carcinoma. J Hepatol 2012;56(2):464–73.

58. Vouche M, Lewandowski RJ, Atassi R, et al. Radiation lobectomy: time-dependent analysis of future liver remnant volume in unresectable liver cancer as a bridge to resection. J Hepatol 2013;59(5):1029–36.

59. Edeline J, Lenoir L, Boudjema K, et al. Volumetric changes after (90)y radioembolization for hepatocellular carcinoma in cirrhosis: an option to portal vein embolization in a preoperative setting? Ann Surg Oncol 2013;20(8):2518–25.

60. Garlipp B, de Baere T, Damm R, et al. Left-liver hypertrophy after therapeutic right-liver radioembolization is substantial but less than after portal vein embolization. Hepatology 2014;59(5):1864–73.

61. Schnitzbauer AA, Lang SA, Goessmann H, et al. Right portal vein ligation combined with in situ splitting induces rapid left lateral liver lobe hypertrophy enabling 2-staged extended right hepatic resection in small-for-size settings. Ann Surg 2012;255(3):405–14.

62. Eshmuminov D, Raptis DA, Linecker M, et al. Meta-analysis of associating liver partition with portal vein ligation and portal vein occlusion for two-stage hepatectomy. Br J Surg 2016;103(13):1768–82.

63. Schadde E, Ardiles V, Slankamenac K, et al. ALPPS offers a better chance of complete resection in patients with primarily unresectable liver tumors compared with conventional-staged hepatectomies: results of a multicenter analysis. World J Surg 2014;38(6):1510–9.

64. Schadde E, Schnitzbauer AA, Tschuor C, et al. Systematic review and meta-analysis of feasibility, safety, and efficacy of a novel procedure: associating liver partition and portal vein ligation for staged hepatectomy. Ann Surg Oncol 2015; 22(9):3109–20.

65. Aloia TA, Vauthey JN. Associating liver partition and portal vein ligation for staged hepatectomy (ALPPS): what is gained and what is lost? Ann Surg 2012;256(3):e9 [author reply: e16–9].

66. Wang Z, Peng Y, Hu J, et al. Associating liver partition and portal vein ligation for staged hepatectomy for unresectable hepatitis B virus-related hepatocellular

carcinoma: a single center study of 45 patients. Ann Surg 2018. [Epub ahead of print].

67. Chia DKA, Yeo Z, Loh SEK, et al. ALPPS for hepatocellular carcinoma is associated with decreased liver remnant growth. J Gastrointest Surg 2018;22(6): 973–80.

68. Vennarecci G, Grazi GL, Sperduti I, et al. ALPPS for primary and secondary liver tumors. Int J Surg 2016;30:38–44.

69. Vennarecci G, Ferraro D, Tudisco A, et al. The ALPPS procedure: hepatocellular carcinoma as a main indication. An Italian single-center experience. Updates Surg 2019;71(1):67–75.

70. D'Haese JG, Neumann J, Weniger M, et al. Should ALPPS be used for liver resection in intermediate-stage HCC? Ann Surg Oncol 2016;23(4):1335–43.

71. Olthof PB, Coelen RJS, Wiggers JK, et al. High mortality after ALPPS for perihilar cholangiocarcinoma: case-control analysis including the first series from the international ALPPS registry. HPB (Oxford) 2017;19(5):381–7.

72. Lang H, de Santibanes E, Clavien PA. Outcome of ALPPS for perihilar cholangiocarcinoma: case-control analysis including the first series from the international ALPPS registry. HPB (Oxford) 2017;19(5):379–80.

73. Oldhafer KJ, Stavrou GA, van Gulik TM, et al. ALPPS–where do we stand, where do we go?: eight recommendations from the First International Expert Meeting. Ann Surg 2016;263(5):839–41.

74. Mazzaferro V, Regalia E, Doci R, et al. Liver transplantation for the treatment of small hepatocellular carcinomas in patients with cirrhosis. N Engl J Med 1996; 334(11):693–9.

75. Marsh JW, Dvorchik I, Bonham CA, et al. Is the pathologic TNM staging system for patients with hepatoma predictive of outcome? Cancer 2000;88(3):538–43.

76. Yao FY, Ferrell L, Bass NM, et al. Liver transplantation for hepatocellular carcinoma: expansion of the tumor size limits does not adversely impact survival. Hepatology 2001;33(6):1394–403.

77. Duffy JP, Vardanian A, Benjamin E, et al. Liver transplantation criteria for hepatocellular carcinoma should be expanded: a 22-year experience with 467 patients at UCLA. Ann Surg 2007;246(3):502–9 [discussion: 509–1].

78. Mazzaferro V, Llovet JM, Miceli R, et al. Predicting survival after liver transplantation in patients with hepatocellular carcinoma beyond the Milan criteria: a retrospective, exploratory analysis. Lancet Oncol 2009;10(1):35–43.

79. Sugawara Y, Tamura S, Makuuchi M. Living donor liver transplantation for hepatocellular carcinoma: Tokyo University series. Dig Dis 2007;25(4):310–2.

80. Zheng SS, Xu X, Wu J, et al. Liver transplantation for hepatocellular carcinoma: Hangzhou experiences. Transplantation 2008;85(12):1726–32.

81. Xu X, Lu D, Ling Q, et al. Liver transplantation for hepatocellular carcinoma beyond the Milan criteria. Gut 2016;65(6):1035–41.

82. Lei J, Yan L. Comparison between living donor liver transplantation recipients who met the Milan and UCSF criteria after successful downstaging therapies. J Gastrointest Surg 2012;16(11):2120–5.

83. Yao FY, Mehta N, Flemming J, et al. Downstaging of hepatocellular cancer before liver transplant: long-term outcome compared to tumors within Milan criteria. Hepatology 2015;61(6):1968–77.

84. Oldhafer KJ, Chavan A, Fruhauf NR, et al. Arterial chemoembolization before liver transplantation in patients with hepatocellular carcinoma: marked tumor necrosis, but no survival benefit? J Hepatol 1998;29(6):953–9.

85. Majno PE, Adam R, Bismuth H, et al. Influence of preoperative transarterial lipiodol chemoembolization on resection and transplantation for hepatocellular carcinoma in patients with cirrhosis. Ann Surg 1997;226(6):688–701 [discussion: 701–3].

86. Chapman WC, Majella Doyle MB, Stuart JE, et al. Outcomes of neoadjuvant transarterial chemoembolization to downstage hepatocellular carcinoma before liver transplantation. Ann Surg 2008;248(4):617–25.

87. Green TJ, Rochon PJ, Chang S, et al. Downstaging disease in patients with hepatocellular carcinoma outside of Milan criteria: strategies using drug-eluting bead chemoembolization. J Vasc Interv Radiol 2013;24(11):1613–22.

88. Yao FY, Kinkhabwala M, LaBerge JM, et al. The impact of pre-operative locoregional therapy on outcome after liver transplantation for hepatocellular carcinoma. Am J Transplant 2005;5(4 Pt 1):795–804.

89. Parikh ND, Waljee AK, Singal AG. Downstaging hepatocellular carcinoma: a systematic review and pooled analysis. Liver Transpl 2015;21(9):1142–52.

90. Kim Y, Stahl CC, Makramalla A, et al. Downstaging therapy followed by liver transplantation for hepatocellular carcinoma beyond Milan criteria. Surgery 2017;162(6):1250–8.

91. Mehta N, Guy J, Frenette CT, et al. Excellent outcomes of liver transplantation following down-staging of hepatocellular carcinoma to within milan criteria: a multicenter study. Clin Gastroenterol Hepatol 2018;16(6):955–64.

92. Goldaracena N, Gorgen A, Sapisochin G. Current status of liver transplantation for cholangiocarcinoma. Liver Transpl 2018;24(2):294–303.

93. Kimura N, Young AL, Toyoki Y, et al. Radical operation for hilar cholangiocarcinoma in comparable Eastern and Western centers: outcome analysis and prognostic factors. Surgery 2017;162(3):500–14.

94. DeOliveira ML, Cunningham SC, Cameron JL, et al. Cholangiocarcinoma: thirty-one-year experience with 564 patients at a single institution. Ann Surg 2007; 245(5):755–62.

95. Hasegawa S, Ikai I, Fujii H, et al. Surgical resection of hilar cholangiocarcinoma: analysis of survival and postoperative complications. World J Surg 2007;31(6): 1256–63.

96. Groot Koerkamp B, Wiggers JK, Gonen M, et al. Survival after resection of perihilar cholangiocarcinoma–development and external validation of a prognostic nomogram. Ann Oncol 2015;26(9):1930–5.

97. Pichlmayr R, Weimann A, Tusch G, et al. Indications and role of liver transplantation for malignant tumors. Oncologist 1997;2(3):164–70.

98. De Vreede I, Steers JL, Burch PA, et al. Prolonged disease-free survival after orthotopic liver transplantation plus adjuvant chemoirradiation for cholangiocarcinoma. Liver Transpl 2000;6(3):309–16.

99. Heimbach JK, Gores GJ, Haddock MG, et al. Liver transplantation for unresectable perihilar cholangiocarcinoma. Semin Liver Dis 2004;24(2):201–7.

100. Rea DJ, Heimbach JK, Rosen CB, et al. Liver transplantation with neoadjuvant chemoradiation is more effective than resection for hilar cholangiocarcinoma. Ann Surg 2005;242(3):451–8 [discussion: 458–1].

101. Darwish Murad S, Kim WR, Harnois DM, et al. Efficacy of neoadjuvant chemoradiation, followed by liver transplantation, for perihilar cholangiocarcinoma at 12 US centers. Gastroenterology 2012;143(1):88–98.e3 [quiz: e14].

102. Ethun CG, Lopez-Aguiar AG, Anderson DJ, et al. Transplantation versus resection for hilar cholangiocarcinoma: an argument for shifting treatment paradigms for resectable disease. Ann Surg 2018;267(5):797–805.

103. Mansour JC, Aloia TA, Crane CH, et al. Hilar cholangiocarcinoma: expert consensus statement. HPB (Oxford) 2015;17(8):691–9.
104. Gores GJ, Gish RG, Sudan D, et al. Model for end-stage liver disease (MELD) exception for cholangiocarcinoma or biliary dysplasia. Liver Transpl 2006; 12(12 Suppl 3):S95–7.
105. Ghali P, Marotta PJ, Yoshida EM, et al. Liver transplantation for incidental cholangiocarcinoma: analysis of the Canadian experience. Liver Transpl 2005; 11(11):1412–6.
106. Sotiropoulos GC, Kaiser GM, Lang H, et al. Liver transplantation as a primary indication for intrahepatic cholangiocarcinoma: a single-center experience. Transplant Proc 2008;40(9):3194–5.
107. Facciuto ME, Singh MK, Lubezky N, et al. Tumors with intrahepatic bile duct differentiation in cirrhosis: implications on outcomes after liver transplantation. Transplantation 2015;99(1):151–7.
108. Sapisochin G, Facciuto M, Rubbia-Brandt L, et al. Liver transplantation for "very early" intrahepatic cholangiocarcinoma: international retrospective study supporting a prospective assessment. Hepatology 2016;64(4):1178–88.
109. Lee DD, Croome KP, Musto KR, et al. Liver transplantation for intrahepatic cholangiocarcinoma. Liver Transpl 2018;24(5):634–44.
110. Lunsford KE, Javle M, Heyne K, et al. Liver transplantation for locally advanced intrahepatic cholangiocarcinoma treated with neoadjuvant therapy: a prospective case-series. Lancet Gastroenterol Hepatol 2018;3(5):337–48.
111. Squires MH 3rd, Hanish SI, Fisher SB, et al. Transplant versus resection for the management of hepatocellular carcinoma meeting Milan Criteria in the MELD exception era at a single institution in a UNOS region with short wait times. J Surg Oncol 2014;109(6):533–41.
112. Koniaris LG, Levi DM, Pedroso FE, et al. Is surgical resection superior to transplantation in the treatment of hepatocellular carcinoma? Ann Surg 2011;254(3): 527–37 [discussion: 537–8].
113. Lee KK, Kim DG, Moon IS, et al. Liver transplantation versus liver resection for the treatment of hepatocellular carcinoma. J Surg Oncol 2010;101(1):47–53.
114. Facciuto ME, Rochon C, Pandey M, et al. Surgical dilemma: liver resection or liver transplantation for hepatocellular carcinoma and cirrhosis. Intention-to-treat analysis in patients within and outwith Milan criteria. HPB (Oxford) 2009; 11(5):398–404.
115. Baccarani U, Isola M, Adani GL, et al. Superiority of transplantation versus resection for the treatment of small hepatocellular carcinoma. Transpl Int 2008;21(3): 247–54.
116. Bellavance EC, Lumpkins KM, Mentha G, et al. Surgical management of early-stage hepatocellular carcinoma: resection or transplantation? J Gastrointest Surg 2008;12(10):1699–708.
117. Del Gaudio M, Ercolani G, Ravaioli M, et al. Liver transplantation for recurrent hepatocellular carcinoma on cirrhosis after liver resection: University of Bologna experience. Am J Transplant 2008;8(6):1177–85.
118. Cillo U, Vitale A, Grigoletto F, et al. Intention-to-treat analysis of liver transplantation in selected, aggressively treated HCC patients exceeding the Milan criteria. Am J Transplant 2007;7(4):972–81.
119. Shah SA, Cleary SP, Tan JC, et al. An analysis of resection vs transplantation for early hepatocellular carcinoma: defining the optimal therapy at a single institution. Ann Surg Oncol 2007;14(9):2608–14.

120. Poon RT, Fan ST, Lo CM, et al. Difference in tumor invasiveness in cirrhotic patients with hepatocellular carcinoma fulfilling the Milan criteria treated by resection and transplantation: impact on long-term survival. Ann Surg 2007; 245(1):51–8.

121. Margarit C, Escartin A, Castells L, et al. Resection for hepatocellular carcinoma is a good option in Child-Turcotte-Pugh class A patients with cirrhosis who are eligible for liver transplantation. Liver Transpl 2005;11(10):1242–51.

122. Bigourdan JM, Jaeck D, Meyer N, et al. Small hepatocellular carcinoma in Child A cirrhotic patients: hepatic resection versus transplantation. Liver Transpl 2003; 9(5):513–20.

123. Adam R, Azoulay D, Castaing D, et al. Liver resection as a bridge to transplantation for hepatocellular carcinoma on cirrhosis: a reasonable strategy? Ann Surg 2003;238(4):508–18 [discussion: 518–9].

124. Shabahang M, Franceschi D, Yamashiki N, et al. Comparison of hepatic resection and hepatic transplantation in the treatment of hepatocellular carcinoma among cirrhotic patients. Ann Surg Oncol 2002;9(9):881–6.

125. De Carlis L, Giacomoni A, Pirotta V, et al. Treatment of HCC: the role of liver resection in the era of transplantation. Transplant Proc 2001;33(1–2):1453–6.

126. Figueras J, Jaurrieta E, Valls C, et al. Resection or transplantation for hepatocellular carcinoma in cirrhotic patients: outcomes based on indicated treatment strategy. J Am Coll Surg 2000;190(5):580–7.

127. Llovet JM, Fuster J, Bruix J. Intention-to-treat analysis of surgical treatment for early hepatocellular carcinoma: resection versus transplantation. Hepatology 1999;30(6):1434–40.

128. Welling TH, Feng M, Wan S, et al. Neoadjuvant stereotactic body radiation therapy, capecitabine, and liver transplantation for unresectable hilar cholangiocarcinoma. Liver Transpl 2014;20(1):81–8.

129. Panjala C, Nguyen JH, Al-Hajjaj AN, et al. Impact of neoadjuvant chemoradiation on the tumor burden before liver transplantation for unresectable cholangiocarcinoma. Liver Transpl 2012;18(5):594–601.

130. Duignan S, Maguire D, Ravichand CS, et al. Neoadjuvant chemoradiotherapy followed by liver transplantation for unresectable cholangiocarcinoma: a single-centre national experience. HPB (Oxford) 2014;16(1):91–8.

UNITED STATES POSTAL SERVICE ® Statement of Ownership, Management, and Circulation
(All Periodicals Publications Except Requester Publications)

1. Publication Title	2. Publication Number	3. Filing Date
SURGICAL ONCOLOGY CLINICS OF NORTH AMERICA	012 – 565	9/18/2019

4. Issue Frequency	5. Number of Issues Published Annually	6. Annual Subscription Price
JAN, APR, JUL, OCT	4	$306.00

7. Complete Mailing Address of Known Office of Publication (Not printer) (Street, city, county, state, and ZIP+4®)

ELSEVIER INC.
230 Park Avenue, Suite 800
New York, NY 10169

Contact Person
STEPHEN R. BUSHING
Telephone (Include area code)
215-239-3688

8. Complete Mailing Address of Headquarters or General Business Office of Publisher (Not printer)

ELSEVIER INC.
230 Park Avenue, Suite 800
New York, NY 10169

9. Full Names and Complete Mailing Addresses of Publisher, Editor, and Managing Editor (Do not leave blank)

Publisher (Name and complete mailing address)

TAYLOR BALL, ELSEVIER INC.
1600 JOHN F KENNEDY BLVD. SUITE 1800
PHILADELPHIA, PA 19103-2899

Editor (Name and complete mailing address)

JOHN VASSALLO, ELSEVIER INC.
1600 JOHN F KENNEDY BLVD. SUITE 1800
PHILADELPHIA, PA 19103-2899

Managing Editor (Name and complete mailing address)

PATRICK MANLEY, ELSEVIER INC.
1600 JOHN F KENNEDY BLVD. SUITE 1800
PHILADELPHIA, PA 19103-2899

10. Owner (Do not leave blank. If the publication is owned by a corporation, give the name and address of the corporation immediately followed by the names and addresses of all stockholders owning or holding 1 percent or more of the total amount of stock. If not owned by a corporation, give the names and addresses of the individual owners. If owned by a partnership or other unincorporated firm, give its name and address as well as those of each individual owner. If the publication is published by a nonprofit organization, give its name and address.)

Full Name	Complete Mailing Address
WHOLLY OWNED SUBSIDIARY OF REED/ELSEVIER, US HOLDINGS	1600 JOHN F KENNEDY BLVD. SUITE 1800 PHILADELPHIA, PA 19103-2899

11. Known Bondholders, Mortgagees, and Other Security Holders Owning or Holding 1 Percent or More of Total Amount of Bonds, Mortgages, or Other Securities. If none, check box ▶ ☐ None

Full Name	Complete Mailing Address
N/A	

12. Tax Status (For completion by nonprofit organizations authorized to mail at nonprofit rates) (Check one)
The purpose, function, and nonprofit status of this organization and the exempt status for federal income tax purposes:
☒ Has Not Changed During Preceding 12 Months
☐ Has Changed During Preceding 12 Months (Publisher must submit explanation of change with this statement)

PS Form 3526, July 2014 [Page 1 of 4 (see instructions page 4)] PSN 7530-01-000-9931 PRIVACY NOTICE: See our privacy policy on www.usps.com.

---

13. Publication Title			14. Issue Date for Circulation Data Below
SURGICAL ONCOLOGY CLINICS OF NORTH AMERICA			JULY 2019

15. Extent and Nature of Circulation			Average No. Copies Each Issue During Preceding 12 Months	No. Copies of Single Issue Published Nearest to Filing Date
a. Total Number of Copies (Net press run)			116	114
b. Paid Circulation (By Mail and Outside the Mail)	(1)	Mailed Outside-County Paid Subscriptions Stated on PS Form 3541 (include paid distribution above nominal rate, advertiser's proof copies, and exchange copies)	39	44
	(2)	Mailed In-County Paid Subscriptions Stated on PS Form 3541 (include paid distribution above nominal rate, advertiser's proof copies, and exchange copies)	0	0
	(3)	Paid Distribution Outside the Mails Including Sales Through Dealers and Carriers, Street Vendors, Counter Sales, and Other Paid Distribution Outside USPS®	28	39
	(4)	Paid Distribution by Other Classes of Mail Through the USPS (e.g. First-Class Mail®)	0	0
c. Total Paid Distribution (Sum of 15b (1), (2), (3), and (4))		▶	67	83
d. Free or Nominal Rate Distribution (By Mail and Outside the Mail)	(1)	Free or Nominal Rate Outside-County Copies included on PS Form 3541	37	16
	(2)	Free or Nominal Rate In-County Copies Included on PS Form 3541	0	0
	(3)	Free or Nominal Rate Copies Mailed at Other Classes Through the USPS (e.g. First-Class Mail)	0	0
	(4)	Free or Nominal Rate Distribution Outside the Mail (Carriers or other means)	0	0
e. Total Free or Nominal Rate Distribution (Sum of 15d (1), (2), (3) and (4))		▶	37	16
f. Total Distribution (Sum of 15c and 15e)		▶	104	99
g. Copies not Distributed (See Instructions to Publishers #4 (page #3))		▶	12	15
h. Total (Sum of 15f and g)		▶	116	114
i. Percent Paid (15c divided by 15f times 100)		▶	64.42%	83.84%

* If you are claiming electronic copies, go to line 16 on page 3. If you are not claiming electronic copies, skip to line 17 on page 3.

PS Form 3526, July 2014 (Page 2 of 4)

16. Electronic Copy Circulation		Average No. Copies Each Issue During Preceding 12 Months	No. Copies of Single Issue Published Nearest to Filing Date
a. Paid Electronic Copies	▶		
b. Total Paid Print Copies (Line 15c) + Paid Electronic Copies (Line 16a)	▶		
c. Total Print Distribution (Line 15f) + Paid Electronic Copies (Line 16a)	▶		
d. Percent Paid (Both Print & Electronic Copies) (16b divided by 16c × 100)	▶		

☒ I certify that 50% of all my distributed copies (electronic and print) are paid above a nominal price.

17. Publication of Statement of Ownership

☒ If the publication is a general publication, publication of this statement is required. Will be printed in the OCTOBER 2019 issue of this publication. ☐ Publication not required.

18. Signature and Title of Editor, Publisher, Business Manager, or Owner

STEPHEN R. BUSHING - INVENTORY DISTRIBUTION CONTROL MANAGER

Date 9/18/2019

I certify that all information furnished on this form is true and complete. I understand that anyone who furnishes false or misleading information on this form or who omits material or information requested on the form may be subject to criminal sanctions (including fines and imprisonment) and/or civil sanctions (including civil penalties).

PS Form 3526, July 2014 (Page 3 of 4) PRIVACY NOTICE: See our privacy policy on www.usps.com

Moving?

Make sure your subscription moves with you!

To notify us of your new address, find your **Clinics Account Number** (located on your mailing label above your name), and contact customer service at:

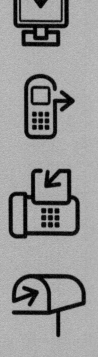

Email: journalscustomerservice-usa@elsevier.com

800-654-2452 (subscribers in the U.S. & Canada)
314-447-8871 (subscribers outside of the U.S. & Canada)

Fax number: 314-447-8029

Elsevier Health Sciences Division
Subscription Customer Service
3251 Riverport Lane
Maryland Heights, MO 63043